AF361890

Dietary Influence on Nutritional Epidemiology, Public Health and Our Lifestyle

Dietary Influence on Nutritional Epidemiology, Public Health and Our Lifestyle

Editor

Lourdes M. Varela

MDPI • Basel • Beijing • Wuhan • Barcelona • Belgrade • Manchester • Tokyo • Cluj • Tianjin

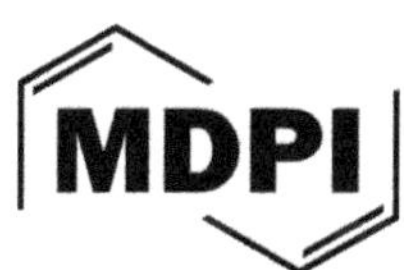

Editor
Lourdes M. Varela
Instituto de Biomedicina
de Sevilla, IBiS/Hospital
Universitario Virgen del
Rocío/CSIC/Universidad de Sevilla
Universidad de Sevilla
Seville
Spain

Editorial Office
MDPI
St. Alban-Anlage 66
4052 Basel, Switzerland

This is a reprint of articles from the Special Issue published online in the open access journal *Nutrients* (ISSN 2072-6643) (available at: https://www.mdpi.com/journal/nutrients/special_issues/dietary_influence_on_nutritional_epidemiology_public_health_and_our_lifestyle).

For citation purposes, cite each article independently as indicated on the article page online and as indicated below:

LastName, A.A.; LastName, B.B.; LastName, C.C. Article Title. *Journal Name* **Year**, *Volume Number*, Page Range.

ISBN 978-3-0365-7712-8 (Hbk)
ISBN 978-3-0365-7713-5 (PDF)

Contents

About the Editor

Lourdes M. Varela

Dr. Lourdes M. Varela graduated in Pharmacy and Ph.D. in Molecular Biology and Biomedicine at the University of Seville (US, Spain). Her Ph.D. received the extraordinary award from the US (2014) and was conducted at the Instituto de la Grasa (CSIC, Seville), the Baylor College of Medicine (Houston, TX, USA), and the Leibniz Institute for Atherosclerosis Research (Münster, Germany). She did postdoc studies at INSERM in France (Paris), at the Instituto Catalán de Ciencias Cardiovasculares in Spain (Barcelona) and at the Andalusian Center for Molecular Biology and Regenerative Medicine (CABIMER, Seville, Spain). Since 2019, she has worked at the Institute of Biomedicine of Seville (IBiS, Spain), and her research focuses primarily on the search for early-stage biomarkers for cardiovascular disease to define potential therapy targets.

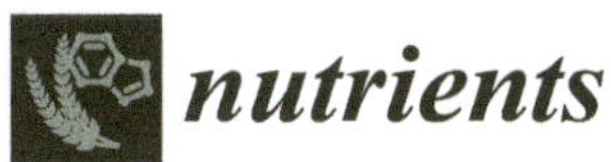

Editorial

Dietary Influence on Nutritional Epidemiology, Public Health and Our Lifestyle

Lourdes M. Varela [1,2]

1 Instituto de Biomedicina de Sevilla, IBiS/Hospital Universitario Virgen del Rocío/CSIC/Universidad de Sevilla, 41013 Sevilla, Spain; lvarela@us.es
2 Departamento de Fisiología Médica y Biofísica, Facultad de Medicina, Universidad de Sevilla, 41009 Sevilla, Spain

Citation: Varela, L.M. Dietary Influence on Nutritional Epidemiology, Public Health and Our Lifestyle. *Nutrients* **2023**, *15*, 2555. https://doi.org/10.3390/nu15112555

Received: 21 May 2023
Accepted: 26 May 2023
Published: 30 May 2023

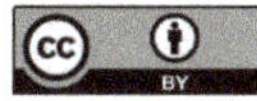

This Special Issue of *Nutrients* "Dietary Influence on Nutritional Epidemiology, Public Health and Our Lifestyle", includes nine original articles and one systematic review related to the associations between some dietary patterns, lifestyle, and socio-demographic factors, analyzed either separately or in combination, with the risk and management of cardiovascular diseases and mental health problems, such as depression and dementia.

Dietary habits differ from person to person and usually are determined by cultural habits and traditions that determine lifestyles linked to the socio-demographic characteristics associated with ethnicity. It is known that dietary habits, lifestyle, and sociodemographic factors impact human health. While individual foods and nutrients are important, overall dietary patterns are more strongly associated with health. The Mediterranean diet is a compilation of the nutritional and dietary habits of the countries of the Mediterranean Basin. There is strong evidence from epidemiological studies that increasing compliance with the Mediterranean diet is associated with a reduction in total and cause-specific mortality. The systematic review by Grao et al. [1] shows that the Mediterranean diet can improve the quality of high-density lipoproteins (HDL) and prevent HDL dysfunctionality, which is a protective factor against cardiovascular disease. The principal product of the Mediterranean Basin is virgin olive oil, which is obtained from different varieties of olives that confer their individual nutritional and organoleptic properties. Epidemiological studies, long- and short-term intervention studies, and postprandial studies have found associations between a diet rich in virgin olive oil and a decrease in cardiovascular risk factors, stroke incidence, and type 2 diabetes. The study by Vazquez-Madrigal et al. [2] suggests that consuming meals enriched in monounsaturated fatty acids (MUFA) from olive oil can protect against dendritic cells postprandial differentiation and potentially prevent the development and progression of inflammatory and autoimmune diseases.

Nowadays, dementia affects about 50 million people globally and is projected to increase to over 130 million by 2050. When this condition affects people under 65, it is called early onset dementia. Epidemiological studies suggest that aging and obesity have negative effects, among other conditions and disease, on cognitive function. Diet is a key modifiable lifestyle factor that may impact on cognitive function as there is no effective treatment for the improvement of cognition or delay decline. The study by Filippini et al. [3] shows that a high intake of cereals and dairy products is associated with an increased risk of early onset dementia, while the intake of some types of fish, vegetables, fruits, and chocolate alongside moderate coffee consumption appears to be beneficial. The study indicates that an increased adherence to the MIND diet (a hybrid of the Mediterranean and DASH—Dietary Approaches to Stop Hypertension—diets) may decrease early onset dementia risk.

In contrast to the beneficial effects associated with an adherence to the Mediterranean and Mediterranean-DASH Intervention for Neurodegenerative Delay (MIND) diets, the study by Llanaj et al. [4] revealed an unhealthy nutrient-based dietary pattern and unsustainable among Hungarian Roma population, which may contribute to Hungarians being one of the most obese and malnourished nations in Europe. The study indicates the identification of nutrient-rich, affordable, healthy, and sustainable dietary patterns for Hungarian population as a foremost public health priority, while also presenting an opportunity to recognize and address social inequalities in nutrition and health. Another study published in this Special Issue also highlighted the importance of a balanced diet that supplies the nutrients our body needs to be healthy, both physically and mentally. The study by Wang et al. [5] suggests that poor diet quality, measured by the Healthy Eating Index (HEI-2015), is associated with elevated depressive symptoms in US adults. This study highlights the importance of a healthy diet in reducing the risk of depression.

In recent years, and in the current climate crisis, the interest in a sustainable diet/lifestyle has increased. Vegetarians and vegans tend to consume more fruits and vegetables, whole grains, legumes, and nuts, and tend to have a lower body mass index and have a lower risk of diabetes, hypertension, and coronary heart disease compared with meat-eaters. However, there is limited understanding of the underlying molecular mechanisms that could help explain the probable ability of vegetarian dietary patterns to prevent chronic diseases. The study by Miles et al. [6] found modest differences in DNA methylation in vegans and non-vegetarians, suggesting that diet can influence DNA methylation patterns, which could have implications for disease risk and prevention linked to lifestyles.

The diet evolves over time, being influenced by food costs, individual preferences and convictions, cultural traditions, and environmental and geographical aspects. However, the constant truth remains that a healthy diet must help protect against malnutrition, as well as prevent noncommunicable diseases. Dietary nutrients play an important role in maintaining the normal physiological function of the body that is dependent on strict control of its blood glucose levels, among other factors. Nutritional management of blood glucose levels is a strategic target in the control of hyperglycemia, a key feature of diabetes. The study by Yin Bai et al. [7] found that daily total vitamin B6 intake could be a possible predictor of recent glycemic control status among non-pregnant American adults older than 20 years of age, supporting its role as a very important molecule necessary for the health and proper functioning of the human body. Closely related to this study, the work by Yeh et al. [8] evaluated the effect of dehulled adlay consumption on blood pressure in spontaneously hypertensive rats and overweight and obese young adults. Hypertension and hyperglycemia are interrelated and strongly predispose to atherosclerotic disease. This study found that the daily intake of dehulled adlay, a grain rich in phenolic compounds popular in Asian cuisine, had beneficial effects in the management of blood pressure, which was more evident in participants with high basal blood pressure.

Previous studies confirm the importance of a healthy diet. However, the consumption of high-caloric foods, fats, sugar, and salt has increased, and many people do not eat enough fruit, vegetables, and fiber in their diets. As a result, obesity has reached epidemic proportions worldwide. Although obesity is not considered an eating disorder, it frequently co-occurs with such disorders. Common risk factors linking obesity and eating disorders include dieting, body dissatisfaction, weight/shape concerns, and unhealthy weight control behaviors. Both conditions have negative health consequences, which worsen when they occur together. In the Special Issue, the study by Pedram et al. [9] found that all-cause mortality of the lifetime self-reported history of eating disorders in the Canadian population was markedly elevated and considerably higher than that of other self-reported disorders, highlighting the seriousness of eating disorders and the urgent need for strategies that can help improve early diagnosis and a long-term plan for adequate interventions.

Finally, the study by Ivey et al. [10] analyzed the influence of the exposome, as a measure of all exposures of an individual in a lifetime, on the cardiometabolic risk profile. The study was carried out on a cohort of US Veterans and found evidence of structural relationships between diet, lifestyle, and demographic exposures and subsequent markers of cardiometabolic health. This study may provide valuable information toward the development of personalized interventions to improve cardiometabolic health outcomes based on the individual's exposome. Additionally, it offers the potential to identify key determinants of cardiometabolic health and guide public health policies toward promoting healthy lifestyle choices.

Funding: Proyectos I + D + i FEDER Andalucía 2014–2020 (US-1381231), VI and VII Plan Propio de la Universidad de Sevilla (2023/00000374).

Conflicts of Interest: The author declares that there are no conflict of interest.

References

1. Grao-Cruces, E.; Varela, L.M.; Martin, M.E.; Bermudez, B.; Montserrat-de la Paz, S. High-Density Lipoproteins and Mediterranean Diet: A Systematic Review. *Nutrients* **2021**, *13*, 955. [CrossRef] [PubMed]
2. Vazquez-Madrigal, C.; Lopez, S.; Grao-Cruces, E.; Millan-Linares, M.C.; Rodriguez-Martin, N.M.; Martin, M.E.; Alba, G.; Santa-Maria, C.; Bermudez, B.; Montserrat-de la Paz, S. Dietary Fatty Acids in Postprandial Triglyceride-Rich Lipoproteins Modulate Human Monocyte-Derived Dendritic Cell Maturation and Activation. *Nutrients* **2020**, *12*, 3139. [CrossRef] [PubMed]
3. Filippini, T.; Adani, G.; Malavolti, M.; Garuti, C.; Cilloni, S.; Vinceti, G.; Zamboni, G.; Tondelli, M.; Galli, C.; Costa, M.; et al. Dietary Habits and Risk of Early-Onset Dementia in an Italian Case-Control Study. *Nutrients* **2020**, *12*, 3682. [CrossRef] [PubMed]
4. Llanaj, E.; Vincze, F.; Kósa, Z.; Bárdos, H.; Diószegi, J.; Sándor, J.; Ádány, R. Deteriorated Dietary Patterns with Regards to Health and Environmental Sustainability among Hungarian Roma Are Not Differentiated from Those of the General Population. *Nutrients* **2021**, *13*, 721. [CrossRef] [PubMed]
5. Wang, K.; Zhao, Y.; Nie, J.; Xu, H.; Yu, C.; Wang, S. Higher HEI-2015 Score Is Associated with Reduced Risk of Depression: Result from NHANES 2005–2016. *Nutrients* **2021**, *13*, 348. [CrossRef] [PubMed]
6. Miles, F.L.; Mashchak, A.; Filippov, V.; Orlich, M.J.; Duerksen-Hughes, P.; Chen, X.; Wang, C.; Siegmund, K.; Fraser, G.E. DNA Methylation Profiles of Vegans and Non-Vegetarians in the Adventist Health Study-2 Cohort. *Nutrients* **2020**, *12*, 3697. [CrossRef] [PubMed]
7. Bai, Y.; Zhang, H.; Yang, J.; Peng, L. The Association between Daily Total Dietary Nutrient Intake and Recent Glycemic Control States of Non-Pregnant Adults 20+ Years Old from NHANES 1999–2018 (Except for 2003–2004). *Nutrients* **2021**, *13*, 4168. [CrossRef] [PubMed]
8. Yeh, W.-J.; Ko, J.; Cheng, W.-Y.; Yang, H.-Y. Dehulled Adlay Consumption Modulates Blood Pressure in Spontaneously Hypertensive Rats and Overweight and Obese Young Adults. *Nutrients* **2021**, *13*, 2305. [CrossRef] [PubMed]
9. Pedram, P.; Patten, S.B.; Bulloch, A.G.M.; Williams, J.V.A.; Dimitropoulos, G. Self-Reported Lifetime History of Eating Disorders and Mortality in the General Population: A Canadian Population Survey with Record Linkage. *Nutrients* **2021**, *13*, 3333. [CrossRef] [PubMed]
10. Ivey, K.L.; Nguyen, X.-M.T.; Posner, D.; Rogers, G.B.; Tobias, D.K.; Song, R.; Ho, Y.-L.; Li, R.; Wilson, P.W.F.; Cho, K.; et al. The Structure of Relationships between the Human Exposome and Cardiometabolic Health: The Million Veteran Program. *Nutrients* **2021**, *13*, 1364. [CrossRef] [PubMed]

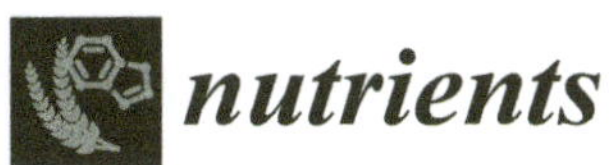

nutrients

Review

High-Density Lipoproteins and Mediterranean Diet: A Systematic Review

Elena Grao-Cruces [1], Lourdes M. Varela [2,3,*], Maria E. Martin [4], Beatriz Bermudez [4] and Sergio Montserrat-de la Paz [1]

[1] Department of Medical Biochemistry, Molecular Biology and Immunology, School of Medicine, University of Seville, 41009 Seville, Spain; egrao@us.es (E.G.-C.); delapaz@us.es (S.M.-d.l.P.)
[2] Institute of Biomedicine of Seville, IBiS, Universitary Hospital Virgen del Rocio/CSIC/University of Seville, 41013 Seville, Spain
[3] Department of Medical Physiology and Biophysics, University of Seville, 41009 Seville, Spain
[4] Department of Cell Biology, Faculty of Biology, University of Seville, 41012 Seville, Spain; mariamartin@us.es (M.E.M.); bbermudez@us.es (B.B.)
* Correspondence: lvarela@us.es; Tel.: +34-955-923-058

Abstract: Cardiovascular disease (CVD) is the leading cause of global mortality and the study of high-density lipoproteins (HDL) particle composition and functionality has become a matter of high interest, particularly in light to the disappointing clinical data for HDL-cholesterol (HDL-C) raising therapies in CVD secondary prevention and the lack of association between HDL-C and the risk of CVD. Recent evidences suggest that HDL composition and functionality could be modulated by diet. The purpose of this systematic review was to investigate the effect of Mediterranean diet (MD) on changes in HDL structure and functionality in humans. A comprehensive search was conducted in four databases (PubMed, Scopus, Cochrane library and Web of Science) and 13 records were chosen. MD showed favorable effects on HDL functionality, particularly by improving HDL cholesterol efflux capacity and decreasing HDL oxidation. In addition, HDL composition and size were influenced by MD. Thus, MD is a protective factor against CVD associated with the improvement of HDL quality and the prevention of HDL dysfunctionality.

Keywords: high-density lipoprotein; lipidome; proteome; Mediterranean diet; olive oil

Citation: Grao-Cruces, E.; Varela, L.M.; Martin, M.E.; Bermudez, B.; Montserrat-de la Paz, S. High-Density Lipoproteins and Mediterranean Diet: A Systematic Review. *Nutrients* **2021**, *13*, 955. https://doi.org/10.3390/nu13030955

Academic Editor: Mario Barbagallo

Received: 23 February 2021
Accepted: 12 March 2021
Published: 16 March 2021

Publisher's Note: MDPI stays neutral with regard to jurisdictional claims in published maps and institutional affiliations.

1. Introduction

Cardiovascular disease (CVD) remains the leading cause of morbidity and mortality worldwide. It is well known that high concentrations of circulating high-density lipoprotein-cholesterol (HDL-C) are inversely correlated with the risk of CVD [1]. While raising HDL-C is a theoretically attractive target, there is no evidence from randomized trials that increasing plasma HDL-C concentrations reduces CVD risk [2].

Several studies have shown that high-density lipoproteins (HDLs) are highly heterogeneous in size, shape, density, lipid and protein composition [3]. HDL particles undergo continuous remodeling through interactions with other circulating lipoproteins and tissues [4]. HDL-associated proteins have been considered until now to predominate in determining the particle structure and biological functions: cholesterol removal, anti-inflammatory, antioxidant and endothelial cell protection [5]. For example, paraoxonase 1 (PON1) is a HDL-associated protein mediating HDL functionality that has been negatively correlated with unfavorable outcome in stroke patients [6]. However, the latest cutting edge lipidomic technology has revealed important roles of lipid components in HDL function. Sphingomielin-1-phosphate (S1P) is the most studied bioactive lipid bound to HDL and it has been negatively correlated with the severity of coronary artery disease [7]. Recent evidence linked increased odds of acute coronary syndrome to low cholesterol efflux capacity (CEC), pro-oxidant and pro-inflammatory HDL particles and low HDL levels of S1P [8]. In addition, HDL-C was found to be highly related to cardiovascular risk when it was carried by small HDLs, suggesting that cardiovascular risk is highly influenced by HDL size [9]. Taken all together, it is becoming clear that circulating HDL-C plasma concentrations is not an appropriate marker of CVD risk and therefore do not represent a reliable therapeutic target. Targeting HDL functionality rather than HDL-C concentrations may represent a more promising therapeutic target.

Different strategies are followed in order to modify plasma HDL-C and cardiovascular health. Healthy diets have beneficial effects on lipid profile, replacing saturated fatty acids (SFA) with either monounsaturated (MUFA) or polyunsaturated fatty acids (PUFA) have been shown to reduce plasma HDL-C [10]. This objective is achieved with Mediterranean diet (MD), rich in olive oil (OO) fruits and vegetables, nuts, legumes and whole cereals, fish and red wine. Data from observational and randomized controlled trials supports that MD protects against CVD, MD has showed capacity to improve lipid profile related to HDL-C [11]. The purpose of this systematic review was to investigate the effect of the MD on changes in HDL structure and functionality in humans.

2. Materials and Methods

This systematic review was conducted following the Preferred Reporting Items for Systematic reviews and Meta-analysis (PRISMA) [12]. This review was registered on PROSPERO (Registration No. CRD42020218784). Available from: https://www.crd.york.ac.uk/prospero/display_record.php?ID=CRD42020218784 (accessed on 23 February 2021).

2.1. Searching Strategy

A comprehensive search was conducted in four databases (PubMed, Scopus, Web of Science and Cochrane Library), searching all years of record up until October 2020. The language restriction was English and Spanish. Search terms were categorized into 3 key concepts: study population, HDL modulation, and nutritional intervention; specific terms used were: (adult OR "middle-aged" OR young OR m?n OR wom?n OR obese OR healthy) AND ("Mediterranean diet" OR "olive oil") AND ("HDL remodel*" or "HDL function*" OR "HDL dysfunction*" OR "HDL change" OR "HDL component"), respectively. Whereas, reference lists of retrieved articles were manually searched for relevant publications (Table 1).

Table 1. Population, intervention, comparator, outcome, and study design (PICOS) model of eligibility criteria.

Criteria	Definition
Population	Human studies: adult men and women, including healthy participants, obese and dyslipidemic patients and not including individuals with genetic diseases
Interventions	MD or MD isolated food interventions
Comparator	Comparison against baseline or comparison against different interventions
Outcomes	HDL composition changes HDL functionality changes HDL components modifications
Study design	Human pilot studies and controlled trials

HDL, high-density lipoprotein; MD, Mediterranean diet.

2.2. Selection Criteria

Published studies included in this review were require to adhere to the following criteria: (1) original research; (2) adult human studies; (3) articles including HDL changes in composition, HDL component modifications or HDL functionality changes; (4) dietary intervention with MD or MD-related foods; (5) obese, dyslipidemic and healthy humans.

2.3. Data Extraction and Reliability

The PRISMA recommendations were followed. Firstly, titles were screened and abstracts were analyzed in order to identify relevant articles. Then, articles chosen were downloaded and reviewed in detail by different researchers.

3. Results

3.1. Search and Selection of Studies

The searching and selection strategies are detailed in Figure 1. A total of 55 records were identified through database searching and 38 through other sources, search of reference list of retrieved articles. Duplicates were removed and a set of 34 records were left to select the ones to be screened. From these 34, 7 records were excluded due to article type and 27 records were susceptible of full-text assessment. Consequently, 13 records were excluded with criteria, and 14 records were assessed for eligibility. Finally, 1 record was excluded because of the methodology used and 13 records were analyzed.

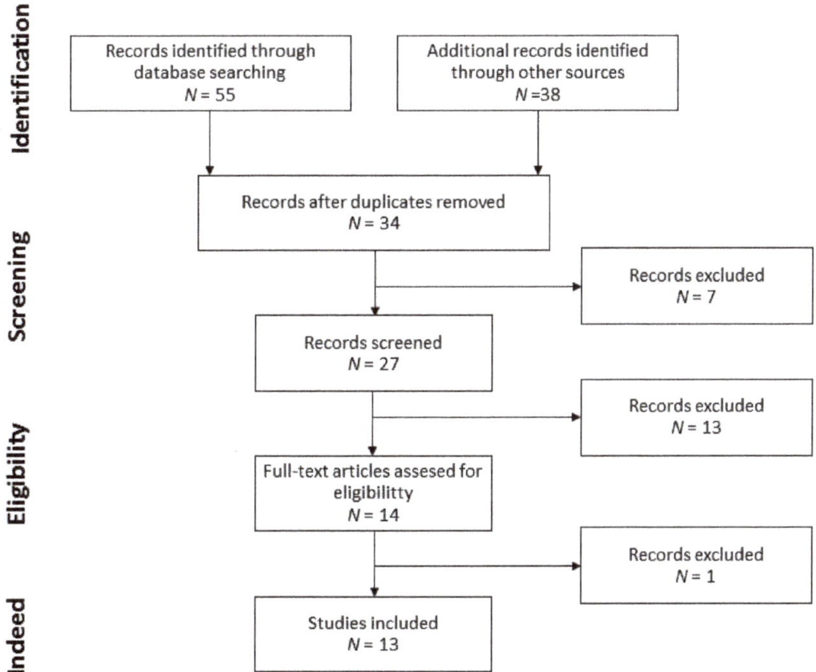

Figure 1. Flow diagram of record selection.

3.2. Comparison between Studies

Nine different study populations have been found in the records chosen, whereas, ten nutritional interventions were studied (Table 2). Two records studied the same 296 individuals with three nutritional interventions [13,14]. Otherwise, after the interventions, Hernaez et al., 2019, made an evaluation of foods consumed by 196 individuals from the initial study population, in order to create different groups [13]. Individuals in each study population were different between studies, healthy individuals were included in a total of 5 study populations [15–19], and the rest of the study populations included high cardiovascular risk individuals, which suffered from dyslipidemia, obesity or hypercholesterolemia [13,14,20–25].

Table 2. Study characteristics.

Authors and Publication Year	Study Characteristic					Intervention
	Sample	Age	Country	Duration	Design	
A. Hernaez et al., 2019 [13]	196 individuals from the PREDIMED study	55–80	Spain	1 year	Randomized controlled trial	Traditional MD—VOO Traditional MD–nuts Traditional MD—fish Traditional MD—legumes Traditional MD—whole grains
A. Hernaez et al., 2017 [14]	296 individuals from the PREDIMED study	55–80	Spain	1 year	Randomized controlled trial	Traditional MD—nuts Traditional MD—VOO Low-fat diet
A. Hernaez et al., 2014 [15]	47 individuals from the EUROLIVE study	20–60	Germany Spain Finland	3 weeks	Randomized controlled trial	HPCOO LPCOO
N. Tanaka et al., 2014 [20]	28 dyslipidemic individuals	50–85	Japan	4 weeks	Randomized trial	Low-fat diet enriched with EPA
R. Sola et al., 2011 [21]	772 individuals from the PREDIMED study	55–80	Spain	3 months	Randomized controlled trial	Traditional MD—VOO Traditional MD—nuts Low-fat diet
J. McEneny et al., 2013 [16]	54 overweight individuals	45–55	UK	12 weeks	Randomized controlled trial	Lycopene rich diet Lycopene supplemented diet
C. Zhu et al., 2019 [17]	10 healthy individuals	18–25	California	4 days	Randomized crossover trial	Fast food diet MD
O. Helal et al., 2013 [18]	26 healthy individuals	18–75	Canada	12 weeks	Randomized trial	Extra VOO
M. Farras et al., 2015 [22] S. Fernandez-Castillejo et al., 2017 [23] M. Farras et al., 2018 [24] A. Pedret et al., 2015 [25]	33 individuals of the VOHF study	35–80	Spain	3 weeks	Randomized controlled trial	VOO FVOO FVOOT
R. Sola et al., 1997 [19]	22 healthy individuals	45–55		8 weeks	Randomized crossover trial	MD rich in oleic MD rich in linoleic

MD, Mediterranean diet; VOO, virgin olive oil; HPCOO, high-polyphenol content olive oil; LPCOO, low-polyphenol content olive oil; EPA, eicosapentaenoic acid; FVOO, functional virgin olive oil; FVOOT, functional olive oil with thyme; UK, United Kingdom.

Intervention time varied between studies. The longest intervention time was 1 year [13,14] and the shortest 4 days [17].

3.3. HDL Functionality Modulation

A set of 7 records measured cholesterol efflux capacity (CEC), CEC measurements were conducted on THP-1 monocyte-derived macrophages [13–15,18,20], on J-774A.1 macrophages [22–25] and on primary cultures [19]. PON, lecithin cholesterol acyl transferase (LCAT), and cholesteryl ester transfer protein (CETP) activities were determined in a set of 5 [13,14,16,20,22–25], 3 [15,16,22–25] and 4 [13–16] populations, respectively, by enzymatic activity measurements.

Specific MD-related foods were able to modulate HDL functions (Table 3). An increase of CEC was showed after virgin OO (VOO), whole grains and nuts [13] eicosapentaenoic acid (EPA) [20] and extra VOO [18] consumption compared to baseline. Enzyme activity was variable after different interventions: CETP activity was decreased by diets enriched with legumes, fish and VOO [13]. PON1 activity was increased by nut, legume and fish enriched diets [13], EPA consumption [20], lycopene rich and supplemented diets [16] and functional VOO with thyme (FVOOT) intervention [22–25]. LCAT activity increased with lycopene supplemented diets [16]. Although there was no change after VOO, functional VOO (FVOO and FVOOT) interventions in LCAT activity, it was significantly higher after FVOOT in comparison with VOO intervention [22–25].

Table 3. High-density lipoprotein (HDL) functionality.

Author(s) and Publication Year		Measurement			
		CEC	CETP	PON1	LCAT
A. Hernaez et al., 2019 [13]	Traditional MD—VOO	Increase	NS	NS	NM
	Traditional MD—nuts	NS	NS	Increase	
	Traditional MD—legumes	NS	Decrease	Increase	
	Traditional MD—whole-grains	Increase	NS	NS	
	Traditional—fish	Decrease	Decrease	Increase	
A. Hernaez et al., 2017 [14]	Traditional MD—VOO	Increase	Decrease	NS [a]	NM
	Traditional MD—nuts	Increase	NS	NS	
A. Hernaez et al., 2014 [15]	LPCOO	NS	NS	NM	NS
	HPCOO	NS [b]	NS		NS
N. Tanaka et al., 2014 [20]	Low fat diet—EPA	Increase	NM	Increase	NM
R. Sola et al., 2011 [21]		NM			
J. McEneny et al., 2013 [16]	Lycopene rich diet	NM	NS	Increase	NS
	Lycopene supplemented diet		NS	Increase	Increase
C. Zhu et al., 2019 [17]		NM			
O. Helal et al., 2013 [18]	Extra VOO	Increase	NM	NM	NM
M. Farras et al., 2015 [22]	VOO	NS		NS	NS
S. Fernandez-Castillejo et al., 2017 [23]	FVOO	NS		NS	NS
			NM		
M. Farras et al., 2018 [24] A. Pedret et al., 2015 [25]	FVOOT	Increase		Increase	NS [c]
R. Sola et al., 1997 [19]	Oleic acid vs. linoleic acid rich MD	NS	NM	NM	NM

MD, Mediterranean diet; VOO, virgin olive oil; LPCOO, low-polyphenol content olive oil; HPCOO, high-polyphenol content olive oil; EPA, eicosapentaenoic acid; FVOO, functional virgin olive oil; FVOOT, functional virgin olive oil with thyme; NS, no significant change; NM, not measured. [a] Significant change compared to traditional MD—nuts; [b] significant change compared to LPCOO; [c] significant change compared to VOO.

3.4. HDL Oxidation

HDLs are affected by oxidative modifications and the fatty acids contained in HDL-associated lipids are the most susceptible components to oxidation. HDL oxidation state (Table 4) is related to HDL functionality. HDL oxidation rate was measured as equivalents of malondialdehyde production [14,19], and other HDL oxidation-related parameters were measured by Hernaez et al. 2017: HDL capacity to prevent low-density lipoprotein (LDL) oxidation and HDL resistance to oxidation in a pro-oxidant environment [14]. After a VOO-enriched traditional MD, HDL antioxidant properties were improved, lower HDL oxidation rate, higher HDL resistance to oxidation and higher prevention of LDL oxidation were found [14]. In addition, linoleic supplemented diet showed capacity to reduce HDL oxidation rate compared to lycopene rich diet [19].

Table 4. High-density lipoprotein (HDL) oxidation.

Author(s) and Publication Year		HDL Oxidation Rate Variation
A. Hernaez et al., 2017 [14]	Traditional MD—VOO	Decreased
	Traditional MD—nuts	NS
M. Farras et al., 2015 [22]	VOO	NS
S. Fernandez-Castillejo et al., 2017 [23]	FVOO	NS
M. Farras et al., 2018 [24]	FVOOT	NS
A. Pedret et al., 2015 [25]		
R. *Sola* et al., 1997 [19]	Oleic acid vs. linoleic acid	Decreased in oleic acid

MD, Mediterranean diet; VOO, virgin olive oil; FVOO, functional virgin olive oil; FVOOT, functional virgin olive oil with thyme; HPCOO, high-polyphenol content olive oil; LPCOO, low-polyphenol content olive oil; EPA, eicosapenthaenoic acid; NS, non-significant change.

HDL antioxidant properties were measured after different VOO interventions (VOO, FVOO and FVOOT) [22–25]. However, no change was found in HDL oxidation rate, HDL resistance to oxidation and glutathione peroxidase activity. To highlight, HDL oxidation rate was measured as white blood cells production of dihydrorhodamine 123 [22].

3.5. HDL Monolayer Fluidity

HDL monolayer fluidity was analyzed by a determination of steady-state anisotropy of 1,6-diphenyl-1,3,4-hexatriene (DHP) (Table 5). High-polyphenol content olive oil (HPCOO) [15] and extra VOO [18] consumption were found to increase HDL monolayer fluidity. However, different VOO interventions (VOO, FVOO and FVOOT) did not show effect over HDL monolayer fluidity [22–25].

Table 5. High-density lipoprotein (HDL) monolayer fluidity.

Author(s) and Publication Year		HDL Monolayer Fluidity Variation
A. Hernaez et al., 2014 [15]	LPCOO	NS
	HPCOO	Increased
O. Helal et al. 2013 [18]	Extra VOO	Increased
M. Farras et al., 2015 [22]		
S. Fernandez-Castillejo et al., 2017 [23]	VOO + FVOO + FVOOT	NS
M. Farras et al., 2018 [24]		
A. Pedret et al., 2015 [25]		
R. Sola et al., 1997 [19]	Oleic acid vs. linoleic acid	NS

LPCOO, low-polyphenol content olive oil; HPCOO, high-polyphenol content olive oil; VOO, virgin olive oil; FVOO, functional virgin olive oil; FVOOT, functional virgin olive oil with thyme; NS, no significant change.

Correlation models between HDL monolayer fluidity and HDL functionality-related parameters found that free HDL-C and triglyceride contents and HDL size were the main determinants of HDL monolayer fluidity [23].

3.6. HDL Composition

HDL lipidome is modulated by diet, even by a short-time dietary intervention. After two 4-day dietary interventions, HDL lipidome was widely modulated and fatty acids contained in HDL phospholipids were the most variable lipids by diet [17]. The 4-day MD intervention increased the quantity of phosphatidylcholine with very long chain and double bonds fatty acids, compared to baseline and to the 4-day fast food diet intervention. Fatty acid length, which was found to increase after the 4-day MD intervention, was directly related to MUFA and PUFA consumption [17]. In addition, an oleic acid rich diet, as MD, increased oleic acid and its derivatives in HDL phospholipids [19,23]. A linoleic acid rich diet increased linoleic HDL quantity, but linoleic acid binding capacity was lower than oleic acid [19].

Phenolic compounds contained in OO were found to present ability to bind to HDL particles. HDL showed higher phenolic compounds after HPCOO intervention [15] and after VOO, FVOO and FVOOT diets [23], specifically α-tocopherol, β-cryptoxanthin and coenzyme Q [23]. Lycopene rich and supplemented diets modulated HDL composition, higher HDL lycopene quantity was found after lycopene interventions [16].

HDL proteome showed to be influenced by nutritional interventions. After three interventions with VOO (VOO, FVOO and FVOOT), the HDL proteome was remodeled: 15 HDL metabolism-related proteins were identified as the most importantly modulated after the interventions, including PON3, apolipoprotein (apo)-AI, apoA-II and apoD [25]. However, no change in apo-AI quantity was found after interventions with HPCOO, LPCOO [15] and lycopene [16]. While, higher apo-AI quantity was found after a traditional MD-enriched diet enriched with nuts and VOO [14] and after three diets with VOO (VOO, FVOO and FVOOT) compared to baseline [25].

3.7. HDL Size

HDL size range between 8–10 nm of diameter and two groups are defined in terms of HDL size: large and small, also named as HDL3 and HDL2, respectively. The effect of different OO interventions on HDL size is shown in Table 6. Large HDL number was found to be increased after a MD enriched with VOO and with nuts [14] and after HPCOO [15] consumption. In addition, HPCOO consumption showed to decrease small HDL number. When HPCOO consumption is compared with LPCOO, large HDL number was increased and small HDL number decreased [15]. However, different VOO enriched with polyphenols (FVOO and FVOOT) showed to decrease large HDL number and to increase small HDL number [22–25]. On the other hand, extra VOO did not show capacity to modulate HDL size [18].

Table 6. High-density lipoprotein (HDL) size variation against baseline.

Author(S) And Publication Year		HDL Size Modifications
A. Hernaez et al., 2017 [14]	Traditional MD—VOO	Increased levels of large HDLs
	Traditional MD—nuts	Increased levels of large HDLs
A. Hernaez et al., 2014 [15]	LPCOO	NS
	HPCOO [a]	Increased levels of large HDLs
		Decreased levels of small HDLs
O. Helal et al. 2013 [18]	Extra VOO	NS
M. Farras et al., 2015 [22]	VOO	NS
S. Fernandez-Castillejo et al., 2017 [23]	FVOO	Increased levels of small HDLs
M. Farras et al., 2018 [24]		
A. Pedret et al., 2015 [25]	FVOOT [b]	Decreased levels of large HDLs

MD, Mediterranean diet; VOO, virgin olive oil; LPCOO, low-polyphenol content olive oil; HPCOO, high-polyphenol content olive oil; FVOO, functional virgin olive oil; FVOOT, functional olive oil with thyme; HDL, high-density lipoprotein; NS, no significant change. [a] Significant change compared to LPCOO. [b] Significant change compared to VOO.

4. Discussion

HDL-C is clinically considered a CVD protective factor. However, pharmacological strategies that led to an increase in HDL-C did not reduce CVD risk [26]. The lack of effect of HDL-C raising strategies puts into question HDL-C concentrations as a protective factor against CVD. HDL-C should be in the spotlight as a CVD lowering risk factor and HDL modulations should be considered in order to predict CVD risk [3].

HDL composition is demonstrated to change in different physiological and pathological conditions [27,28]. Diseases associated to higher CVD risk, such as obesity and diabetes, remodel HDL composition and functionality. Diabetic people showed glycosylated and oxidized HDLs that presented lower HDL CEC, antioxidant and anti-inflammatory activities [29]. Moreover, lifestyle remodels HDLs and influences on their biological activities. In particular, unhealthy diets contribute to the development of dysfunctional HDLs, even in people without diseases [27]. In addition, healthy diets such as MD, have shown capacity to remodel HDL functionality even in pathological conditions, like obesity [28].

In a whole view of the data analyzed in this review, MD showed capacity to produce changes in HDL by modulating HDL functionality, oxidation, composition, and size. MD-induced changes in HDL are variable between records analyzed and not all data were comparable because the same measurements were not always performed. This variability could be influenced by population differences, healthy and high cardiovascular risk populations. Moreover, despite all records performed interventions with MD, different foods or dietary patterns were used in each record, which may contribute to different changes in HDLs, highlighting the need for greater consistency between studies in the amount of foods and nutrients administered as part of a MD. Interestingly, intervention time in the studies included in this review was found not to be a limiting factor, because even after short interventions HDL were remodeled. Several studies were conducted over different samples of the PREDIMED population, which demonstrated that HDL are widely altered by diet and that MD improves HDL quality [13,14,21].

A set of 5 studies made an intervention with VOO [13,14,18], OO or components isolated from OO, specifically polyphenols [15,22–25] and oleic acid [19]. HDL CEC was the most OO-enhanced HDL function [13–15,18,22–25], due, at least in part, to OO polyphenols [15,22–25]. CETP was not significantly decreased after OO interventions, with the exception of a traditional MD-enriched with VOO [14]. However, when the study population was subdivided, the new VOO group did not show changes in CETP activity [13]. LCAT activity showed significant change only after FVOOT when compared to VOO [22–25], which suggests that LCAT activity is specially modulated by polyphenols. However, a HPCOO diet did not increase LCAT activity, against baseline neither against LPCOO [15]. In addition, lycopene rich and supplemented diets were the only interventions that showed an improvement of LCAT activity compared to baseline [16]. FVOOT differs from FVOO and HPCOO in that it is enriched in thyme polyphenols. Thus, LCAT activity may be susceptible to thyme polyphenols when compared to other OO and OO polyphenols.

In regards to antioxidant functions of HDL, a traditional MD enriched with VOO and an oleic acid enriched diet lowered HDL oxidation [14,19], but no significant change in oxidation rate was found after phenol enriched VOO diets (FVOO and FVOOT). However, PON1 activity was higher after a FVOOT intervention [22–25], but no significant change was found after a traditional MD enriched with VOO [14]. FVOOT was demonstrated to increase HDL antioxidant function but not to alter HDL oxidation rate. On one hand, a traditional MD enriched with VOO decreased HDL oxidation but did not change PON1 activity. PON1 is not the only HDL antioxidant component, so the reduction on HDL oxidation rate described after a traditional MD-enriched with VOO could be due to other HDL antioxidant components, or to a MD-induced lower pro-oxidant environment, which in addition to VOO leads to lower HDL oxidation rate. On the other hand, PON1 activity could be increased by the higher presence of polyphenols on FVOOT, not altering other HDL oxidation parameters or the environment. The study population is not widely differential between interventions, since high cardiovascular risk people were included in both. However, the number of participants in the traditional MD enriched with VOO intervention was higher compared to the intervention with FVOOT, and the HDL oxidation rate was differently measured. It would be necessary to determine HDL oxidation rate after FVOO and FVOOT interventions as malondialdehyde production to be able to compare.

A HPCOO diet and an extra VOO intervention increased HDL fluidity [15,18]. There was no change in HDL monolayer fluidity in phenol enriched VOO (FVOOT and FVOO) and VOO diets [22–25]. Opposed evidences are exposed in terms of VOO and polyphenols influence on HDL monolayer fluidity. However, it is important to highlight that there were differences between the study populations. When the study population was healthy, HDL monolayer fluidity was increased by OO, but no change was found when the study population was hypercholesterolemic. OO does not benefit HDL monolayer fluidity when hypercholesterolemia is present.

Taken all data together, OO showed ability to modulate HDL functionality, and polyphenols may be very influencing components. Despite controversial results were found in HDL oxidation and monolayer fluidity, and the missing data of some enzyme activities, HDL functions could be modulated by OO. The remodeling pattern needs to be clarified, suggesting the need for further research.

EPA is an essential fatty acid, which has showed anti-inflammatory functions (complete). Fish is an EPA-rich food highly consumed in MD. An EPA enriched diet showed ability to increase HDL CEC and PON1 activity [20]. In addition, a traditional MD enriched with fish increased HDL CEC and PON1 activity and decreased CETP activity [13]. Dyslipidemia did not alter EPA-related HDL functionality improvement. Whereas, the data is not contradictory compared to interventions with VOO enriched with polyphenols (FVOO and FVOOT) in hypercholesterolemia, because PON1 activity and CEC were improved after FVOOT intervention and VOO, FVOO and FVOOT, respectively. It would be interesting to study the effect of EPA in hypercholesterolemic population over HDL oxidation rate as malondialdehyde production, to clarify if high CVD risk population is not susceptible to improve HDL oxidation rate by diet.

All records in which HDL compositional change was analyzed, HDL composition was modulated by a MD. HDL seem to be susceptible to the kind of lipid consumed. HDL lipid composition was enriched on dietary lipids. However, there is not a HDL composition change pattern by MD and no correlations could be made between HDL composition and HDL functionality.

HDL do not only vary in composition and functionality, they are subdivided by size in different types of HDLs. HDL size is variable due to HDL metabolism, since HDLs bind different components and modulate their size, as a result of HDL synthesis and catabolism, and it is also reflected in the HDL functions. HDL type in terms of size seems to influence CVD risk. Owing to the relation between HDL size and HDL functionality development, MD could change HDL size distribution. Results found by different researches are controversial, since VOO and nuts enriched diets increased large HDL quantity [14], and a HPCOO intervention increased large HDL quantity and decreased small HDL quantity, compared to baseline and to a LPCOO diet [15]. Nevertheless, two diets based on VOO enriched with polyphenols (FVOO and FVOOT) showed to have the contrary effect [22–25]. HDL size could be differently modulated when the study population is hypercholesterolemic, since hypercholesterolemia could alter OO benefits over HDL functionality.

5. Conclusions

In conclusion, this systematic review shows that MD influences HDL functionality, composition, and size. HDL functionality is improved by MD, in terms of enzymatic activity and CEC, also HDL antioxidant properties are improved, as HDL oxidation is reduced. There is a need to clarify MD-derived modulation of HDL size to determine HDL components which fundamentally are influenced by MD. In addition, further research is needed to determine MD specific food HDL-modulating abilities and the effect of the global MD. While, it would be interesting to clarify the MD abilities over healthy and hypercholesterolemic or dyslipidemic population separately. Taken together, MD has demonstrated to be an influencing factor over HDL quality, which indicate that MD could be a target to improve cardiovascular health via HDL modulation.

Author Contributions: Conceptualization, E.G.-C., L.M.V., M.E.M., B.B., S.M.-d.l.P.; data collection and analysis: E.G.-C.; data interpretation: E.G.-C., L.M.V., M.E.M., B.B., S.M.-d.l.P.; writing-original draft preparation: E.G.-C. with the assistance from S.M.-d.l.P. and L.M.V.; writing-review and editing, E.G.-C., L.M.V., M.E.M., B.B., S.M.-d.l.P.; funding acquisition, B.B. and S.M.-d.l.P. All authors have read and agreed to the published version of the manuscript.

Funding: This study was supported by the research Grant US-1263458 (Andalusian Ministry of Economy, Knowledge, Business, and University, Government of Andalusia, Spain) into the European Regional Development Fund Operational Programme—2014 to 2020.

Institutional Review Board Statement: This research was exempt from ethics approval because the work was carried out on published documents.

Informed Consent Statement: Not applicable.

Data Availability Statement: Not applicable.

Acknowledgments: L.M.V. acknowledges financial support from VI PPIT-US (University of Seville).

Conflicts of Interest: The authors state no conflict of interest.

References

1. Kontush, A.; Lindahl, M.; Lhomme, M.; Calabresi, M.; Chapman, M.J.; Davidson, W. Structure of HDL: Particle subclases and molecular components. *Handb. Exp. Pharmacol.* **2015**, *224*, 3–51. [CrossRef]
2. March, F.; Baigent, C.; Catapano, A.L.; Koskinas, K.C.; Casula, M.; Badimon, L.; Chapman, M.J.; de Backer, G.G.; Delgado, V.; Ference, B.A.; et al. 2019 ESC/EAS Guidelines for the management of dyslipidaemias: Lipid modification to reduce cardiovascularrisk. *Eur. Heart J.* **2020**, *41*, 111–181. [CrossRef]
3. Ronsein, G.E.; Heinecke, J.W. Time to ditch HDL-C as a measure of HDL function. *Curr. Opin. Lipidol.* **2017**, *28*, 414–418. [CrossRef] [PubMed]
4. Lim, G.B. Dyslipidaemia: Effect of hypercholesterolaemia on HDL particle remodelling. *Nat. Rev. Cardiol.* **2017**, *14*, 505. [CrossRef] [PubMed]
5. Choi, H.Y.; Hafiane, A.; Schwertani, A.; Genest, J. High-Density Lipoproteins: Biology, Epidemiology, and Clinical Management. *Can. J. Cardiol.* **2017**, *33*, 325–333. [CrossRef] [PubMed]
6. Varela, L.M.; Mesenguer, E.; Apergue, B.; Couret, D.; Amarenco, P.; Meilhac, O. Changes in High-density Lipoproteins Related to Outcomes in Patients with Acute Stroke. *J. Clin. Med.* **2020**, *9*, 2269. [CrossRef] [PubMed]
7. Sattler, K.; Lehmann, L.; Graler, M.; Brocker-Preuss, M.; Erbel, R.; Heusch, G.; Levkau, B. HDL-bound sphingosine 1-phosphate (S1P) predicts the severity of coronary artery atherosclerosis. *Cell Physiol. Biochem.* **2014**, *34*, 172–184. [CrossRef]
8. Soria-Florido, M.T.; Castañer, O.; Lassale, C.; Estruch, R.; Salas-Salvado, J.; Martinez-Gonzalez, M.A.; Corella, D.; Ros, E.; Arós, F.; Elosua, R.; et al. Dysfunctional High-Density lipoproteins Are Associated With a Greater Incidence of Acute Coronary Syndrome in a Population at High Cardiovascular Risk. A Nested Case-Control Study. *Circulation* **2020**, *141*, 444–453. [CrossRef]
9. Prats-Uribe, A.; Sayols-Baixeras, S.; Fernandez-Sanles, A.; Subirana, I.; Carreras-Torres, R.; Vilahur, G.; Civeira, F.; Marrugat, J.; Fitó, M.; Hernáez, Á.; et al. High-density lipoprotein characteristics and coronary artery disease: A Mendelian randomization study. *Metabolism* **2020**, *112*, 154351. [CrossRef]
10. Hisham, M.D.B.; Aziz, Z.; Huin, W.K.; Teoh, C.H.; Jamil, A.H.A. The effects of palm oil on serum lipid profiles: A systematic review and meta-analysis. *Asia Pac. J. Clin. Nutr.* **2020**, *28*, 523–536. [CrossRef]
11. Di Renzo, L.; Cinelli, G.; Dri, M.; Gualtieri, P.; Attina, A.; Leggeri, C.; Cenname, G.; Esposito, E.; Pujia, A.; Chiricolo, G.; et al. Mediterranean personalized diet combined with physical activity therapy for the prevention of cardiovascular diseases in Italian women. *Nutrients* **2020**, *12*, 3456. [CrossRef] [PubMed]
12. Moher, D.; Liberati, A.; Tetzlaff, J.; Altman, D.G.; PRISMA Group. Preferred reporting items for systematic reviews and meta-analyses. The PRISMA statement. *PLoS Med.* **2009**, *6*, e1000097. [CrossRef] [PubMed]
13. Hernaez, A.; Sanllorente, A.; Castañer, O.; Martinez-Gonzalez, M.; Ros, E.; Pinto, X.; Estruch, R.; Salas-Salvado, J.; Corella, D.; Alonso-Gomez, A.M.; et al. Increased Consumption of Virgin Olive Oil, Nuts, Legumes, Whole Grains, and Fish Promotes HDL Functions in Humans. *Mol. Nutr. Food Res.* **2019**, *63*, 1–5. [CrossRef] [PubMed]
14. Hernaez, A.; Castañer, O.; Elosua, R.; Pinto, X.; Estruch, R.; Salas-Salvado, J.; Corella, D.; Aros, F.; Serra-Majem, L.; Fiol, M.; et al. Mediterranean Diet Improves High-Density Lipoprotein Function in High-Cardiovascular-Risk Individuals. *Circulation* **2017**, *135*, 633–643. [CrossRef] [PubMed]
15. Hernaez, A.; Fernandez-Castillejo, A.; Farras, M.; Catalan, U.; Subirana, I.; Montes, R.; Sola, R.; Muñoz-Aguayo, D.; Gelabert-Gorges, A.; Diaz-Gil, O.; et al. Olive oil polyphenols enhance high-density lipoprotein function in humans: A randomized controlled trial. *Arterioscler. Thromb. Vasc. Biol.* **2014**, *34*, 2115–2119. [CrossRef]
16. McEneny, J.; Wade, L.; Young, I.S.; Masson, L.; Duthie, G.; McGinty, A.; Duthie, G.; McGinty, A.; McMaster, C.; Thies, F. Lycopene intervention reduces inflammation and improves HDL functionality in moderately overweight middle-aged individuals. *J. Nutr. Biochem.* **2013**, *24*, 163–168. [CrossRef]
17. Zhu, C.; Sawrey-Kubicek, L.; Beals, E.; Hughes, R.L.; Rhodes, C.H.; Sacchi, R.; Zivkovic, A.M. The HDL lipidome is widely remodelled by fast food versus Mediterranean diet in 4 days. *Metabolomics* **2019**, *15*, 1–11. [CrossRef] [PubMed]
18. Helal, O.; Berrougui, H.; Loued, A.; Khalil, A. Extra-virgin olive oil consumption improves the capacity of HDL to mediate cholesterol efflux and increases ABCA1 and ABCG1 expression in human macrophages. *Br. J. Nutr.* **2013**, *109*, 1844–1855. [CrossRef]

19. Sola, R.; la Ville, A.E.; Richard, J.L.; Motta, C.; Bargallo, M.T.; Girona, J.; Masana, L.; Bernard, J. Oleic acid rich diet protects against the oxidative modification of high density lipoprotein. *Free Radic. Biol. Med.* **1997**, *22*, 1037–1045. [CrossRef]
20. Tanaka, N.; Ishida, T.; Nagao, M.; Mori, T.; Monguchi, T.; Sasaki, M.; Mori, K.; Kondo, K.; Nakajima, H.; Honjo, T.; et al. Administration of high dose eicosapentaenoic acid enhances anti-inflammatory properties of high-density lipoprotein in Japanese patients with dyslipidemia. *Atherosclerosis* **2014**, *237*, 577–583. [CrossRef]
21. Sola, R.; Fito, M.; Estruch, R.; Salas-Salvado, J.; Corella, D.; de la Torre, R.; Muñoz, M.A.; Lopez-Sabater, M.C.; Martinez-Gonzalez, M.A.; Aros, F.; et al. Effect of a traditional Mediterranean diet on apolipoproteins B, A-I, and their ratio: A randomized controlled trial. *Atherosclerosis* **2011**, *218*, 174–180. [CrossRef]
22. Farras, M.; Castañer, O.; Martin-Pelaez, S.; Hernaez, A.; Schroder, H.; Subirana, I.; Muñoz-Aguayo, D.; Gaixas, S.; de la Torre, R.; Farre, M.; et al. Complementary phenol-enriched olive oil improves HDL charasteristic in hypercholesterolemic subjects. A randomized, double-blind, crossover, controlled trial. The VOHF Study. *Mol. Nutr. Food Res.* **2015**, *59*, 1758–1770. [CrossRef]
23. Fernandez-Castillejo, S.; Rubio, L.; Hernaez, A.; Catalan, U.; Pedret, A.; Valls, R.M.; Mosele, J.I.; Covas, M.I.; Remaley, A.T.; Castañer, O.; et al. Determinants of HDL Cholesterol Efflux Capacity after Virgin Olive Oil Ingestion: Interrelationships with Fluidity of HDL Monolayer. *Mol. Nutr. Food Res.* **2017**, *61*, 1–21. [CrossRef]
24. Farras, M.; Fernandez-Castillejo, S.; Rubio, L.; Arranz, S.; Catalan, U.; Subirana, I.; Romero, M.P.; Castañer, O.; Pedret, A.; Blanchart, A.; et al. Phenol-enriched olive oils improve HDL antioxidant content in hypercholesterolemic subjects. A randomized double-blind, cross-over, controlled trial. *J. Nutr. Biochem.* **2018**, *51*, 99–104. [CrossRef] [PubMed]
25. Pedret, A.; Catalan, U.; Fernandez-Castillejo, S.; Farras, M.; Valls, R.M.; Rubio, L.; Canela, N.; de la Torre, R.; Covas, M.I.; Fito, M.; et al. Impact of virgin olive oil and phenol-enriched virgin olive oils on the HDL proteome in hypercholesterolemic subjects: A double blind, randomized, controlled, cross-over clinical trial (VOHF study). *PLoS ONE* **2015**, *10*, 1–19. [CrossRef] [PubMed]
26. Cimmino, G.; Ciccarelli, G.; Morello, A.N.; Ciccarelli, M.; Golino, P. High Density Lipoprotein Cholesterol Increasing Therapy: The Unmet Cardiovascular Need. *Transl. Med. UniSa* **2015**, *12*, 29–40. [PubMed]
27. Morgantini, C.; Trifiro, S.; Trico, D.; Meriwether, D.; Baldi, S.; Mengozzi, A.; Reddy, S.T.; Natali, A. A short-term increase in dietary cholesterol and fat intake affects high-density lipoprotein composition in healthy subjects. *Nutr. Metab. Cardiovasc. Dis.* **2018**, *28*, 575–581. [CrossRef] [PubMed]
28. Andraski, A.B.; Singh, S.A.; Lee, H.L.; Higashi, H.; Smith, N.; Zhang, B.; Aikawa, M.; Sacks, F.M. Effects of Replacing Dietary Monounsaturated Fat with Carbohydrate on HDL (High-Density Lipoprotein) Protein Metabolism and Proteome Composition in Humans. *Arterioscler. Thromb. Vasc. Biol.* **2019**, *39*, 2411–2430. [CrossRef]
29. Kashyap, S.R.; Osme, A.; Ilchenko, S.; Golizeh, M.; Lee, K.; Wang, S.; BENA, J.; Previs, S.F.; Smith, J.D.; Kasumov, T. Glycation reduces the stability of apoai and increases HDL dysfunction in diet-controlled type 2 diabetes. *J. Clin. Endocrinol Metab.* **2018**, *103*, 388–396. [CrossRef]

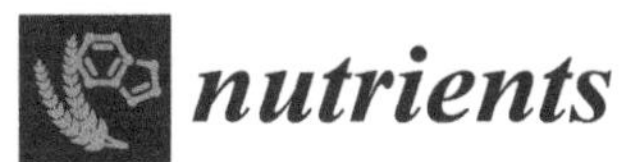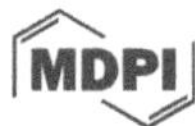

Article

Dietary Fatty Acids in Postprandial Triglyceride-Rich Lipoproteins Modulate Human Monocyte-Derived Dendritic Cell Maturation and Activation

Carlos Vazquez-Madrigal [1,†], Soledad Lopez [1,†], Elena Grao-Cruces [1], Maria C. Millan-Linares [2], Noelia M. Rodriguez-Martin [2], Maria E. Martin [3], Gonzalo Alba [1], Consuelo Santa-Maria [4], Beatriz Bermudez [3] and Sergio Montserrat-de la Paz [1,*]

[1] Department of Medical Biochemistry, Molecular Biology and Immunology, School of Medicine, Universidad de Sevilla, 41009 Seville, Spain; vazquezmadrigal@gmail.com (C.V.-M.); slopez9@us.es (S.L.); egrao@us.es (E.G.-C.); galbaj@us.es (G.A.)
[2] Department of Food & Health, Instituto de la Grasa, CSIC, 41013 Seville, Spain; mcmillan@ig.csic.es (M.C.M.-L.); noe91rm@gmail.com (N.M.R.-M.)
[3] Department of Cell Biology, Faculty of Biology, Universidad de Sevilla, 41012 Seville, Spain; mariamartin@us.es (M.E.M.); bbermudez@us.es (B.B.)
[4] Department of Biochemistry and Molecular Biology, School of Pharmacy, Universidad de Sevilla, 41012 Seville, Spain; csm@us.es
* Correspondence: delapaz@us.es; Tel.: +34-954-559-850
† These authors contributed equally to this work.

Received: 13 August 2020; Accepted: 12 October 2020; Published: 14 October 2020

Abstract: Dietary fatty acids have been demonstrated to modulate systemic inflammation and induce the postprandial inflammatory response of circulating immune cells. We hypothesized that postprandial triglyceride-rich lipoproteins (TRLs) may have acute effects on immunometabolic homeostasis by modulating dendritic cells (DCs), sentinels of the immunity that link innate and adaptive immune systems. In healthy volunteers, saturated fatty acid (SFA)-enriched meal raised serum levels of granulocyte/macrophage colony-stimulating factor GM-CSF (SFAs > monounsaturated fatty acids (MUFAs) = polyunsaturated fatty acids (PUFAs)) in the postprandial period. Autologous TRL-SFAs upregulated the gene expression of DC maturation (*CD123* and *CCR7*) and DC pro-inflammatory activation (*CD80* and *CD86*) genes while downregulating tolerogenic genes (*PD-L1* and *PD-L2*) in human monocyte-derived DCs (moDCs). These effects were reversed with oleic acid-enriched TRLs. Moreover, postprandial SFAs raised IL-12p70 levels, while TRL-MUFAs and TRL-PUFAs increased IL-10 levels in serum of healthy volunteers and in the medium of TRL-treated moDCs. In conclusion, postprandial TRLs are metabolic entities with DC-related tolerogenic activity, and this function is linked to the type of dietary fat in the meal. This study shows that the intake of meals enriched in MUFAs from olive oil, when compared with meals enriched in SFAs, prevents the postprandial production and priming of circulating pro-inflammatory DCs, and promotes tolerogenic response in healthy subjects. However, functional assays with moDCs generated in the presence of different fatty acids and T cells could increase the knowledge of postprandial TRLs' effects on DC differentiation and function.

Keywords: fatty acids; postprandial state; chylomicron; olive oil; dendritic cells; myeloid lineage; triglyceride-rich lipoprotein

---

1. Introduction

The emerging research topic called immunometabolism investigates mutual interactions between the immune system and the metabolism [1]. Chronic low-grade inflammation and disturbances in immune cell population participate in metabolic disorders such as non-alcoholic fatty liver disease, type 2 diabetes mellitus, atherosclerosis, and metabolic syndrome [2]. Contrariwise, the dysfunctional remodeling of intracellular metabolic pathways plays a critical role for the functions of immune cells [3].

Dendritic cells (DCs) are the major antigen-presenting cells, which link the innate and adaptive immunity, maintaining tolerance to self-antigens. The human-derived DC family are typically classified into two phenotypically and functionally subsets, plasmacytoid DCs (pDCs) and myeloid DCs (mDCs) [4]. In bloodstream, in vitro homologous monocyte-derived DCs (moDCs), require the influence of granulocyte/macrophage colony-stimulating factor (GM-CSF) and interleukin-4 (IL-4) for differentiation [5]. Upon differentiation, moDCs undergo an activation process that, depending on their membrane receptors and secreted cytokines, means that moDCs may have either a pro-inflammatory or tolerogenic function. Pro-inflammatory activation is with CD80 and CD86 surface marker expression and IL-12p70 cytokine secretion, whereas PD-L1 and PD-L2 surface marker expression and IL-10 cytokine secretion are considered to prompt tolerogenic or anti-inflammatory activation of moDCs [6]. Any microenvironmental disturbance produces dysfunctional mDCs that may initiate inflammatory or autoimmune diseases. However, all the causes of mDC dysfunction have not been completely unraveled. One of the recognized causes is lipid accumulation, specifically triglycerides (TGs), in DCs from patients with cancer and autoimmune diseases, which may disturb DC function [7,8].

Owing to their hydrophobic nature, dietary fatty acids are transported in the form of postprandial TG-rich lipoproteins (TRLs, mainly chylomicrons) [9]. In healthy subjects, serum TG levels reach a peak over 1-3 h after eating a fatty meal, resulting in postprandial TRL accumulation in the bloodstream [10]. In previous studies, our research team has demonstrated the superiority of dietary oleic acid (i.e., monounsaturated fatty acid, MUFA) over palmitic and stearic acid (i.e., saturated fatty acids, SFAs) in buffering silent alterations postprandially [11–13]. Postprandial disturbances have been markedly interconnected with oxidative and inflammatory process linked to the differentiation and activation of circulating myeloid cells [14]. The binding of postprandial TRLs with their receptor, the ApoB48 receptor (ApoB48R), modulates TG accumulation in myeloid lineage [13,15], proposing that activation of immune cells may be the result of TRL uptake via ApoB48R. However, it is scarcely known whether dietary fatty acids in postprandial TRLs play a role in lipid accumulation in moDCs.

In this study, we assessed the potential role of TRLs rich in MUFAs (olive oil) without or with omega-3 long-chain polyunsaturated fatty acids (PUFAs)—olive oil + eicosapentaenoic acid (EPA) and docosahexaenoic acid (DHA)—compared to TRLs rich in SFAs (cow's milk cream) in regulating moDC differentiation and whether dietary fatty acids are implicated in this process.

2. Materials and Methods

This study was conducted according to good clinical practice guidelines and in line with the principles outlined in the Helsinki Declaration of the World Medical Association. Ethics approval was obtained from the Human Clinical Research and Ethics Committee of the University Hospital Virgen Macarena (PI00082017) and all subjects gave written, informed consent.

2.1. Human Postprandial Study and TRL Isolation

Six volunteers, aged 25 to 35 years, non-smokers, with no medical history of disease known, nor any abnormality of hematological or biochemical parameters, were recruited in Clinical Biochemistry Unit at the University Hospital Virgen Macarena (UHVM, Seville). After an overnight fasting period of 12 h, all of them were given, over three different occasions, an oral fat emulsion containing cow's milk cream (meal rich in SFAs), refined olive oil (meal rich in MUFAs) or refined olive oil plus a dose of omega-3 long-chain PUFAs, which consisted of 920 mg of EPA and 760 mg of DHA (a meal rich in PUFAs). They also consumed the same test meal without fat as a control meal. Oral fat emulsions were prepared according to the method described by our Patent WO/2014/191597. They consisted of water, sucrose, fat (50 g/m^2 body surface area), emulsifier, and flavoring. At fasting (0 min) and after the ingestion of the meals within 10 min, blood samples were collected each hour into K3EDTA-containing Vacutainer tubes (Becton Dickinson, NJ, USA) over 6 h. Postprandial TRLs were isolated, pooled, and dialyzed against cold phosphate-buffered saline (PBS) [16]. TRLs were then immediately stored at −80 °C. Lipid oxidizability of postprandial TRL was checked (Thiobarbituric acid reactive substances level) during isolation and storage, but oxidation of lipids was not detected. TRLs were tested for lipopolysaccharide (LPS) contamination using the Pierce LAL Chromogenic Endotoxin Quantification kit (Thermo Scientific, Madrid, Spain). LPS contamination was always <0.2 EU/mL. TG concentration in postprandial TRLs was determined by colorimetric assay kit TG GPO-POD (Bioscience Medical, Madrid, Spain).

2.2. Fat and TRL Fatty Acid Composition

The fatty acid composition of cow's milk cream, refined olive oil, and refined olive oil plus omega-3 long-chain PUFAs was determined, in triplicate from the same lot, by the method described in EEC/796/2002 [17] using a gas chromatography system (HP-5890, Hewlett-Packard, Waldbronn, Germany) equipped with flame ionization detector and a SP-2380 capillary column (Supelco, 30 m × 0.32 mm) packed with cyanopropylsiloxane (0.25 μm) (Supplementary Materials Table S1). The initial column temperature was 165 °C, which was held for 10 min, then programmed from 165 °C to 200 °C at 1.5 °C/min. Injector and detector temperature were 250 °C, with the carrier gas H_2.

For fatty acid composition in postprandial TRLs (named TRL-SFAs from cow's milk cream, TRL-MUFAs from refined olive oil, and TRL-PUFAs from refined olive oil plus omega-3 long-chain PUFAs), aliquots of 100 μL were lyophilized [18]. A solution composed of methanol: toluene: dimethoxypropane: sulphuric acid (16.5:5:1:1) and heptane was added on the lyophilized residue. After shaking and incubating the mixture at 80 °C for 1 h, the upper phase was transferred to another vial and dried with a stream of N_2 gas. The resulting extract was dissolved in heptane and the FA methyl esters were analyzed into a gas chromatography system as described above (Table 1).

Table 1. Fatty acid composition of postprandial TRLs.

Fatty Acid	TRL-SFAs	TRL-MUFAs	TRL-PUFAs
	g/100 g of Fatty Acid		
4:0, butyric	0.26 ± 0.03	-	-
6:0, caproic	0.19 ± 0.02	-	-
8:0, caprylic	0.38 ± 0.14	-	-
10:0, capric	1.62 ± 0.52	-	-
12:0, lauric	3.52 ± 1.01	-	-
14:0, myristic	8.76 ± 1.63	-	-
16:0, palmitic	38.10 ± 1.87	11.2 ± 1.52	11.98 ± 1.21
16:1(n-7), palmitoleic	1.03 ± 0.10	0.79 ± 0.21	1.42 ± 0.61
18:0, stearic	18.8 ± 1.32	5.71 ± 0.73	5.54 ± 0.78
18:1(n-9), oleic	20.7 ± 1.76	67.2 ± 2.97	61.3 ± 3,87
18:2(n-6), linoleic	4.04 ± 0.98	8.95 ± 1.32	9,06 ± 1.03
18:3(n-3), α-linolenic	1.96 ± 0.57	3.29 ± 0.74	3.03 ± 0.98
20:4(n-6), arachidonic	0.49 ± 0.09	1.18 ± 0.37	1.79 ± 0.42
20:5(n-3), eicosapentaenoic	-	0.78 ± 0.19	2.82 ± 0.29
22:6(n-3), docosahexaenoic	-	0.70 ± 0.28	2.63 ± 0.14
Others	0.51 ± 0.13	0.34 ± 0.07	0.56 ± 0.07

Data are expressed as mean ± SD, *n* = 18. TRL: triglyceride-rich lipoprotein; SFAs:saturated fatty acids; MUFAs: monounsaturated fatty acids; PUFAs: polyunsaturated fatty acids.

2.3. Monocyte Isolation

The same six volunteers who took part as donors of postprandial TRLs participated as donors of monocytes. After an overnight fasting period of 12 h, peripheral blood samples were drawn from a large antecubital vein and collected into K_3EDTA-containing tubes (BD). Peripheral blood mononuclear cells (MNCs) were isolated by centrifugation over a Ficoll–Histopaque (Sigma, Madrid, Spain) gradient [19]. Monocytes were isolated from peripheral blood MNCs using anti-CD14 microbeads and LS columns on a midiMACS system (MiltenyiBiotec, Madrid, Spain). Monocyte ($CD14^+$) purity was routinely >90% by flow cytometry analysis (FACSCanto II flow cytometer and FACSDiva software, BD) and cell viability >95% by trypan blue exclusion (Sigma). The monocytes were seeded in 24-well culture plates at a density of 1×10^6 cells/mL and cultured in ultra-low attachment flasks in RPMI 1640 medium supplemented with L-glutamine, penicillin, streptomycin, and 10% heat-inactivated fetal bovine serum (complete culture medium).

2.4. MonocyteDerived Dendritic Cell Maturation and Activation

Monocytes were seeded in 24-well plates (1×10^6 cells/well) and induced to differentiate for 6 days in the presence of human recombinant GM-CSF (50 ng/mL) and IL-4 (20 ng/mL) to obtain moDCs. Degree of differentiation of the resulting population was determined for CD123 antigen using anti-human CD123 monoclonal antibody (Miltenyi Biotec) by flow cytometry analysis (more than 95% of cells were positive for CD123) [20–22]. Complete culture medium was replaced every 2 days with fresh medium and the cytokines. To study the effect of TRLs on moDC differentiation, monocytes were treated for 6 days with TRL-SFAs, TRL-MUFAs, or TRL-PUFAs at 100 µg TG/mL in presence of GM-CSF and IL-4.

2.5. Monocyte-Derived Dendritic Cell Viability

For cell viability, monocytes were seeded in 96-well plates (1×10^5 cells/well) and differentiated into moDCs as indicated above. At days 1, 2, 4, and 6, 3-(4,5-dimethylthiazol-2-yl)-2,5-diphenyltetrazolium bromide (MTT) solution (Sigma) was added to cells for 2 h until a purple precipitate was visible. MTT–formazan crystals were then solubilized with dimethyl sulfoxide (DMSO) (Sigma) and measured with a microplate reader at 570 nm corrected to 650 nm. Cell survival was expressed as the percentage of absorbance compared with that of the control, non-treated cells.

2.6. Triglyceride Quantification

Cellular lipids were extracted using hexane/isopropanol (3:2, *v/v*). The supernatant was obtained after centrifugation at $500 \times g$ for 5 min. The TG content was measured using the assay kits GPO/PAP (Axiom Diagnostics, Burstadt and Worms, Germany). To determine the protein content, cells were sonicated in radioimmunoprecipitation assay (RIPA) buffer, and the lysate was measured using the Bradford protein assay (Bio-Rad Laboratories, Madrid, Spain).

2.7. RNA Isolation and RT-qPCR

Total RNA was extracted by using Trisure Reagent (Bioline). RNA quality was assessed by A_{260}/A_{280} ratio in a NanoDrop ND-1000 Spectrophotometer (Thermo Scientific). Briefly, RNA (1 µg) was subjected to reverse transcription (iScript, Bio-Rad, Madrid, Spain). An amount of 10 ng of the resulting cDNA was used as a template for real-time PCR amplifications. The mRNA levels for specific genes were determined in a CFX96 system (Bio-Rad). For each PCR reaction, cDNA template was added to Brilliant SYBR green QPCR Supermix (Bio-Rad) containing the primer pairs for either gene or for glyceraldehyde 3-phosphate dehydrogenase (*GAPDH*) and hypoxanthine phosphoribosyltransferase (*HPRT*) as housekeeping genes (Supplementary Materials Table S2). All amplification reactions were performed in triplicate and average threshold cycle (Ct) numbers of the triplicates were used to calculate the relative mRNA expression of candidate genes. The magnitude of change of mRNA expression for candidate genes was calculated by using the standard $2^{-(\Delta\Delta Ct)}$ method. All data were normalized to endogenous reference (*GAPDH* and *HPRT*) gene content and expressed as relative fold-change of control.

2.8. Cytokine Quantification

The cytokines GM-CSF, IL-12p70, and IL-10 were determined by enzyme-linked immunosorbent assay (ELISA), following the indications of the manufacturer (Diaclone, Besançon, France). Cytokine concentration was expressed in *pg*/mL, as calculated from the calibration curves from serial dilution of human recombinant standards in each assay.

2.9. Statistical Analysis

All values are expressed as arithmetic means ± standard deviations (SD). Data were evaluated with Graph Pad Prism Version 5.01 software (San Diego, CA, USA). The statistical significance of any difference in each parameter among the groups was evaluated by one-way analysis of variance following Tukey's multiple comparisons test as a post hoc test. The Pearson *r* value was used to analyze the statistical significance of correlation test. *p* values less than 0.05 were considered statistically significant.

3. Results

3.1. Dietary Saturated Fatty Acids Acutely Increase Serum GM-CSF Levels in the Postprandial State of Healthy Volunteers

Serum from healthy volunteers was collected at fasting (TG concentration 0.42 ± 0.1 mmol/L) and at the postprandial hypertriglyceridemic peak (1–3 h) after SFA-enriched (TG concentration 1.54 ± 0.4 mmol/L), MUFA-enriched (TG concentration 0.65 ± 0.2 mmol/L), or PUFA-enriched (TG concentration 0.63 ± 0.2 mmol/L) meal ingestion. As depicted in Figure 1a, only the meal rich in SFAs postprandially increased serum GM-CSF levels when compared to the other fatty acid-enriched and no-fat meals. Thus, the total area under the curve (AUC_{TOTAL}) values for serum GM-CSF were significantly higher ($p = 0.0170$) only after the ingestion of the high-fat meal enriched in SFAs in healthy volunteers (Figure 1b). Interestingly, serum GM-CSF levels, which is a DC maturation factor, were acutely increased by the SFA-enriched meal at the postprandial hypertriglyceridemic peak, suggesting that dietary fatty acids present in TRLs modulate the DC maturation process. In addition, serum TG correlated with the levels of serum GM-CSF in healthy volunteers (R^2 0.9977, $p = 0.0308$, Figure 1c).

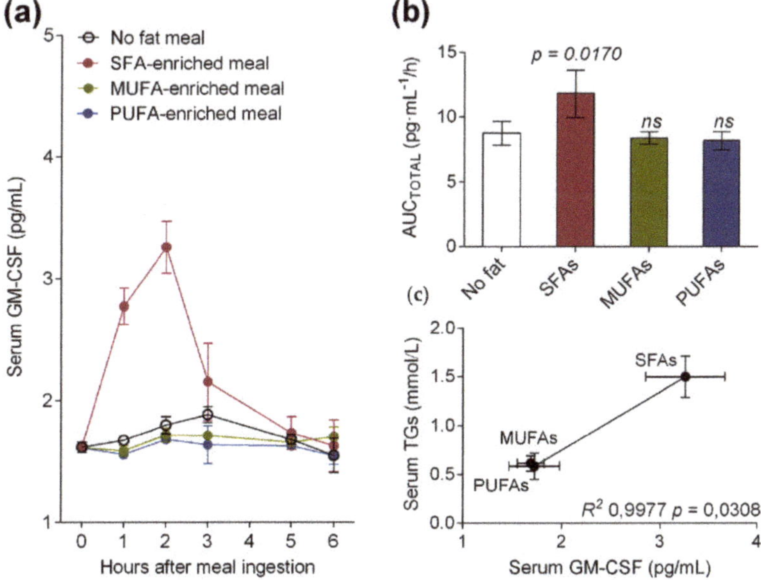

Figure 1. (**a**) Serum granulocyte/macrophage colony-stimulating factor (GM-CSF) levels at fasting and at the postprandial period after the administration of a control meal (with no fat) or high-fat meals enriched in saturated fatty acids (SFAs), monounsaturated fatty acids (MUFAs) or MUFAs + omega-3 long-chain polyunsaturated fatty acids (PUFAs) in healthy subjects. (**b**) Area under the curve of serum GM-CSF during postprandial period in response to test meals. (**c**) Correlation between postprandial serum GM-CSF levels and serum triglycerides (TGs) in healthy subjects after administration of test meals. Values are presented as means ± SD ($n = 6$).

3.2. Triglyceride Rich-Lipoproteins Modulate Maturation and Activation Markers in Human Monocyte-Derived Dendritic Cells

In gaining deeper insight into the role of postprandial TRLs in DC maturation and activation, marker gene expressions during human monocyte differentiation into moDCs were studied. Postprandial TRLs at 100 µg TGs/mL added to the differentiation medium that contained GM-CSF and IL-4 for 6 days did not induce cytotoxicity (data not shown). In previous reports, postprandial TRLs were not cytotoxic to human monocyte-derived osteoclasts [9] and macrophages [15] at similar concentrations. As shown in Figure 2, both transcriptional activity of *CD123* (Figure 2a) and *CCR7* (Figure 2b), key regulators of DC maturation, were upregulated by TRL-MUFAs and TRL-PUFAs but more markedly by TRL-SFAs, suggesting that postprandial fatty acids present in TRLs, in a saturation degree-dependent manner, modulate the DC maturation process. To further explore the possible pro-inflammatory or tolerogenic effects of postprandial TRLs in human moDCs, gene expression of CD80 (Figure 2c) and CD86 (Figure 2d) pro-inflammatory activation markers and PD-L1 (Figure 2e) and PD-L2 (Figure 2f) tolerogenic activation markers were analyzed. Postprandial TRLs affected the activation status of moDCs. Interestingly, TRL-SFAs upregulated the postprandial-TRL-induced transcriptional activity of CD80 and CD86 pro-inflammatory gene markers in moDCs. In contrast, TRL-MUFAs and TRL-PUFAs induced an upregulation in PD-L1 and PD-L2 gene expression, whereas TRL-SFAs did not induce any changes compared to control gene expression.

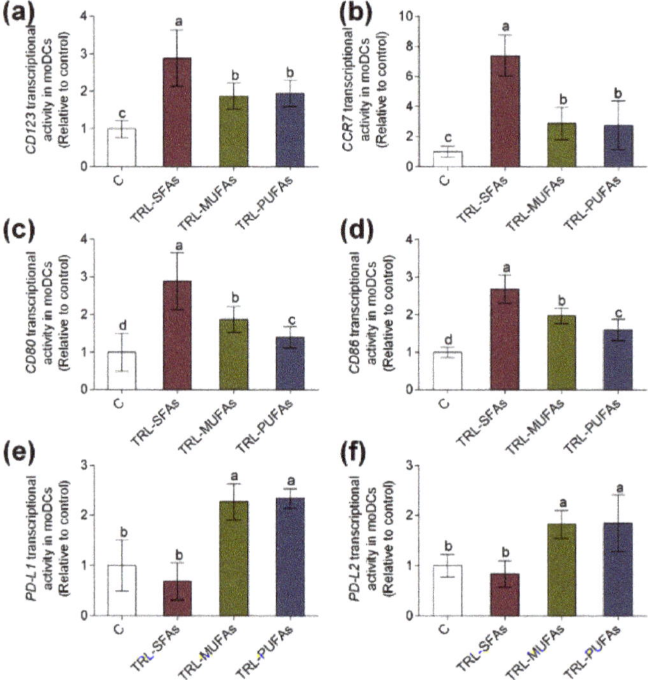

Figure 2. In vitro expression of dendritic cell (DC) gene markers in monocyte-derived DCs (moDCs) after stimulation with TRL-SFAs, TRL-MUFAs and TRL-PUFAs (TRL, triglyceride-rich lipoprotein) at 100 µg of TGs/mL for 6 days and in presence of GM-CSF and interleukin-4 (IL-4). DC maturation markers: (**a**) CD123 and (**b**) CCR7. DC pro-inflammatory activation markers: (**c**) CD80 and (**d**) CD86. DC tolerogenic activation markers: (**e**) PD-L1 and (**f**) PD-L2. Control means non-treated cells in the presence of GM-CSF and IL-4. Values are presented as means ± SD (*n* = 6) and those marked with different letters are significantly different ($p < 0.05$).

3.3. Fatty Acid-Enriched Meals Modulate Serum IL-12p70 and IL-10 Postprandial Secretion and Triglyceride-Rich Lipoproteins Regulate Cytokine Levels and Gene Expression in Human Monocyte-Derived Dendritic Cells

We also investigated the secretion levels of pro-inflammatory IL-12p70 and tolerogenic IL-10 in postprandial serum of healthy volunteers. After meal ingestion, postprandial serum levels of IL-12p70 (Figure 3a) were increased by the SFA meal but not by the MUFA or PUFA meal when compared to the control meal with no fat. Remarkably, IL-12p70 AUC_{TOTAL} was particularly increased by the SFA meal ($p = 0.0125$, Figure 3b) over postprandial 6 h. In contrast, IL-10 levels were postprandially lower after the SFA meal (Figure 3c) and higher after the MUFA and PUFA meal ingestion. Thus, AUC_{TOTAL} values for serum IL-10 were significantly lower ($p = 0.0039$) only after the ingestion of the high-fat meal enriched in SFAs and higher after the ingestion of the MUFA- ($p = 0.0054$) and PUFA- ($p = 0.0170$) enriched meals in healthy volunteers when compared to the control meal with no fat (Figure 3d).

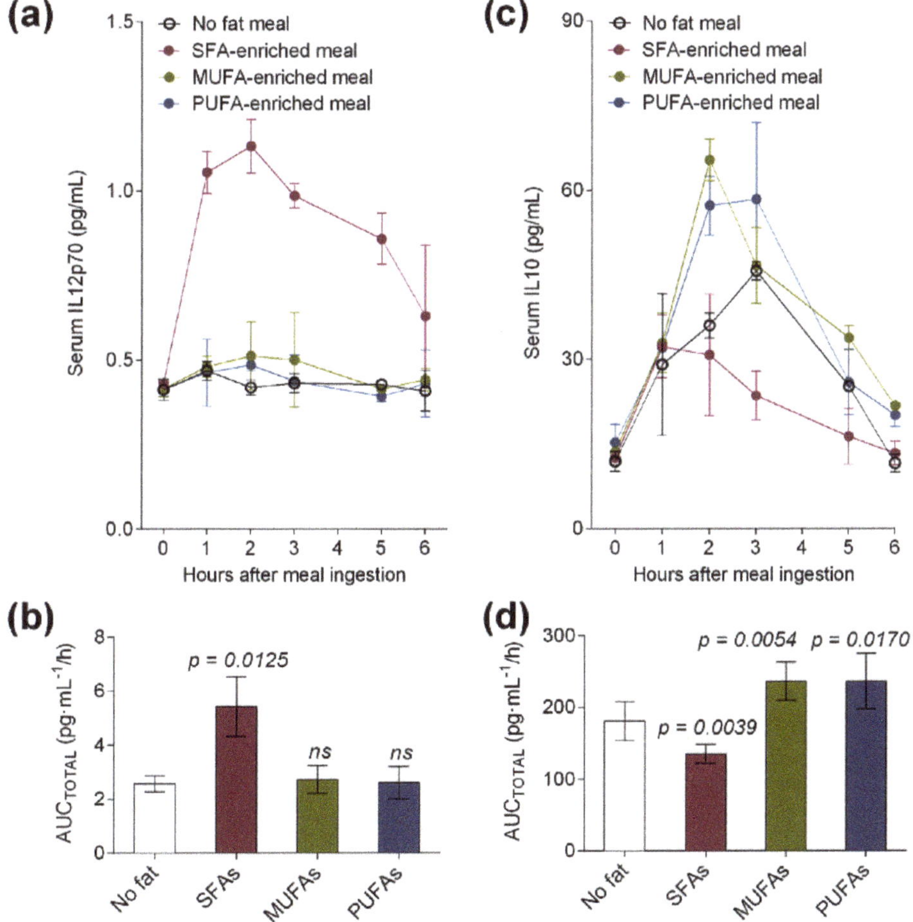

Figure 3. (**a**) Serum and (**b**) area under the curve of pro-inflammatory IL12p70 levels and (**c**) serum and (**d**) area under the curve of tolerogenic IL10 levels at fasting and at postprandial period after the administration of a control meal (with no fat) or high-fat meals enriched in SFAs, MUFAs, or MUFAs + omega-3 LCPUFAs (PUFAs) in healthy subjects. Values are presented as means ± SD ($n = 6$) and those marked with different letters are significantly different ($p < 0.05$). AUC: area under the curve.

In line with these results, in vitro experiments showed that TRL-SFAs promoted the secretion and transcriptional activity of *IL12p70* (Figures 4a and 4b, respectively). On the other hand, no changes were observed on the IL-10 secretion in moDCs (Figure 4c); however, TRL-SFAs downregulated *IL10* transcriptional activity in moDCs (Figure 4d). Contrary to SFAs, TRL-MUFAs and TRL-PUFAs upregulated tolerogenic *IL10* transcriptional activity in moDCs.

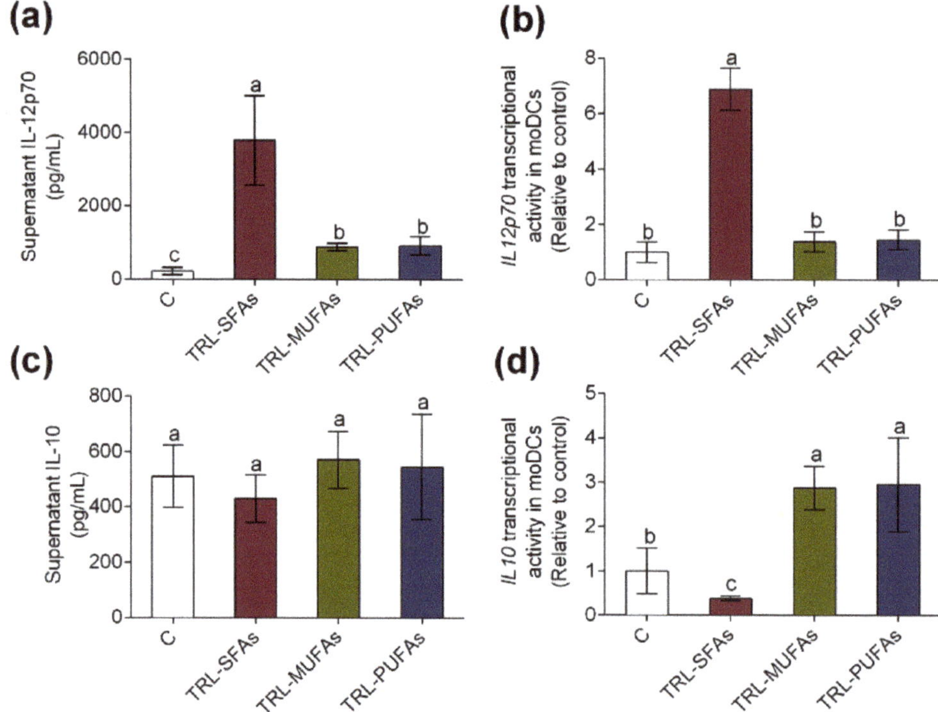

Figure 4. In vitro expression and secretion of proinflammatory and tolerogenic cytokines in moDCs after stimulation with TRL-SFAs, TRL-MUFAs, and TRL-PUFAs at 100 µg of TGs/mL for 6 days and in presence of GM-CSF and IL-4. (**a**) IL-12p70 secretion and (**b**) mRNA expression. (**c**) IL-10 secretion and (**d**) mRNA expression. Values are presented as means ± SD ($n = 6$) and those marked with different letters are significantly different ($p < 0.05$).

3.4. Triglyceride-Rich Lipoproteins Induce Lipid Accumulation and ApoB48R Transcriptional Activity in Monocyte-Derived Dendritic Cells in a Fatty Acid-Dependent Manner

Finally, we want to establish whether lipid accumulation would function to induce moDC activation. TRL-SFAs induced higher increase in TG accumulation (Figure 5a) and *ApoB48R* transcriptional activity (Figure 5b) compared those induced by TRL-MUFAs and TRL-PUFAs in moDCs. In addition, intracellular TG correlated with the expression of the ApoB48R (R^2 0.9998, $p = 0.0093$, Figure 5c) and *CD80* (R^2 0.9991, $p = 0.0192$, Figure 5d) activation marker, suggesting that dietary FAs present in TRLS, in a saturation degree-dependent manner, intervene in the activation process of moDCs.

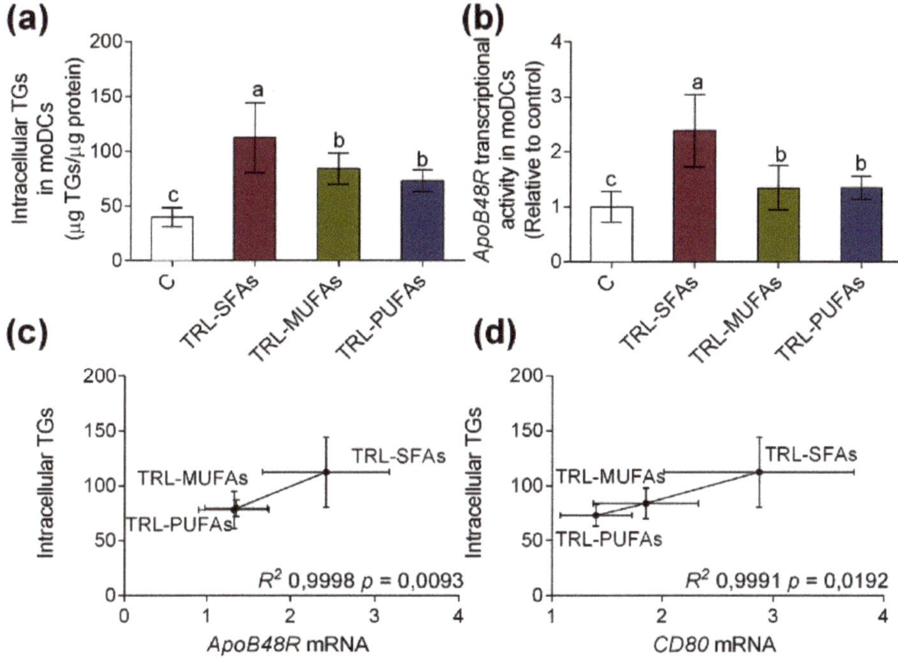

Figure 5. (**a**) Intracellular TGs accumulation and (**b**) In vitro *apoB48R* mRNA induced in moDCs after stimulation with TRL-SFAs, TRL-MUFAs and TRL-PUFAs at 100 µg of TGs/mL for 6 days and in presence of GM-CSF and IL-4. (**c**) Correlation between *apoB48R* mRNA and (**d**) *CD80* mRNA (DC activation marker) with intracellular TGs in moDCs. Control means non-treated cells in presence of GM-CSF and IL-4. Values are presented as means ± SD ($n = 6$) and those marked with different letters are significantly different ($p < 0.05$). TGs: triglycerides.

4. Discussion

The literature often suggests that lifestyle and traditional dietary habits unique to the Mediterranean region play a role in the prevention of oxidative- and inflammatory-related pathologies, such as cardiometabolic diseases and cancer [23]. Olive oil, the main dietary fat in the Mediterranean diet, due to its content of oleic acid (MUFA) and minor constituents, modulate different processes linked to chronic low-grade inflammation [24]. This view is in contrast to diets rich in SFAs, such as the "meat-based" or "Westernized" diets, which are inductive of inflammatory states [25]. One of the key processes of inflammation is the maturation and activation of circulating myeloid cells. These leukocytes are the first immune cells that respond quickly to injury and their activation, if permanent or chronic, may cause the increase of the inflammatory response, the perpetuation of the inflammatory state and the development of obesity or autoimmune disease [26,27]. DCs are professional antigen-presenting cells within the immune system, that are uniquely capable of priming naïve T cells, and once activated they have a pivotal ability to induce primary innate and adaptive immune response [28]. However, little is known about the effect of dietary fatty acids on human moDC [29]. The experimental use of primary human DCs is limited by their rarity in peripheral blood (less than 1% of MNCs), so to avoid this, in vitro moDCs are generally selected as a pragmatic model [30].

The postprandial period, the state that comprises and follows a meal, has an important, yet underrated, role in the onset of several pathologies. After fatty meal intake, dietary fatty acids are largely integrated into nascent TRLs, which are liberated from the small intestine into the bloodstream. It has been previously reported that dietary fatty acids have divergent postprandial effects on chronic disease-related events [31], suggesting that acute outcomes in response to dietary SFA-, MUFA-

or PUFA-adjustment may be helpful to lightly attenuate, even for preventing, diet-related chronic diseases [10]. It is essential to mention that the postprandial period is defined by a large number of metabolic transformations that comprise the raise of circulating TRLs. In response to fatty meal intake, earlier human studies have demonstrated the association of activated myeloid cells with postprandial hyperlipidemia [32,33]. Notwithstanding the relevance, studies during the postprandial period on interaction between human postprandial TRLs and moDCs are still unknown. Our results show for the first time that, after SFA-enriched meal intake, postprandial hypertriglyceridemia is associated with an increase of serum GM-CSF in healthy subjects. This effect was regulated by the main fatty acids in dietary fats, being significantly raised after the ingestion of an SFA-enriched meal when compared to the ingestion of MUFA-enriched meals. In line with these results, McFarlin et al. demonstrated that high-calorie meals significant increased postprandial GM-CSF and G-CSF levels in humans [34].

In gaining deeper insight into the role of dietary fatty acids on differentiation of moDCs, we obtained fresh monocytes from the fasting blood samples of healthy volunteers. Then, cells were differentiated into moDCs (GM-CSF + IL4 treatment for 6 days) in the absence or the presence of TRL-SFAs, TRL-MUFAs, and TRL-PUFAs isolated from postprandial serum samples of the same volunteers. In these experimental setting of autologous interaction, we observed an upregulation of DC maturation (CD123 and CCR7) and pro-inflammatory activation (CD80 and CD86) markers, and a downregulation of tolerogenic activation (PD-L1 and PD-L2) markers in human moDCs in response to postprandial TRL-SFAs. These effects support the notion that dietary saturated fats promote pro-inflammatory functions in mature DCs through metabolic pathways involving lipoproteins. In line with these results, Nicholas et al. demonstrated that palmitic acid-stimulated moDCs upregulated the expression of CD83 and CD86 [35]. Additionally, palmitic acid induced TLR4-dependent secretion of IL-1β, generated reactive oxygen species, and activated the NFκB canonical pathway in moDCs [35]. Importantly, our study showed a significant attenuation of incremental DC maturation and activation following the treatment with TRL-MUFAs and TRL-PUFAs, suggesting that the replacement of dietary SFAs by MUFAs (in combination or not with omega-3 long-chain PUFAs) could be helpful to prevent excessive DC-associated with postprandial events. Our new data extend the previous in vitro studies with PUFAs, and emphasize their acute benefits on TRLs to a healthy population. In line with this notion, moDCs stimulated with DHA and EPA show a reduction in the expression of CD80 and CD86 and in the secretion of IL-12p70 [36]. To our best knowledge, for the first time, the current study demonstrates that oleic acid from olive oil decreases, even abrogates, the gene expression of DC maturation and activation gene markers and the pro-inflammatory cytokine release. However, functional assays with moDCs generated in the presence of different fatty acids and T cells could increase the knowledge of postprandial TRLs' effects on DC differentiation and function.

Finally, in line with previous data in human neutrophils [37], monocytes [15,38], and murine microglia [13], our study have showed that postprandial TRLs induced DC activation through ApoB48R upregulation in a FA-dependent manner. Dietary oleic acid, EPA, and DHA attenuated ApoB48R gene expression while triggering a depletion in intracellular TG accumulation compared to palmitic acid.

5. Conclusions

In conclusion, these findings suggest that dietary fatty acids play a relevant and interrelated role in protecting against DC postprandial differentiation. Our results open new opportunities for developing novel nutritional strategies with olive oil as the principal dietary source of MUFAs, notably oleic acid, to prevent development and progression of inflammatory- and autoimmune-related diseases.

Supplementary Materials: The following are available online at http://www.mdpi.com/2072-6643/12/10/3139/s1, Table S1: Fatty acid composition of dietary fats, Table S2: Detailed information about primers' sequences used in this study.

Author Contributions: Conceptualization, C.V.-M., B.B., and S.M.d.l.P.; methodology, C.V.-M., E.G.-C., M.C.M.-L., and N.M.R.-M.; formal analysis, S.L.; investigation, M.E.M., G.A., and C.S.-M.; writing—original draft preparation,

S.L. and S.M.-d.l.P.; project administration, S.M.-d.l.P.; funding acquisition, B.B. and S.M.-d.l.P. All authors have read and agreed to the published version of the manuscript.

Funding: This study was supported by the research Grant US-1263458 (Andalusian Ministry of Economy, Knowledge, Business, and University, Government of Andalusia, Spain) into the European Regional Development Fund Operational Programme 2014 to 2020.

Conflicts of Interest: The authors state no conflicts of interest.

Abbreviations

DC	dendritic cell
GM-CSF	granulocyte/macrophage colony stimulating factor
IL	interleukin
mDC	myeloid dendritic cell
moDC	monocyte-derived dendritic cell
MUFA	monounsaturated fatty acid
pDC,	plasmacytoid dendritic cell
SFA	saturated fatty acid
TG	triglyceride
TRL	triglyceride-rich lipoprotein

References

1. Ayres, J.S. Immunometabolism of infections. *Nat. Rev. Immunol.* **2020**, *20*, 79–80. [CrossRef] [PubMed]

2. Luque-Sierra, A.; Alvarez-Amor, L.; Kleemann, R.; Martin, F.; Varela, L.M. Extra-Virgin Olive Oil with Natural Phenolic Content Exerts an Anti-Inflammatory Effect in Adipose Tissue and Attenuates the Severity of Atherosclerotic Lesions in Ldlr-/-.Leiden Mice. *Mol. Nutr. Food Res.* **2018**, *62*, 1800295. [CrossRef] [PubMed]

3. Salvatore, G.; Bernoud-Hubac, N.; Bissay, N.; Debard, C.; Daira, P.; Meugnier, E.; Proamer, F.; Hanau, D.; Vidal, H.; Arico, M.; et al. Human monocyte-derived dendritic cells turn into foamy dendritic cells with IL-17A. *J. Lipid Res.* **2015**, *56*, 1110–1122. [CrossRef]

4. Villar, J.; Segura, E. Recent advances towards deciphering human dendritic cell development. *Mol. Immunol.* **2020**, *122*, 109–115. [CrossRef]

5. Sander, J.; Schmidt, S.; Cirovic, B.; McGovern, N.; Papantonopoulou, O.; Hardt, A.L.; Aschenbrenner, A.C.; Kreer, C.; Quast, T.; Xu, A.M.; et al. Cellular Differentiation of Human Monocytes Is Regulated by Time-Dependent Interleukin-4 Signaling and the Transcriptional Regulator NCOR2. *Immunity* **2017**, *47*, 1051–1066. [CrossRef]

6. Zhang, J.A.; Lu, Y.B.; Wang, W.D.; Liu, G.B.; Chen, C.; Shen, L.; Luo, H.L.; Xu, H.; Peng, Y.; Luo, H.; et al. BTLA-Expressing Dendritic Cells in Patients with Tuberculosis Exhibit Reduced Production of IL-12/IFN-α and Increased Production of IL-4 and TGF-β, Favoring Th2 and Foxp3+ Treg Polarization. *Front. Immunol.* **2020**, *11*, 518. [CrossRef] [PubMed]

7. Herber, D.L.; Cao, W.; Nefedova, Y.; Novitskiy, S.V.; Nagaraj, S.; Tyurin, V.A.; Corzo, A.; Cho, H.I.; Celis, E.; Lennox, B. Lipid accumulation and dendritic cell dysfunction in cancer. *Nat. Med.* **2010**, *16*, 880–886. [CrossRef] [PubMed]

8. Ryu, H.; Kim, J.; Kim, D.; Lee, J.E.; Chung, Y. Cellular and Molecular Links between Autoimmunity and Lipid Metabolism. *Mol. Cells* **2019**, *42*, 747–754. [CrossRef]

9. Naranjo, M.C.; Garcia, I.; Bermudez, B.; Lopez, S.; Cardelo, M.P.; Abia, R.; Muriana, F.J.G.; Montserrat-de la Paz, S. Acute effects of dietary fatty acids on osteclastogenesis via RANKL/RANK/OPG system. *Mol. Nutr. Food Res.* **2016**, *60*, 2505–2513. [CrossRef]

10. Montserrat-de la Paz, S.; Bermudez, B.; Cardelo, M.P.; Lopez, S.; Abia, R.; Muriana, F.J.G. Olive Oil and postprandial hyperlipidemia: Implications for atherosclerosis and metabolic syndrome. *Food Funct.* **2016**, *7*, 4734–4744. [CrossRef]

11. Montserrat-de la Paz, S.; Bermudez, B.; Lopez, S.; Naranjo, M.C.; Romero, Y.; Bando-Hidalgo, M.J.; Abia, R.; Muriana, F.J.G. Exogenous fatty acids and niacin on acute prostaglandin D2 production in human myeloid cells. *J. Nutr. Biochem.* **2017**, *39*, 22–31. [CrossRef] [PubMed]

12. Montserrat-de la Paz, S.; Lopez, S.; Bermudez, B.; Guerrero, J.M.; Abia, R.; Muriana, F.J.G. Effects of immediate-release niacin and dietary fatty acids on acute insulin and lipid status in individuals with metabolic syndrome. *J. Sci. Food Agric.* **2018**, *98*, 2194–2200. [CrossRef]

13. Toscano, R.; Millan-Linares, M.C.; Lemus-Conejo, A.; Claro, C.; Sanchez-Margalet, V.; Montserrat-de la Paz, S. Postprandial triglyceride-rich lipoproteins promote M1/M2 microglia polarization in a fatty-acid-dependent manner. *J. Nutr. Biochem.* **2020**, *75*, 108248. [CrossRef]

14. Alipour, A.; Van Oostrom, A.J.; Izraeljan, A.; Verseyden, C.; Collins, J.M.; Frayn, K.N.; Plokker, T.W.M.; Elte, J.W.F.; Castro Cabezas, M. Leukocyte activation by triglyceride-rich lipoproteins. *Arterioscler. Thromb. Vasc. Biol.* **2008**, *28*, 792–797. [CrossRef]

15. Varela, L.M.; Ortega-Gomez, A.; Lopez, S.; Abia, R.; Muriana, F.J.G.; Bermudez, B. The effects of dietary fatty acids on the postprandial triglyceride-rich lipoprotein/apoB48 receptor axis in human monocyte/macrophage cells. *J. Nutr. Biochem.* **2013**, *24*, 2031–2039. [CrossRef] [PubMed]

16. Varela, L.M.; Bermudez, B.; Ortega-Gomez, A.; Lopez, S.; Sanchez, R.; Villar, J.; Muriana, F.J.G.; Abia, R. Postprandial triglyceride-rich lipoproteins promote invasion of human coronary artery smooth muscle cells in a fatty-acid manner through Pl3k-Rac1-JNK signalling. *Mol. Nutr. Food Res.* **2014**, *58*, 1349–1364. [CrossRef] [PubMed]

17. EEC. Comision regulation (EEC) no. 796/02 of 6 May 2002 amending regulation EEC2568/91 on the characteristics of olive oil and olive residue oil and on the relevant methodology analysis. *Off. J. Eur. Commun.* **2002**, *128*, 8–28.

18. Montserrat-de la Paz, S.; Naranjo, M.C.; Bermudez, B.; Lopez, S.; Moreda, W.; Abia, R.; Muriana, F.J.G. Postprandial dietary fatty acids exert divergent inflammatory response in retinal-pigmented epithelium cells. *Food Funct.* **2016**, *7*, 1345–1353. [CrossRef]

19. Montserrat-de la Paz, S.; de la Puerta, R.; Fernandez-Arche, A.; Quilez, A.M.; Muriana, F.J.G.; Garcia-Gimenez, M.D.; Bermudez, B. Pharmacological effects of mitraphylline from Uncaria tomentosa in primary human monocytes: Skew toward M2 macrophages. *J. Ethnopharmacol.* **2015**, *170*, 128–135. [CrossRef]

20. Shi, J.; Ikeda, K.; Maeda, Y.; Shinagawa, K.; Ohtsuka, A.; Yamamura, H.; Tanimoto, M. Identification of CD123+ myeloid dendritic cells as an early-stage immature subset with strong tumoristatic potential. *Cancer Let.* **2008**, *270*, 19–29. [CrossRef]

21. Collin, M.; Bigley, V. Human dendritic cell subsets: An update. *Immunology* **2018**, *154*, 3–20. [CrossRef]

22. Sugimoto, C.; Hasegawa, A.; Saito, Y.; Fukuyo, Y.; Chiu, K.B.; Cai, Y.; Breed, M.W.; Mori, K.; Roy, C.J.; Lackner, A.A.; et al. Differentiation Kinetics of Blood Monocytes and Dendritic Cells in Macaques: Insights to Understanding Human Myeloid Cell Development. *J. Immunol.* **2015**, *1954*, 1774–1781. [CrossRef]

23. Roncero-Ramos, I.; Rangel-Zuñiga, O.A.; Lopez-Moreno, J.; Alcala-Diaz, J.F.; Perez-Martinez, P.; Jimenez-Lucena, R.; Castaño, J.P.; Roche, H.M.; Delgado-Lista, J.; Ordovas, J.M.; et al. Mediterranean Diet, Glucose Homeostasis, and Inflammasome Genetic Variants: The CORDIOPREV Study. *Mol. Nutr. Food Res.* **2018**, *62*, e1700960. [CrossRef]

24. Hernaez, A.; Sanllorente, A.; Castañer, O.; Martinez-Gonzalez, M.A.; Ros, E.; Pinto, X.; Estruch, R.; Salas-Salvado, J.; Corella, D.; Alonso-Gomez, A.M.; et al. Increased Consumption of Virgin Olive Oil, Nuts, Legumes, Whole Grains, and Fish Promotes HDL Functions in Humans. *Mol. Nutr. Food Res.* **2019**, *63*, e1800847. [CrossRef]

25. Montserrat-de la Paz, S.; Naranjo, M.C.; Millan-Linares, M.C.; Lopez, S.; Abia, R.; Biessen, E.A.L.; Muriana, F.J.G.; Bermudez, B. Monounsaturated Fatty Acids in a High-Fat Diet and Niacin Protect from White Fat Dysfunction in the Metabolic Syndrome. *Mol. Nutr. Food Res.* **2019**, *63*, 1900425. [CrossRef]

26. Lopez, S.; Garcia-Serrano, S.; Gutierrez-Repiso, C.; Rodriguez-Pacheco, F.; Ho-Plagaro, E.; Santiago-Fernandez, C.; Alba, G.; Cejudo-Guillen, M.; Rodrigue-Cañete, A.; Valdes, S.; et al. Tissue-Specific Phenotype and Activation of iNKT Cells in Morbidly Obese Subjects: Interaction with Adipocytes and Effect of Bariatric Surgery. *Obes. Surg.* **2018**, *28*, 2774–2782. [CrossRef]

27. Ganguly, D.; Haak, S.; Sisirak, V.; Reizis, B. The role of dendritic cells in autoimmunity. *Nat. Rev. Immunol.* **2013**, *13*, 566–577. [CrossRef]

28. Mraz, M.; Cinkajzlova, A.; Klouckova, J.; Lacinova, Z.; Kratochvilova, H.; Lips, M.; Porizka, M.; Kopecky, P.; Lindner, J.; Kotulak, T.; et al. Dendritic Cells in Subcutaneous and Epicardial Adipose Tissue of Subjects with Type 2 Diabetes, Obesity, and Coronary Artery Disease. *Mediators Inflamm.* **2019**, *2019*, 5481725. [CrossRef]

29. Radzikowska, U.; Rinaldi, A.O.; Sozener, Z.C.; Karaguzel, D.; Wojcik, M.; Cypryk, K.; Akdis, M.; Akdis, C.A.; Sokolowska, M. The Influence of Dietary Fatty Acids on Immune Responses. *Nutrients* **2019**, *11*, 2990. [CrossRef]

30. Nastasi, C.; Candela, M.; Bonefeld, C.M.; Geisler, C.; Hansen, M.; Krejsgaard, T.; Biagi, E.; Andersen, M.H.; Brigidi, P.; Odum, N.; et al. The effect of short-chain fatty acids on human monocyte-derived dendritic cells. *Sci. Rep.* **2015**, *5*, 16148. [CrossRef]

31. Lopez, S.; Bermudez, B.; Ortega, A.; Varela, L.M.; Pacheco, Y.M.; Villar, J.; Abia, R.; Muriana, F.J.G. Effects of meals rich in either monounsaturated or saturated fat on lipid concentrations and on insulin secretion and action in subjects with high fasting triglyceride concentrations. *Am. J. Clin. Nutr.* **2011**, *93*, 494–499. [CrossRef]

32. Khan, I.M.; Pokharel, Y.; Dadu, R.T.; Lewis, D.E.; Hoogeveen, R.C.; Wu, H.; Ballantyne, C.M. Postprandial Monocyte Activation in Individuals with Metabolic Syndrome. *J. Clin. Endocrinol. Metab.* **2016**, *101*, 4195–4204. [CrossRef]

33. Montserrat-de la Paz, S.; Rodriguez, D.; Cardelo, M.P.; Naranjo, M.C.; Bermudez., B.; Abia, R.; Muriana, F.J.G.; Lopez, S. The effects of exogenous fatty acids and niacin on human monocyte-macrophage plasticity. *Mol. Nutr. Food Res.* **2017**, *61*, 1600824. [CrossRef]

34. McFarlin, B.K.; Carpenter, K.C.; Henning, A.L.; Venable, A.S. Consumption of a high-fat breakfast on consecutive days alters preclinical biomarkers for atherosclerosis. *Eur. J. Clin. Nutr.* **2017**, *71*, 239–244. [CrossRef]

35. Nicholas, D.A.; Zhang, K.; Hung, C.; Glasgow, S.; Aruni, A.W.; Unternaehrer, J.; Payne, K.J.; Langridge, W.H.R.; De Leon, M. Palmitic acid is a toll-like receptor 4 ligand that induces human dendritic cell secretion of IL-1beta. *PLoS ONE* **2017**, *12*, e0176793. [CrossRef]

36. Kong, W.; Yen, J.H.; Vassiliou, E.; Adhikary, S.; Toscano, M.G.; Ganea, D. Docosahexaenoic acid prevents dendritic cell maturation and in vitro and in vivo expression of the IL-12 cytokine family. *Lipids Health Dis.* **2010**, *9*, 12. [CrossRef] [PubMed]

37. Ortega-Gomez, A.; Varela, L.M.; Lopez, S.; Montserrat-de la Paz, S.; Sanchez, R.; Muriana, F.J.G.; Bermudez, B.; Abia, R. Postprandial triglyceride-rich lipoproteins promote lipid accumulation and apolipoprotein B-48 receptor transcriptional activity in human circulating and murine bone marrow neutrophils in a fatty acid-dependent manner. *Mol. Nutr. Food Res.* **2017**, *61*, 1600879. [CrossRef]

38. Varela, L.M.; Ortega, A.; Bermudez, B.; Lopez, S.; Pacheco, Y.M.; Villar, J.; Abia, R.; Muriana, F.J.G. A high-fat meal promotes lipid-load and apolipoprotein B-48 receptor transcriptional activity in circulating monocytes. *Am. J. Clin. Nutr.* **2011**, *93*, 918–925. [CrossRef]

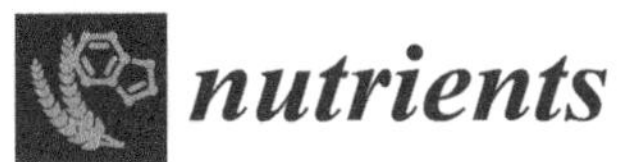 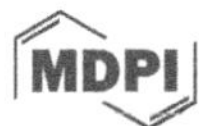

Article

Dietary Habits and Risk of Early-Onset Dementia in an Italian Case-Control Study

Tommaso Filippini [1], Giorgia Adani [1], Marcella Malavolti [1], Caterina Garuti [1], Silvia Cilloni [1], Giulia Vinceti [2,3], Giovanna Zamboni [2,3], Manuela Tondelli [3,4], Chiara Galli [3,4,5], Manuela Costa [6], Annalisa Chiari [3] and Marco Vinceti [1,7,*]

[1] Environmental, Genetic and Nutritional Epidemiology Research Center (CREAGEN), Department of Biomedical, Metabolic and Neural Sciences, University of Modena and Reggio Emilia, 41125 Modena, Italy; tommaso.filippini@unimore.it (T.F.); giorgia.adani@unimore.it (G.A.); marcella.malavolti@unimore.it (M.M.); caterina.garuti@gmail.com (C.G.); silvia.cilloni@unimore.it (S.C.)

[2] Center for Neurosciences and Neurotechnology, Department of Biomedical, Metabolic, and Neural Sciences, University of Modena and Reggio Emilia, 41126 Modena, Italy; giulia.vinceti@unimore.it (G.V.); giovanna.zamboni@unimore.it (G.Z.)

[3] Neurology Unit, Modena Policlinico-University Hospital, 41126 Modena, Italy; manuelatondelli@gmail.com (M.T.); ch.galli@ausl.mo.it (C.G.); chiari.annalisa@aou.mo.it (A.C.)

[4] Primary care Department, Modena Local Health Authority, 41124 Modena, Italy

[5] Department of Neuroscience, Psychology, Pharmacology and Child Health (NeuroFARBA), University of Florence, 50139 Florence, Italy

[6] Neurology Unit of Carpi Hospital, Modena Local Health Authority, 41012 Carpi, Italy; m.costa@ausl.mo.it

[7] Department of Epidemiology, Boston University School of Public Health, Boston, MA 02118, USA

* Correspondence: marco.vinceti@unimore.it; Tel.: +39-059-2055481

Received: 29 October 2020; Accepted: 27 November 2020; Published: 29 November 2020

Abstract: Risk of early-onset dementia (EOD) might be modified by environmental factors and lifestyles, including diet. The aim of this study is to evaluate the association between dietary habits and EOD risk. We recruited 54 newly-diagnosed EOD patients in Modena (Northern Italy) and 54 caregivers as controls. We investigated dietary habits through a food frequency questionnaire, assessing both food intake and adherence to dietary patterns, namely the Greek-Mediterranean, the Dietary Approaches to Stop Hypertension (DASH), and the Mediterranean-DASH Intervention for Neurodegenerative Delay (MIND) diets. We modeled the relation between dietary factors and risk using the restricted cubic spline regression analysis. Cereal intake showed a U-shaped relation with EOD, with risk increasing above 350 g/day. A high intake (>400 g/day) of dairy products was also associated with excess risk. Although overall fish and seafood consumption showed no association with EOD risk, we found a U-shaped relation with preserved/tinned fish, and an inverse relation with other fish. Similarly, vegetables (especially leafy) showed a strong inverse association above 100 g/day, as did citrus and dry fruits. Overall, sweet consumption was not associated with EOD risk, while dry cake and ice-cream showed a positive relation and chocolate products an inverse one. For beverages, we found no relation with EOD risk apart from a U-shaped relation for coffee consumption. Concerning dietary patterns, EOD risk linearly decreased with the increasing adherence to the MIND pattern. On the other hand, an inverse association for the Greek-Mediterranean and DASH diets emerged only at very high adherence levels. To the best of our knowledge, this is the first study that explores the association between dietary factors and EOD risk, and suggests that adherence to the MIND dietary pattern may decrease such risk.

Keywords: early-onset dementia; dietary habits; MIND diet; DASH diet; Mediterranean diet; risk; prevention

---

1. Introduction

Dementia is a syndrome, usually of a chronic or progressive nature, characterized by impairment of cognitive functions beyond what might be expected from normal ageing [1,2]. Early-onset dementia (EOD) is a heterogeneous group of cognitive disorders characterized by an onset of dementia symptoms before the age of 65 [3]. Such an age cut-point has not been established based on biological differences between younger and older subjects, but mainly on the socio-economic implications of dementia diagnosis at a younger age [3,4]. Indeed, the main feature of EOD compared to late-onset forms is a higher impact at two levels: First, on affected people, particularly in terms of their social functioning and working life [5]; second, on family members, especially when young children are still present [6].

EOD prevalence has been estimated to range between 38 and 420 cases per 100,000 inhabitants, with an annual incidence between 2.4 and 22.6 new cases per 100,000 inhabitants [4], the most common forms being Alzheimer's dementia (AD), frontotemporal dementia (FTD), and vascular dementia [7].

Little is known about EOD etiology, not least in comparison with the determinants of late-onset dementia. Genetic mutations apparently only account for a small percentage of EOD, around 10% [8,9]. Therefore, the role of environmental factors and modifiable lifestyles including diet seems particularly relevant [10–14]. Among the dietary habits involved, a high consumption of vegetables, fruit, and fish [15–17], and adherence to the Mediterranean diet or other dietary patterns (e.g., the Dietary Approaches to Stop Hypertension (DASH) and the Mediterranean-DASH Intervention for Neurodegenerative Delay (MIND) diet) have been associated with a slower cognitive decline and decreased risk of all-age dementia [12,18–21]. Interestingly, recent studies have evaluated the correlation between AD brain biomarkers and dietary patterns characterized by a higher intake of fresh fruit and vegetables, whole grains, fish and low-fat dairies, along with a lower intake of sweets, fried potatoes, high-fat dairies, and meat. Data provided evidence of protective effects against the risk of developing AD, suggesting that dietary interventions may play a role in the prevention of cognitive decline [22,23].

In this study, we investigated EOD risk in an Italian population in relation to dietary habits, including food consumption and adherence to dietary patterns.

2. Methods

Following approval by the Modena Ethics Committee (*n.* 186/2016), we performed a case-control study on environmental and lifestyle risk factors for EOD in the province of Modena, Northern Italy. We recruited EOD cases from newly-diagnosed patients referred to the Cognitive Neurology Network of Modena province, including the Modena Policlinico-University Hospital Memory Center (Modena, Italy) and the Carpi Hospital Neurology Department (Carpi, Italy), in the period October 2016–2019 [7,24]. Cases are referred to this Network by either Neurology Units, primary care services, or general practitioners through specific pathways activated by the Modena Local Health Authority to identify and care for subjects with dementia. Inclusion criteria encompassed EOD diagnosis, residence in the Modena province, and presence of a reliable caregiver. The diagnosis of EOD subtypes has been established according to the most recent clinical criteria, as previously described [7]. The gene mutation status was not available for all participants since it is not routinely part of the clinical workflow. Among those tested, one subject was a carrier of *SP1* gene mutation. We recruited controls from caregivers of subjects with a diagnosis of early or late-onset dementia referred to the same Cognitive Neurology Network. All subjects provided a written informed consent.

We administered a questionnaire tailored to collect personal characteristics and clinical, occupational, and environmental factors potentially affecting the central nervous system [25], and a detailed food frequency questionnaire (FFQ). The latter is a validated semi-quantitative FFQ developed within the European Prospective Investigation in Cancer (EPIC) project, in a version specifically validated for the population of Northern Italy [26,27]. The EPIC-FFQ was designed to estimate the intake of 188 food items over the previous year in terms of frequency and amount. Photos of serving sizes were also used to assist with proper completion by participants.

Foods and beverages were categorized into major food groups and subgroups based on the common EPIC-SOFT classification, as previously reported in detail [28,29]. The final list of food categories included the following items and subcategories: Cereals and cereal products, meat and meat products, milk and dairy products, eggs, fish and seafood, vegetables, mushrooms, legumes, potatoes, fresh and dry fruits, sweet products, oils and fats, and beverages. We also computed alcohol (ethanol) intake by conversion of all quantities of alcoholic beverages into grams of ethanol per day using a methodology previously described [30]. We also computed scores for three diet quality patterns defined *a priori*: The Greek Mediterranean (GM) diet [31], the Dietary Approaches to Stop Hypertension (DASH) diet [32,33], based on a methodology described elsewhere [34], and the Mediterranean-DASH Intervention for Neurodegenerative Delay (MIND) diet [19,35]. In more detail, the GM diet is based on Mediterranean diet scales [31], and scoring is calculated on median intake levels of nine items: Vegetables, legumes, fruit and nuts, dairy products, cereals, meat and meat products, fish, alcohol, and the monounsaturated/saturated fatty acid ratio [34,36]. The range of possible scores was 0–9, with higher scores indicating higher adherence. The DASH diet was originally designed to reduce blood pressure [32,33], and it has been suggested to be neuroprotective [37]. DASH diet adherence scores were calculated according to previous studies [34,38] based on eight components: Fruits, vegetables, nuts and legumes, low-fat dairy products, whole grains, sodium, sweetened beverages, red and processed meats. Overall, possible scores ranged from 8 to 40, with higher scores indicating higher adherence. Eventually, the MIND diet was developed as a hybrid of the Mediterranean and DASH diets associated with slower cognitive decline and decreased incidence of Alzheimer's dementia [19,35]. MIND diet scores were based on the intake of 15 items, namely whole grains, green leafy and other vegetables, berries, red meat, poultry, fish, legumes, nuts, fast/fried food, olive oil and other fats, cheese, sweets and alcohol/wine. Scores ranged from 0 to 15, with higher scores meaning higher adherence.

In data analysis, we used a multivariable unconditional logistic regression model to estimate the EOD risk associated with dietary factors and patterns. We performed an analysis on the overall population for risk of EOD, also performing a stratified analysis according to the type of diagnosis, namely early-onset Alzheimer's dementia (EO-AD) and early-onset frontotemporal dementia spectrum (EO-FTD). Regarding dietary factors, we calculated the odds ratio (ORs) and 95% confidence intervals (CIs) according to the increasing tertiles based on the distribution in the control group using the lowest tertile as a reference category. We also modeled the relation between dietary factors and EOD risk using the restricted cubic spline model with three knots (10, 50, and 90 percentiles). We included in the multivariable model as potential confounders and effect-modifiers sex, age, educational attainment (as years of education), and total energy intake (kcal/day). We used "logit", "mkspline", and "xblc" routines of the Stata-16.1 statistical package (Stata Corp., College Station, TX, USA, 2020) for statistical analyses.

3. Results

3.1. Characteristics of the Study Population

Of the 150 eligible participants, only 144 could be contacted. We recruited 112 subjects, 58 EOD cases, and 54 controls with an average response rate of 78%. Reasons for non-participation were unwillingness to contribute to the research and lack of time to fill out the questionnaire. In addition, four cases were excluded as they did not return a reliable and complete FFQ, leaving 54 cases and 54 controls for the final analysis. Table 1 reports the characteristics of the study participants. The average age at the questionnaire filling date was 65 years (66 for EOD cases and 64 years for referents), with a higher proportion of women (57%). The mean age of EOD onset was 59.8 years (59.7 years for EO-AD and 59.8 for EO-FTD), ranging from 45 to 65 years. Alzheimer's dementia (EO-AD) was the most frequent diagnosis (*n* = 30), followed by frontotemporal dementia spectrum disorders (EO-FTD, *n* = 18), vascular dementia (*n* = 4), or other rarer diseases (Supplemental Table S1).

Table 1. Characteristics of the study participants. Early-onset dementia (EOD), early-onset Alzheimer's dementia (EO-AD), and early-onset frontotemporal dementia spectrum (EO-FTD).

	Controls	All EOD Cases	EO-AD Cases	EO-FTD Cases
	n (%)	*n* (%)	*n* (%)	*n* (%)
All subjects	54 (100)	54 (100)	30 (100)	18 (100)
Age at questionnaire filling				
Mean (standard deviation)	63.8 (9.6)	66.2 (4.6)	65.9 (4.5)	66.6 (4.7)
<65 years	28 (51.8)	19 (35.2)	11 (36.7)	5 (27.8)
≥65 years	26 (48.2)	35 (64.8)	19 (63.3)	13 (72.2)
Sex				
Men	23 (42.6)	24 (44.4)	11 (36.7)	10 (55.6)
Women	31 (57.4)	30 (55.6)	19 (63.3)	8 (44.4)
Educational attainment				
Primary or less	11 (20.4)	13 (24.1)	6 (20.0)	5 (27.8)
Middle school	11 (20.4)	20 (37.0)	10 (33.3)	8 (44.4)
High school	21 (38.9)	18 (33.3)	12 (40.0)	4 (22.2)
College or more	11 (20.4)	3 (5.6)	2 (6.7)	1 (5.6)
Marital status				
Married/unmarried partner	48 (88.9)	45 (83.3)	23 (76.7)	16 (88.9)
Single	3 (5.6)	1 (1.9)	1 (3.3)	0 (0.0)
Separated/divorced	2 (3.7)	2 (3.7)	0 (0.0)	2 (11.1)
Widowed	1 (1.9)	6 (11.1)	6 (20.0)	0 (0.0)

3.2. Assessment of Dietary Habits

Supplemental Tables S2 and 3 show the average intake of food and beverages for the study participants. No subjects reported a special dietary regimen for medical purposes. The total energy intake was slightly higher in cases compared to controls. In regards to cereal products, cases were shown to have a higher intake compared to controls, in particular EO-FTD subjects. Cases had a slightly higher intake of meat products compared with controls, including red and white meat, and a higher intake of dairy products, particularly milk and yogurt, especially in EO-AD compared to EO-FTD cases. Cases also showed a substantially similar intake of fish and seafood, but a higher consumption of preserved and tinned fish particularly for EO-FTD cases, a lower intake of piscivorous fish and crustaceans/molluscs, especially in EO-FTD cases. Cases also showed a lower intake of overall vegetables, with similar results for all vegetable types but cabbage, and a lower intake of potatoes and legumes. Overall, fresh fruit intake was somewhat higher in cases than controls, although the former showed a lower intake of citrus fruits yet a higher intake of all other fruits, with similar results across EO-AD and EO-FTD. Dry fruit intake was lower in cases than in controls, particularly for nuts and seeds and especially in EO-FTD, characterized by a much lower intake of both overall dry fruit, nuts, and seeds. Sweet intake was higher in cases, particularly due to a higher consumption of ice-cream, biscuits, and dry cakes, while consumption of chocolate-based products was lower. Cases consumed less oils and fats, with a lower intake of both vegetable oils and olive oil. Concerning beverages, cases had a lower intake of coffee and tea, but results were the opposite in the subgroup analysis according to an EOD diagnosis, with a higher intake in EO-AD cases and a much lower one in EO-FTD cases, who showed very low tea consumption. Wine consumption was substantially similar in cases and controls, with EO-AD cases reporting a lower intake and EO-FTD a higher one, mainly due to the higher consumption of white wine. A higher intake of aperitif wines and beers was reported for controls. The overall alcohol intake was comparable in cases and controls, although EO-FTD cases showed a much higher intake compared to EO-AD cases. Concerning non-alcoholic beverages, cases reported a higher intake of fruit juices and a lower consumption of soft drinks.

3.3. Assessment of the Relation between Dietary Habits and Dementia Risk

In Supplemental Table S4, we report risk estimates associated with increasing tertiles of food and beverage intake. Overall, about cereals products, we found an inverse association with EOD risk, although a positive association can be noted for subjects in the third tertile for both pasta and rice consumption. For meat products, we found a direct association with EOD, with a higher risk in the second tertile compared to the third one. In the subgroup analyses, however, red, white, and processed meat showed a very imprecise inverse association in the second tertile, but a null/positive association in the third tertile. On the other hand, offal intake seemed inversely associated with EOD risk, especially for subjects in the third tertile. Milk and dairy products were in general positively associated with EOD, particularly in the third tertile of exposure. Both piscivorous and non-piscivorous fish seemed inversely associated with EOD risk. For preserved and tinned fish, crustaceans and molluscs, conversely, we found an inverse association in the second tertile, but a positive one in the third tertile. In general, vegetables were inversely associated with EOD risk, particularly leafy, root, and other vegetables as well as mushrooms and potatoes, and an almost substantial null association for legumes. In regards to fruits, we found an inverse association for fresh fruits, especially citrus fruits, as well as dry fruits. Conversely, the intake of all other fruits showed a negative association in the second tertile and a positive one in the third tertile. For overall sweets, we found a positive association with EOD risk, mainly due to ice-cream, cakes, pies/pastries, and biscuits/dry cakes, while chocolate and other (non-chocolate) confectionery showed an inverse association. Overall, oils and fats showed an inverse association, mainly due to the intake of olive and non-olive oils, while we found a positive association with butter and other animal fats. Concerning beverages, coffee and tea, aperitif wines/beers, and spirits/liqueurs showed an inverse association with EOD risk. Red wine showed an inverse association for subjects in the second tertile, and a positive one in the third tertile. Conversely, white wine and soft drinks showed a higher risk in the second tertile and lower one in the third tertile. Finally, fruit juices seemed positively associated with disease risk, especially in the second tertile.

In general, we found similar results in the analysis based on the EOD diagnosis, with a few exceptions (Supplemental Table S4). Bread intake was inversely associated with EOD risk and this was also true for EO-AD. However, a direct/null association is present in EO-FDT. Fresh cheese intake showed a positive association with EO-FTD, but a null association for EO-AD. Conversely, aged cheese intake did not show such an association with EO-FTD and a slight positive association emerged for EO-AD in the third tertile of exposure. With regard to fish intake, EO-FTD showed a positive association with preserved and tinned fish, while an inverse one can be noted for EO-AD. In regards to fresh fruit intake, both EO-AD and EO-FTD showed an inverse association, but we found a positive association for citrus fruit in EO-FTD and a negative one in EO-AD. In relation to sweet intake, the increased risk for biscuits and dry cakes was confirmed in EO-AD, while we found a decreased risk for EO-FTD. Finally, alcohol intake was associated with a slightly increased risk in EO-FTD, but not in EO-AD.

3.4. Assessment of the Relation between Dietary Patterns and Dementia Risk

Moving on to the analysis of adherence to the investigated dietary patterns, cases (overall and both EO-AD and EO-FTD) generally showed slightly lower mean scores (Table 2). In the risk analysis according to the tertile distribution (Table 3), we found a lower EOD risk at increasing adherence in all three dietary patterns, especially for high adherence to MIND dietary patterns.

Table 2. Adherence to dietary patterns (Greek-Mediterranean (GM) diet; DASH: Dietary Approaches to Stop Hypertension (DASH) diet); Mediterranean-DASH Intervention for Neurodegenerative Delay (MIND) diet) in the study population (Early-onset dementia (EOD), early-onset Alzheimer's dementia (EO-AD), and early-onset frontotemporal dementia spectrum (EO-FTD). Values reported as mean and standard deviation.

Dietary Pattern	Controls	EOD Cases	EO-AD Cases	EO-FTD Cases
GM diet (range 0–9)	4.4 (1.7)	4.1 (1.5)	4.1 (1.5)	4.1 (1.5)
DASH diet (rang 8–40)	23.7 (5.5)	23.1 (5.0)	23.5 (5.4)	23.6 (4.4)
MIND diet (range 0–15)	7.8 (1.3)	7.1 (1.4)	7.2 (1.4)	7.2 (1.3)

Table 3. Odds ratio (OR) and 95% confidence intervals (CI) of early-onset dementia (EOD), early-onset Alzheimer's dementia (EO-AD), and early-onset frontotemporal dementia spectrum (EO-FTD) for increasing tertiles of adherence to dietary patterns. Greek-Mediterranean (GM) diet, Dietary Approaches to Stop Hypertension (DASH) diet, and Mediterranean-DASH Intervention for Neurodegenerative Delay (MIND) diet. A linear trend for 1-unit increase is reported.

			All EOD			EO-AD			EO-FTD	
Food Items	Median	Cases/ Controls	OR	(95% CI)	Cases/ Controls	OR	(95% CI)	Cases/ Controls	OR	(95% CI)
GM diet										
1st tertile (ref.)	3	24/19	1.00	-	14/19	1.00	-	7/19	1.00	-
2nd tertile	5	18/18	0.76	(0.30–1.96)	10/18	0.73	(0.24–2.17)	6/18	0.87	(0.22–3.35)
3nd tertile	6	12/17	0.45	(0.16–1.26)	6/17	0.40	(0.12–1.35)	5/17	0.60	(0.14–2.61)
Linear trend			0.84	(0.65-1.09)		0.84	(0.62–1.13)		0.83	(0.57–1.20)
DASH diet										
1st tertile (ref.)	18	21/19	1.00	-	10/19	1.00	-	7/19	1.00	-
2nd tertile	25	22/19	0.87	(0.35–2.15)	13/19	1.08	(0.37–3.17)	7/19	0.80	(0.22–3.00)
3nd tertile	29	11/16	0.60	(0.21–1.72)	7/16	0.79	(0.23–2.74)	4/16	0.71	(0.14–3.52)
Linear trend			0.98	(0.90–1.06)		0.99	(0.91–1.08)		1.01	(0.89–1.14)
MIND diet										
1st tertile (ref.)	6.5	30/16	1.00	-	16/16	1.00	-	9/16	1.00	-
2nd tertile	7.5	15/22	0.32	(0.12–0.83)	9/22	0.39	(0.13–1.15)	5/22	0.31	(0.07–1.28)
3nd tertile	9.0	9/16	0.31	(0.11–0.90)	5/16	0.32	(0.09–1.13)	4/16	0.45	(0.10–2.00)
Linear trend			0.66	(0.47–0.91)		0.67	(0.46–0.98)		0.66	(0.41–1.08)

In Figures 1–10, we present data based on the spline regression analysis adjusted for sex, age, educational attainment, and total energy intake. Due to the very high number of non-consumers, the spline analysis was not feasible for some offal and several beverages, namely tea, red and white wine, aperitif wines and beers, and soft drinks. Overall, cereal products showed a U-shaped relation with EOD, with a lower risk at around 200 g/day, yet a higher one above 350 g/day (Figure 1). A similar relation was found for bread and rice intake. Conversely, pasta and other grains showed a linear relation with decreased risk at low intake levels and an increasing one from 50–60 g/day. On the other hand, pizza, crackers, and other salty snacks showed increased risk in the case of null exposure, with decreased risk from 40 g/day after which a plateau was reached. Overall meat consumption did not seem to be associated with EOD (Figure 2), although an increase in risk can be noted for a high intake of both red (>100/120 g/day) and white meat (>40/50 g/day). In regards to dairy products, we found null/decreased risk for all products, except for an increase in risk at very high intake levels, namely >400 g/day for overall dairy products or >350 g/day for milk and yogurt (Figure 3). Similarly, we found null risk in association with the intake of eggs (Figure 3) and overall fish and seafood (Figure 4). Interestingly, we found a U-shaped relation with fish intake, with increased risk for null consumption and above 20 g/day for preserved and tinned fish (Figure 4). Conversely, a high intake (>20 g/day) of other fish, especially piscivorous fish, appeared to the decreased EOD risk. All vegetables showed an inverse association with EOD, with increased risk in the case of null intake and decreasing risk starting from 100 g/day, above which a plateau seems to have been reached (Figure 5). Such pattern of association can also be noted in all vegetable subgroups, especially leafy vegetables showing a slight continuous decrease, while cabbages showed a null association at all intake levels. Mushrooms showed a U-shape relation, with a lower risk at around 4 g/day. On the other hand, we found a slight inverse association for potatoes and legumes, albeit a very imprecise one (Figure 6). In spite of the substantially linear inverse correlation of citrus fruit intake with EOD risk, we found a U-shaped relation with fresh fruit and all other fruit intake, with a lower risk at approximately 250 and 200 g/day, respectively (Figure 7). Conversely, dry fruit intake showed an increased risk for subjects reporting null consumption and a decreased risk from 4 g/day of dry fruits and nuts and from 1 g/day of dry fruits, above which a plateau was reached (Figure 7). Sweet products showed an inverse-U relation with EOD risk, mainly driven by the lower risk associated with a high intake of chocolate and other chocolate-based products (Figure 8). However, sugar and other confectionery showed a null association, while ice-cream, biscuits, and dry cakes showed a positive correlation, with null risk for non-consumers and an increased risk for intake above 20–30 g/day for both ice-cream and dry cakes, respectively (Figure 8). In general, oils and fats showed that a linear inverse association with increased risk starting from null intake, soon reversed above 20 g/day especially for olive oil and other vegetable oils and fats (Figure 9). For beverages, we found a U-shaped relation with coffee consumption, with a lower risk at 70 g/day (Figure 10). Conversely, we found almost a null relation with wine and alcohol intake, while risk increased with fruit juice consumption exceeding 100 g/day (Figure 10).

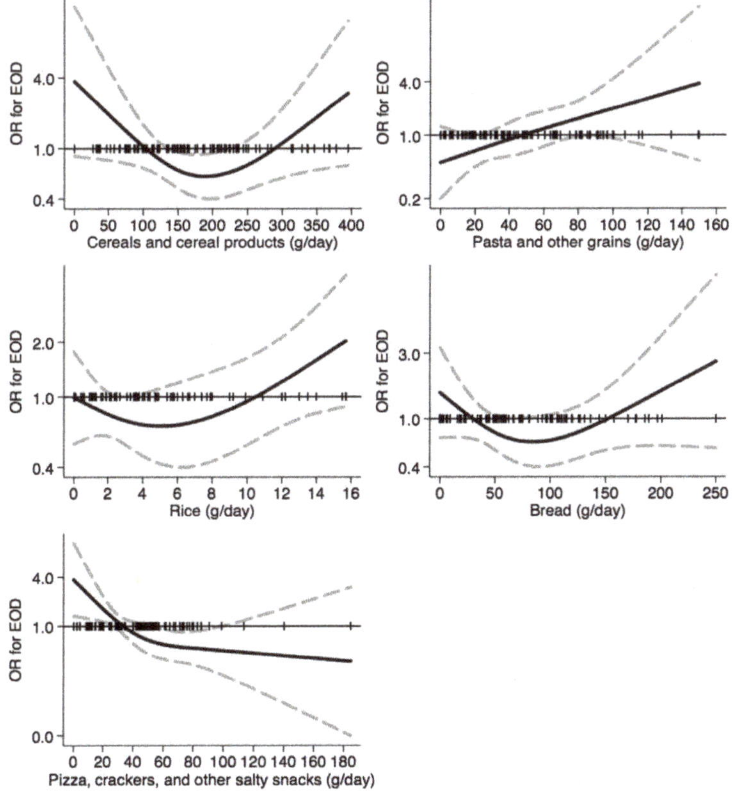

Figure 1. Spline regression analysis of early-onset dementia (EOD) risk for increasing intake of cereals and cereal products. The black line indicates odds ratios for dementia risk; dash gray lines are 95% confidence limits; the reference line at 1.0 with black spikes indicates the distribution of participant intake.

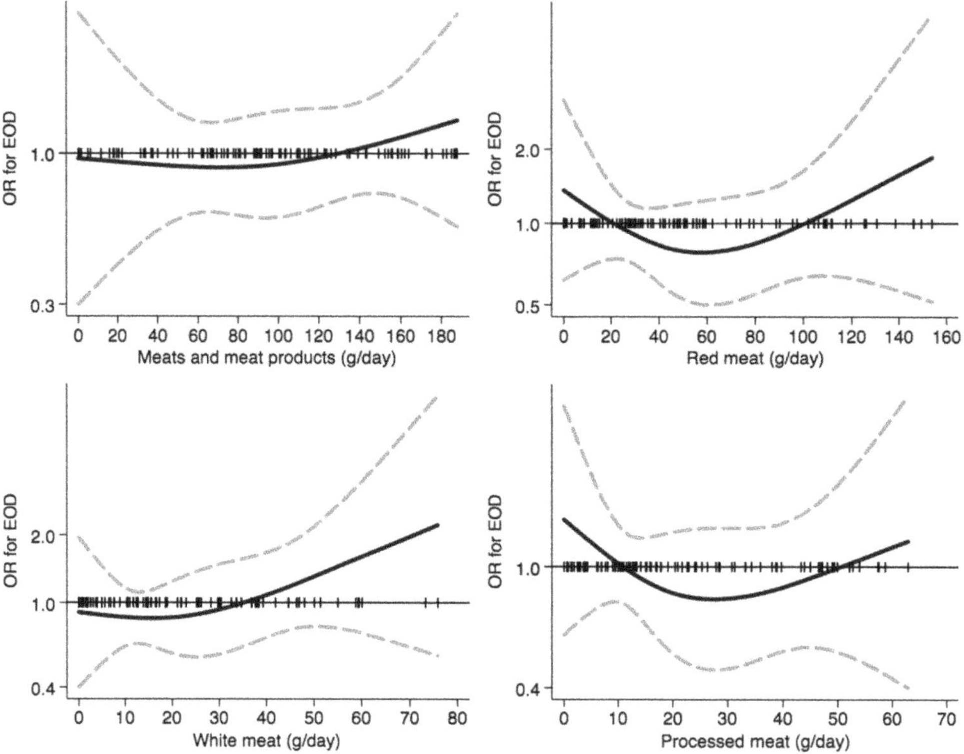

Figure 2. Spline regression analysis of early-onset dementia (EOD) risk for increasing intake of meats and meat products. The black line indicates odds ratios for dementia risk; dash gray lines are 95% confidence limits; the reference line at 1.0 with black spikes indicates the distribution of participant intake. Note: spline analysis was not possible for offal due to a few subjects reporting consumption which is different from a null value.

Spline regression analyses stratified by the EOD clinical type are reported in Supplemental Figures S1–S10 for EO-AD and in Supplemental Figures S11–S20 for EO-FTD. We generally found comparable results across EOD forms. Nonetheless, there was evidence of a U-shaped relation between red meat intake and EO-AD (Supplemental Figure S2), and between processed meat and EO-FTD (Supplemental Figure S12), with the lowest risk ratio occurring at 60 and at 25 g/day, respectively. In regards to dairy products, the shape of the relation with cheese intake seemed opposite for EO-AD and EO-FTD, with an inverse U-shaped relation for EO-AD, especially for fresh-cheese intake (Supplemental Figure S3), and a U-shaped relation for EO-FTD, especially for overall cheese intake (Supplemental Figure S13). Moreover, egg intake seemed to establish an inverse-U relation for EO-AD only (Supplemental Figure S3). In addition, mushroom intake showed a linear inverse association for EO-AD (Supplemental Figure S6), and a U-shaped one with EO-FTD (Supplemental Figure S16).

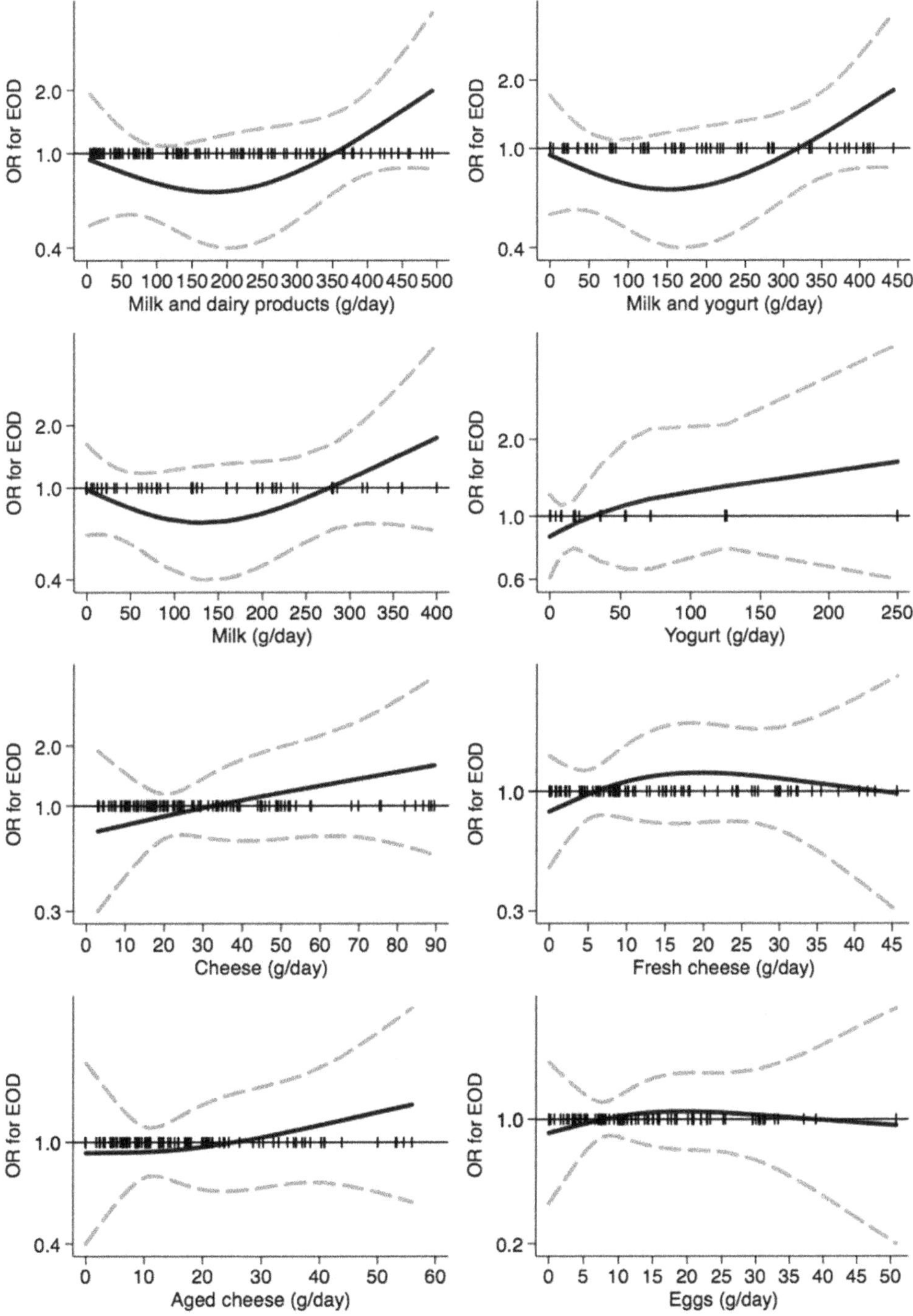

Figure 3. Spline regression analysis of early-onset dementia (EOD) risk for increasing intake of milk, dairy products, and eggs. The black line indicates odds ratios for dementia risk; dash gray lines are 95% confidence limits; the reference line at 1.0 with black spikes indicates the distribution of participant intake.

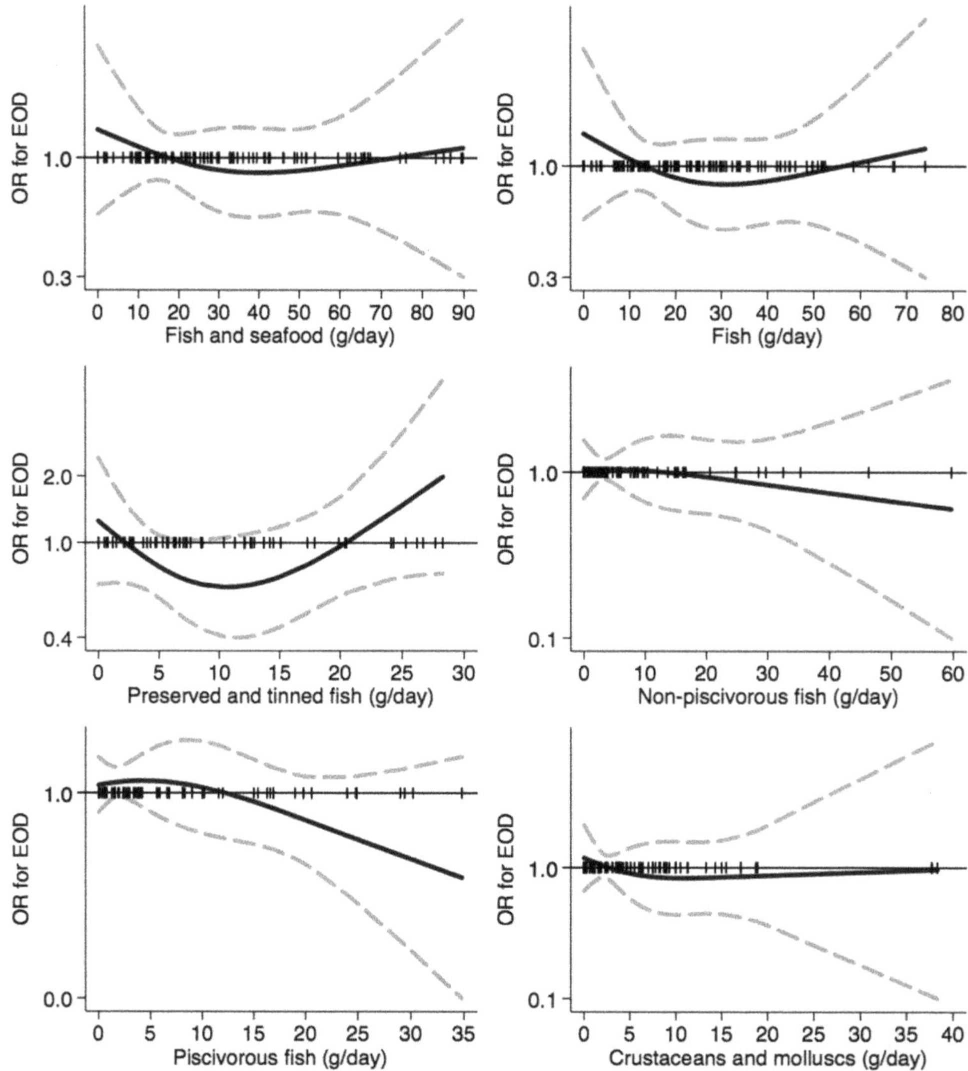

Figure 4. Spline regression analysis of early-onset dementia (EOD) risk for increasing intake of fish and seafood. The black line indicates odds ratios for dementia risk; dash gray lines are 95% confidence limits; the reference line at 1.0 with black spikes indicates the distribution of participant intake.

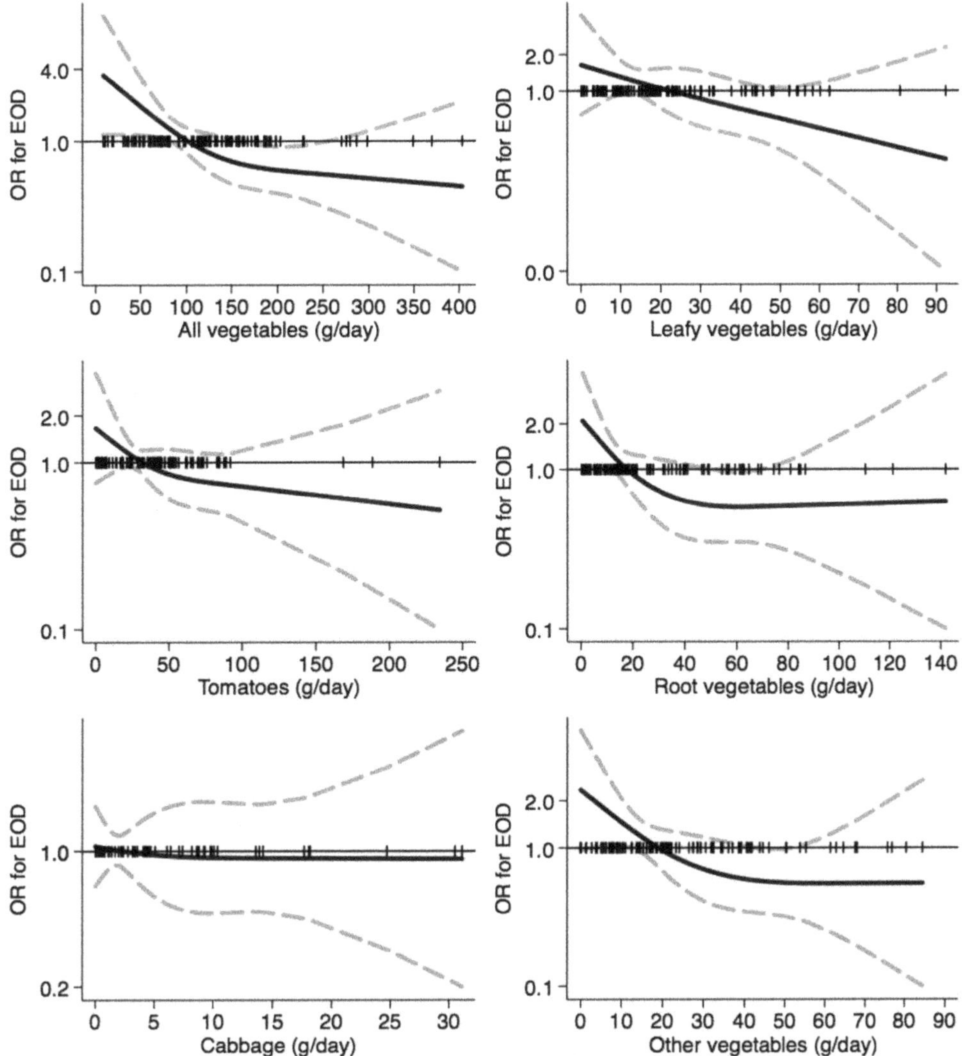

Figure 5. Spline regression analysis of early-onset dementia (EOD) risk for increasing intake of vegetables. The black line indicates odds ratios for dementia risk; dash gray lines are 95% confidence limits; the reference line at 1.0 with black spikes indicates the distribution of participant intake.

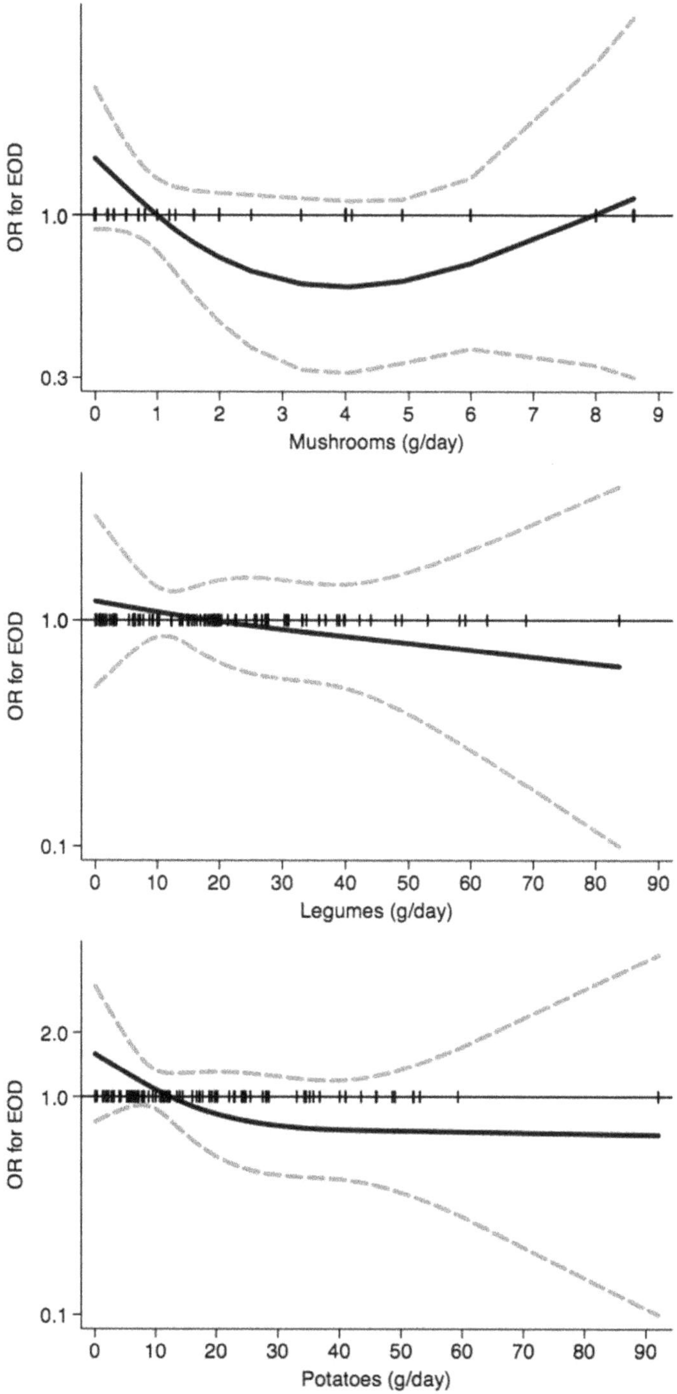

Figure 6. Spline regression analysis of early-onset dementia (EOD) risk for increasing intake of mushrooms, legumes, and potatoes. The black line indicates odds ratios for dementia risk; dash gray lines are 95% confidence limits; the reference line at 1.0 with black spikes indicates the distribution of participant intake.

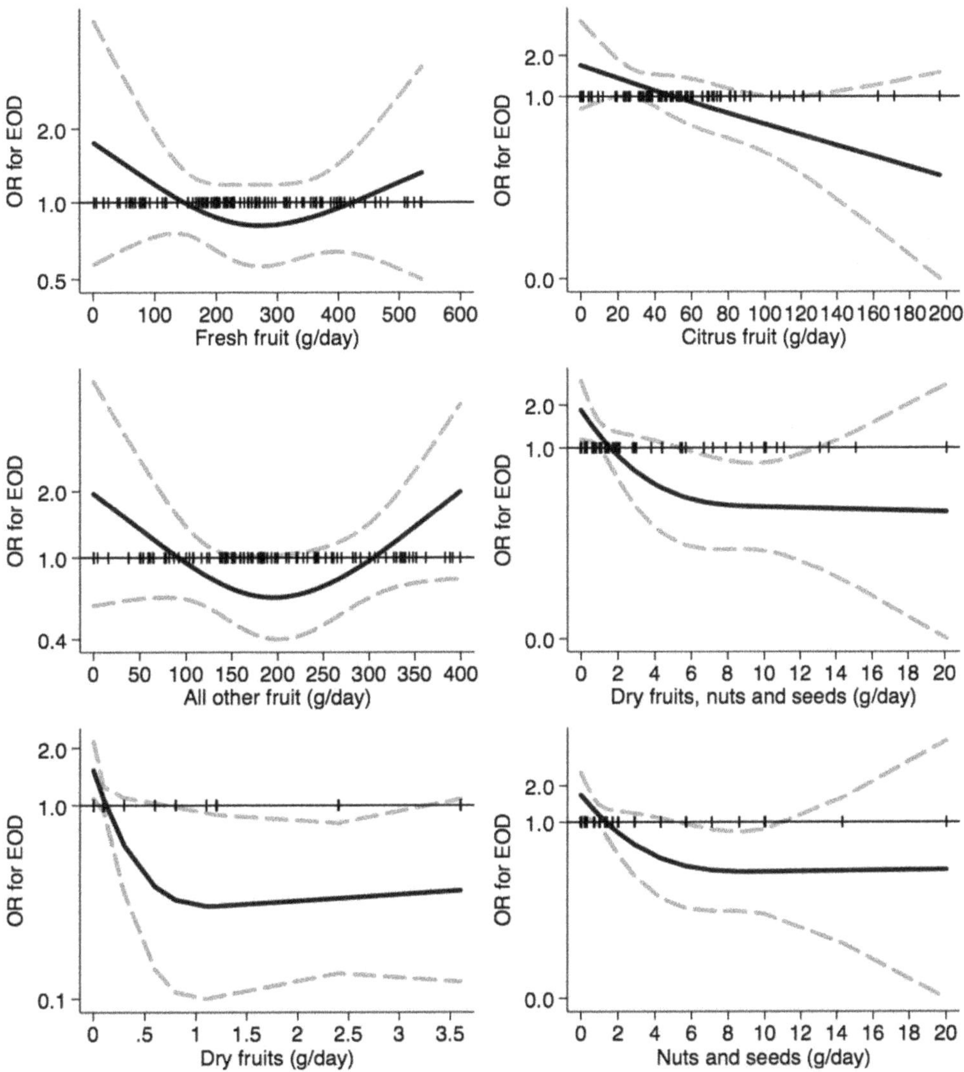

Figure 7. Spline regression analysis of early-onset dementia (EOD) risk for increasing intake of fresh and dry fruits. The black line indicates odds ratios for dementia risk; dash gray lines are 95% confidence limits; the reference line at 1.0 with black spikes indicates the distribution of participant intake.

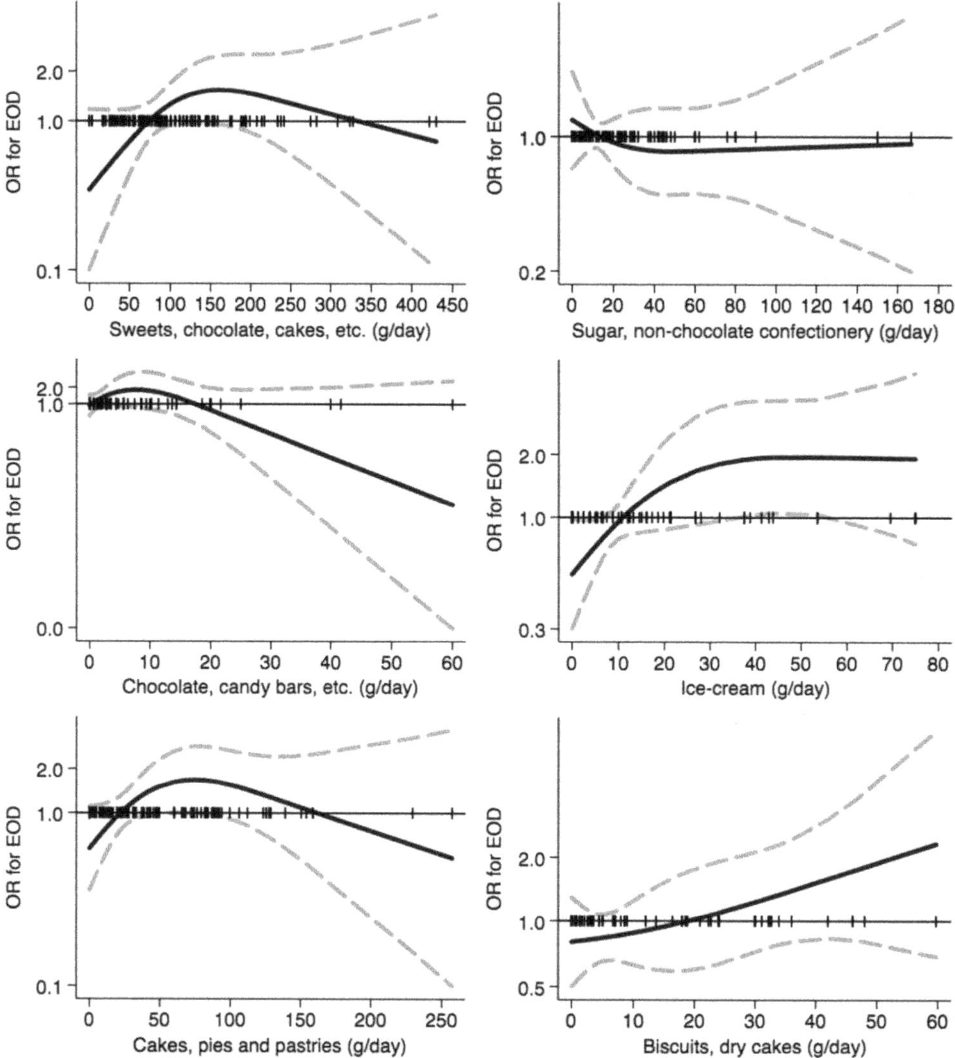

Figure 8. Spline regression analysis of early-onset dementia (EOD) risk for increasing intake of sweets products. The black line indicates odds ratios for dementia risk; dash gray lines are 95% confidence limits; the reference line at 1.0 with black spikes indicates the distribution of participant intake.

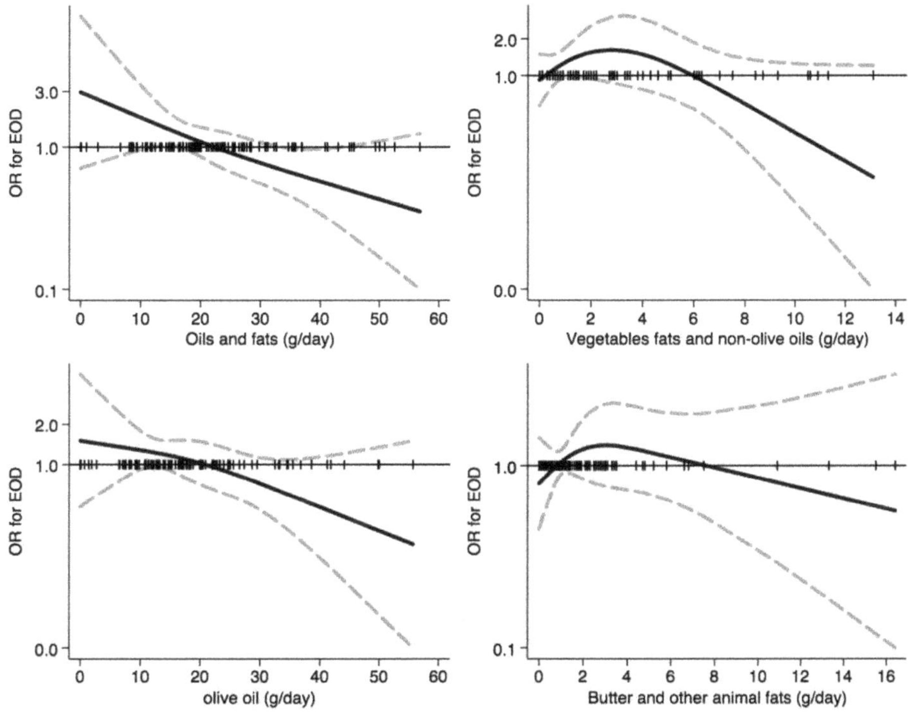

Figure 9. Spline regression analysis of early-onset dementia (EOD) risk for increasing intake of oils and fats. The black line indicates odds ratios for dementia risk; dash gray lines are 95% confidence limits; the reference line at 1.0 with black spikes indicates the distribution of participant intake.

The spline regression analysis carried out for dietary pattern adherence showed no substantial association between EOD risk and both GM and DASH diets, with a reduction in risk from a score of ≥6 and ≥28, respectively (Figure 11). Conversely, a substantially linear inverse association emerged for the MIND diet, with a higher risk at very low adherence and decreasing risk above a total score around 8/9. We found comparable results in the analyses performed by the EOD subtype (Supplemental Figures S21 and 22), with the exception of adherence to the DASH diet. This dietary pattern showed an inverse U-shaped relation with EO-FTD risk, with a decreased risk for subjects at very low and very high adherence levels (Supplemental Figure S22), while no association emerged for EO-AD (Supplemental Figure S21).

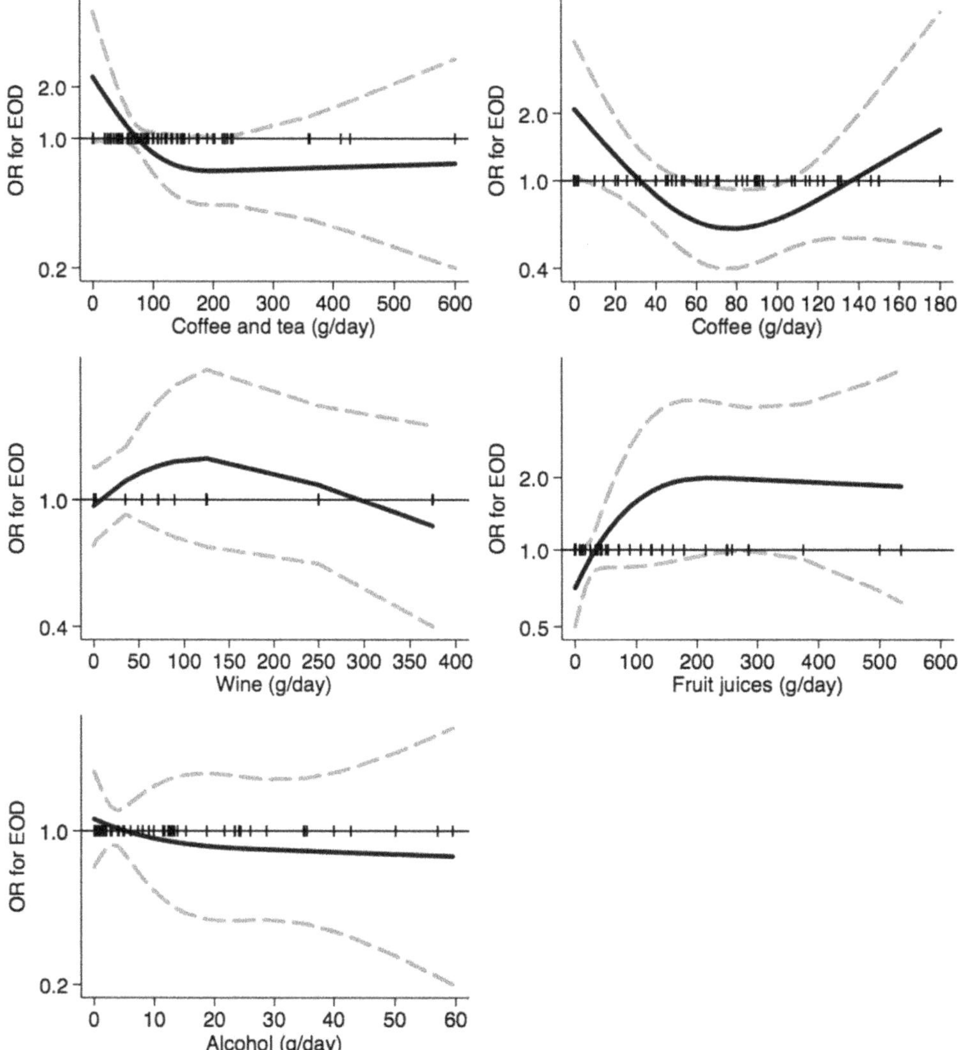

Figure 10. Spline regression analysis of early-onset dementia (EOD) risk for increasing intake of beverages. The black line indicates odds ratios for dementia risk; dash gray lines are 95% confidence limits; the reference line at 1.0 with black spikes indicates the distribution of participant intake. Note: Spline analysis was not possible for most of the beverages (namely tea, red, white and aperitif wines and beers, spirits and soft drinks) due to a few subjects reporting consumption which is different from a null value.

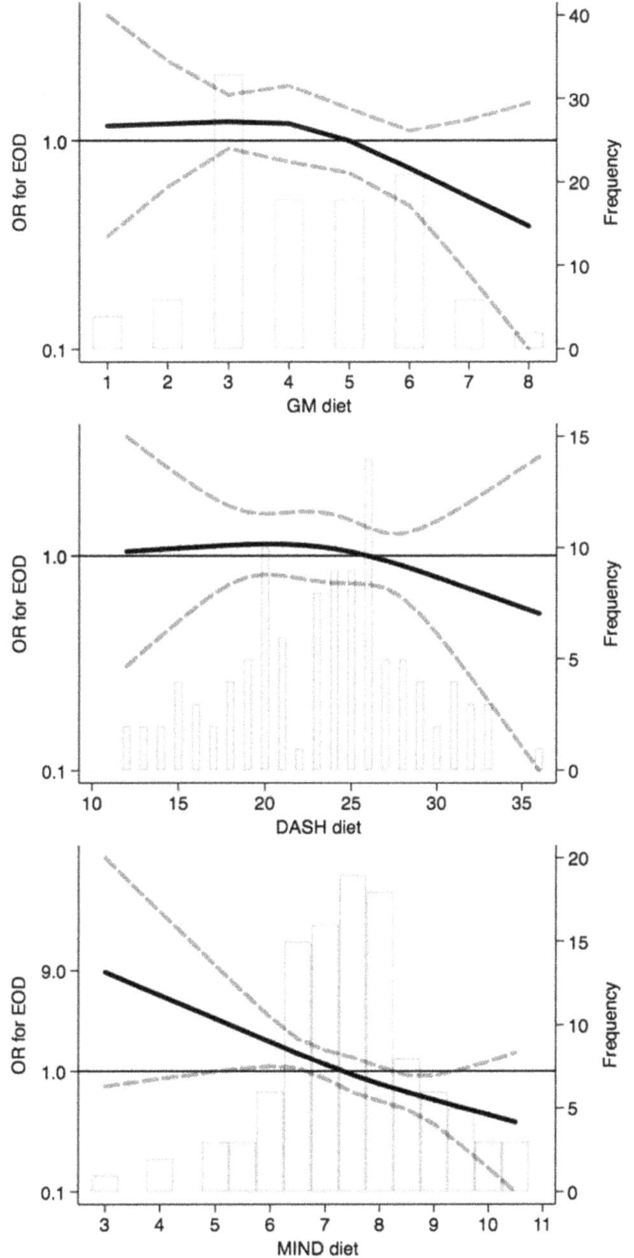

Figure 11. Spline regression analysis for dietary patterns. Greek-Mediterranean (GM) diet, Dietary Approaches to Stop Hypertension (DASH) diet, and Mediterranean-DASH Intervention for Neurodegenerative Delay (MIND) diet. The black line indicates odds ratios for dementia risk; dash gray lines are 95% confidence limits; the reference line at 1.0 with gray bars shows the dietary-pattern score distribution.

4. Discussion

In this study, we found detrimental effects of consumption of high amounts of cereals, dairy products, and some types of sweets on EOD risk, while the intake of vegetables, dry fruits, and chocolate appeared to be beneficial, as was a specific dietary pattern, the MIND diet.

The role of dietary habits on cognitive decline has been investigated in previous studies [39], but the real association between diet and dementia, along with the mechanisms involved in beneficial and detrimental effects, are still unclear and thoroughly debated. In addition, it should be noted that previous studies were generally performed among individuals with late-onset dementia, while the present study specifically focused on younger subjects. Consistent with previous findings, we found a protective effect on EOD particularly with a higher consumption of leafy vegetables and fresh fruit. This protective effect on cognitive decline could be linked to the consumption of foods rich in bioactive substances such as polyphenols, highly present in fruits, vegetables, cereals, coffee/tea, cacao, and wine [40–42]. In the studies suggesting that vegetable intake showed an inverse association with cognitive decline [43,44], an apparent beneficial role of consumption of leafy and root vegetables has been reported [17,45]. Conversely, fruit intake showed contrasting results with null [17,44] or an inverse association [42], with the latter mainly emerging from the analysis evaluating dry fruit intake [17,40,46].

Similarly, the intake of omega-3 fatty acids due to fish consumption has been linked to improved cognition capacities [41,43,47–50]. Interestingly, we found a null association when overall fish and seafood intake was considered, whereas a slight decrease in risk could be found when considering fish, particularly fresh fish, only. The association we detected between a high daily intake of preserved and tinned fish and EOD is of interest, since such an intake in Italy is mainly due to the consumption of canned tuna [51], a source of heavy metals such as mercury, lead, cadmium, and a metalloid of potential neurotoxicity such as selenium [51–56].

Contrasting results with detrimental [57,58] or null effects [31,59] have been reported for dairy products. However, a preventive role has not yet been entirely ruled out, especially considering the different types of dairy products [60,61]. In particular, we found a dose-dependent association between dairy products and EOD risk. In addition, a null to negative association was observed for subjects reporting an intake of up to 350 g/day, when EOD risk starts to increase, thus suggesting adverse effects only at very high intake levels. A possible beneficial role in the cognitive function of substances released during fermentation processes, such as oleamide and dehydroergosterol, has been suggested, following suppression of microglial inflammation, as well as promotion of synaptic extension and neuronal survival [62].

A high cereal intake seems associated with a sharper cognitive decline [58]. In our study, we found an optimum cereal intake at approximately 200 g/day with reference to EOD risk. This is not surprising in that cereals (particularly bread) are fundamental components of the Mediterranean diet [63]. This mainly relates to a beneficial effect of whole grain consumption [64], possibly due to high concentrations of dietary fiber, resistant starch, and oligosaccharides, as well as several phytochemicals (phytates and phenolic compounds) characterized by antioxidant activities [65].

Sweets are generally associated with adverse cognitive effects [66,67]. Possible biological mechanisms of that association may involve generally high fat contents, especially high in saturated and trans-fats and lower in polyunsaturated and monounsaturated fats leading to blood brain barrier dysfunction and increased amyloid beta protein aggregation [68]. However, we observed an indication of beneficial effects from moderate consumption of chocolate products, consistent with previous studies [69,70]. Such beneficial effects, if real, may be due to the cocoa polyphenol intake [71] that might slow MCI progression to dementia [72].

We found a clear inverse association between coffee consumption and EOD risk. A recent dose-response meta-analysis of prospective studies [73] showed a statistically imprecise U-shaped relation between coffee intake and all-cause dementia risk, with the lowest dementia risk at two cups/day (RR = 0.90, 95% CI 0.95 to 1.08) and increased risk at and above five cups/day (RR = 1.11,

95% CI 0.94 to 1.30). Estimate imprecision might be due to the heterogeneity of exposure assessment methods (i.e., cups), which may correspond to different coffee amounts depending on country. Nonetheless, we also found a U-shaped association with a lowest risk at 70 g/day, corresponding to approximately two small (i.e., 'espresso type') cups, according to typically Italian habits as assessed in the EPIC-FFQ [74,75]. Contrary to our expectations based on the epidemiologic literature, we found no clear and meaningful relation between wine or alcohol intake and disease risk. No consumption and excessive consumption of wine or alcohol have both been associated with increased dementia risk [76,77]. In particular, a J-shaped relation has been proposed where low-to-moderate intake was associated with reduced risk, while both null and elevated intakes were correlated with increased risk [78–80].

Concerning dietary patterns, our results for EOD are fully consistent with previous studies, although these were generally carried out in older individuals, suggesting a beneficial effect on the overall cognitive function at higher adherence levels [19,35,81–86]. In particular, we found an indication of protective effects on EOD risk only at high adherence levels to the Greek-Mediterranean Diet (≥6) and DASH index (≥28). On the other hand, the only diet which was strongly and linearly associated with EOD risk was the MIND pattern. This was not entirely unexpected, since the MIND pattern has been shown to better predict an incidence of cognitive impairment or cognitive decline as compared to the Mediterranean Diet and DASH index [87,88]. In addition, the MIND diet has shown beneficial effects on other neurological diseases [89–91], while a clinical trial about the role of the diet on cognitive decline and brain neurodegeneration is ongoing [92].

The three dietary patterns under investigation have some similarities, since they emphasize natural plant-based foods and limit the intake of animal-derived products and high saturated-fats. Nevertheless, MIND has a distinctive pattern. It was developed as a hybrid of the DASH and Mediterranean diets with modifications, by reflecting the most compelling scientific evidence on foods and nutrients that protect the brain [93]. The MIND pattern attributes beneficial effects to the intake of cheese (<1 serving/week), green leafy vegetables (≥6 servings/week), berries (>1 serving/week), and fast fried food (<1 time/week) [35,83]. In addition, a high adherence to the investigated dietary patterns is generally associated with high levels of physical activity and other diet-related lifestyle factors [63] having beneficial effects on cognitive function [94,95]. These factors were not taken into account in our study. They might have contributed to a lower EOD risk and to masking the effect of the diet, which becomes evident only at high adherence levels.

To the best of our knowledge, our study is the first to investigate the role of dietary factors on early-onset dementia risk. In fact, previous studies focused on late-onset dementia or did not implement a specific restriction to EOD cases. The use of the validated EPIC-FFQ also allowed for a comprehensive assessment of dietary habits, including the investigation of single food categories and overall dietary-pattern adherence. In addition, we included recently-diagnosed EOD cases, thus limiting the risk of bias related to a long duration of the disease due to disease progression and increasing disability. Another strength of the present study was the ability to apply stratified analyses to the investigation of possible selective associations between diet and EOD risk according to the clinical dementia type.

Some limitations of our study should also be noted. First, the small samples of EOD participants, mainly due to the low incidence of the disease, affected the statistical precision of the risk estimates, especially for those food categories characterized by a large number of non-consumers. As a consequence, such a limited number of subjects hampered our ability to reliably identify weak associations. This was the case especially in subgroup analyses, which suggest caution in the interpretation of estimates characterized by a high imprecision, as well as the need to plan larger studies on the relations between diet and EOD. Secondly, although the EPIC-FFQ was designed and validated to collect dietary information at least over the previous year, we cannot rule out a possible misclassification due to changes of dietary habits of study participants, especially with reference to life-long habits. However, a recent survey comparing adherence to the Mediterranean diet over a long time period (1997–2012) showed similar values for the Emilia Romagna population [96], suggesting a general stability over time of dietary habits. In addition, the use of caregivers as controls could have led to a risk of overmatching and downplayed the real associations between dietary factors and disease risk. As a matter of fact, some controls (particularly cases' family members) may have shared lifestyle habits including dietary patterns with EOD cases, thus reducing the strength of the associations we estimated. Finally, a genetic status was unavailable for almost all study participants. In particular, no data about the referent population could be retrieved, thus hampering the ability to assess their role in modifying EOD risk in relation to dietary factors.

5. Conclusions

This case-control study provides insights on the role of dietary factors in EOD risk. In particular, our findings suggest a detrimental effect on EOD risk due to a high intake of cereals, dairy products, and some types of sweets. Conversely, the intake of some types of fish, vegetables, dry fruits, and chocolate alongside moderate coffee consumption appear to be beneficial. Finally, our study indicates that an increasing adherence to the Mediterranean-DASH Intervention for Neurodegenerative Delay (MIND) may decrease EOD risk.

Supplementary Materials: The following are available online at http://www.mdpi.com/2072-6643/12/12/3682/s1. Supplemental Table S1: Clinical diagnosis of early-onset dementia cases; Supplemental Table S2: Food and beverages mean (standard deviation (SD)) intake and number (%) of consumers in the study population. Early-onset dementia (EOD); Supplemental Table S3: Food and beverages mean (standard deviation (SD)) intake and number (%) of consumers according to the EOD subtype. Early-onset Alzheimer's dementia (EO-AD) and early-onset frontotemporal dementia spectrum (EO-FTD); Supplemental Table S4: Odds ratio (OR) and 95% confidence intervals (CI) for early-onset dementia (EOD), early-onset Alzheimer's dementia (EO-AD), and early-onset frontotemporal dementia spectrum (EO-FTD) for increasing tertiles of food and beverage intake; Supplemental Figures S1–S10: Spline regression analysis of risk of early-onset Alzheimer's dementia (EO-AD) for an increasing intake of food: Cereals and cereal products (1); meats and meat products (2); milk, dairy products, and eggs (3); fish and seafood (4); vegetables (5); mushrooms, legumes, and potatoes (6); fresh and dry fruits (7); sweets, chocolate, cakes, etc. (8); oils and fats (9); beverages (10). The black line indicates the odds ratio for dementia risk; the dash gray lines are 95% confidence limits; the reference line at 1.0 with black spikes indicates the distribution of intake of participants. Note: Spline analysis was not possible for offal and most beverages due to a few subjects reporting consumption which is different from the null value (tea, red, white, aperitif wines and beers, spirits and soft drinks); Supplemental Figures S11–S20: Spline regression analysis of risk of early-onset frontotemporal dementia spectrum (EO-FTD) for an increasing intake of food: Cereals and cereal products (1); meats and meat products (2); milk, dairy products, and eggs (3); fish and seafood (4); vegetables (5); mushrooms, legumes, and potatoes (6); fresh and dry fruits (7); sweets, chocolate, cakes, etc. (8); oils and fats (9); beverages (10). The black line indicates the odds ratio for dementia risk; the dash gray lines are 95% confidence limits; the reference line at 1.0 with black spikes indicates the distribution of intake of participants. Note: Spline analysis was not possible for offal and most beverages due to a few subjects reporting consumption which is different from the null value (tea, red, white, aperitif wines and beers, spirits, fruit juices, and soft drinks); Supplemental Figure S21: Spline regression analysis of risk of early-onset Alzheimer's dementia (EO-AD) for increasing adherence to the Greek-Mediterranean (GM) diet, Dietary Approaches to Stop Hypertension (DASH) diet, and Mediterranean-DASH Intervention for Neurodegenerative Delay (MIND) diet. The black line indicates the odds ratio for dementia risk; the dash gray lines are 95% confidence limits; the reference line at 1.0 with gray bars shows the distribution of dietary pattern scores; Supplemental Figure S22: Spline regression analysis of risk of frontotemporal dementia spectrum (EO-FTD) for increasing adherence to dietary patterns. Greek-Mediterranean (GM) diet, Dietary Approaches to Stop Hypertension (DASH) diet, and Mediterranean-DASH Intervention for Neurodegenerative Delay (MIND) diet. The black line indicates the odds ratio for dementia risk; the dash gray lines are 95% confidence limits; the reference line at 1.0 with gray bars shows the distribution of dietary pattern scores.

Author Contributions: Conceptualization, A.C., T.F., and M.V.; data curation, T.F., G.A., C.G., (Caterina Garuti), M.M., and S.C.; formal analysis, G.A., T.F., and M.V.; participant recruitment, A.C., M.C., C.G. (Caterina Garuti), C.G. (Chiara Galli), M.T., G.V., and G.Z.; writing—original draft, G.A., T.F., and M.V.; writing—review and editing, all authors. All authors have read and agreed to the published version of the manuscript.

Funding: This study was supported by the grant "Dipartimenti di Eccellenza 2018–2022, MIUR, Italy" awarded to the Department of Biomedical, Metabolic and Neural Sciences of the University of Modena and Reggio Emilia, and by a grant from the Airalzh ONLUS & Coop Italia.

Acknowledgments: We are grateful to all the patients and their families for participating in this study. We also thank Martha Clare Morris who was the lead creator of the MIND pattern and originally inspired the analysis of the effect of dietary patterns in this research.

Conflicts of Interest: The authors declare no conflict of interest.

References

1. WHO. Dementia. 2019. Available online: https://www.who.int/news-room/fact-sheets/detail/dementia (accessed on 15 November 2020).
2. Wolters, F.J.; Ikram, M.A. Epidemiology of dementia: The burden on society, the challenges for research. *Methods Mol. Biol.* **2018**, *1750*, 3–14.
3. Rossor, M.N.; Fox, N.C.; Mummery, C.J.; Schott, J.M.; Warren, J.D. The diagnosis of young-onset dementia. *Lancet Neurol.* **2010**, *9*, 793–806. [CrossRef]
4. Vieira, R.T.; Caixeta, L.; Machado, S.; Silva, A.C.; Nardi, A.E.; Arias-Carrion, O.; Carta, M.G. Epidemiology of early-onset dementia: A review of the literature. *Clin. Pract. Epidemiol. Ment. Health* **2013**, *9*, 88–95. [CrossRef] [PubMed]
5. Sakata, N.; Okumura, Y. Job loss after diagnosis of early-onset dementia: A matched cohort study. *J. Alzheimers Dis.* **2017**, *60*, 1231–1235. [CrossRef]
6. Sikes, P.; Hall, M. The impact of parental young onset dementia on children and young people's educational careers. *Br. Educ. Res. J.* **2018**, *44*, 593–607. [CrossRef] [PubMed]
7. Chiari, A.; Vinceti, G.; Adani, G.; Tondelli, M.; Galli, C.; Fiondella, L.; Costa, M.; Molinari, M.A.; Filippini, T.; Zamboni, G.; et al. Epidemiology of early onset dementia and its clinical presentations in the province of Modena, Italy. *Alzheimer's Dement.* **2020**. [CrossRef] [PubMed]
8. Jarmolowicz, A.I.; Chen, H.Y.; Panegyres, P.K. The patterns of inheritance in early-onset dementia: Alzheimer's disease and frontotemporal dementia. *Am. J. Alzheimers Dis. Other Demen.* **2015**, *30*, 299–306. [CrossRef] [PubMed]
9. Koedam, E.L.; Lauffer, V.; van der Vlies, A.E.; van der Flier, W.M.; Scheltens, P.; Pijnenburg, Y.A. Early-versus late-onset Alzheimer's disease: More than age alone. *J. Alzheimers Dis.* **2010**, *19*, 1401–1408. [CrossRef]
10. Cations, M.; Withall, A.; Low, L.F.; Draper, B. What is the role of modifiable environmental and lifestyle risk factors in young onset dementia? *Eur. J. Epidemiol.* **2016**, *31*, 107–124. [CrossRef]
11. Cations, M.; Withall, A.; Draper, B. Modifiable risk factors for young onset dementia. *Curr. Opin. Psychiatry* **2019**, *32*, 138–143. [CrossRef]
12. Angeloni, C.; Businaro, R.; Vauzour, D. The role of diet in preventing and reducing cognitive decline. *Curr. Opin. Psychiatry* **2020**, *33*, 432–438. [CrossRef] [PubMed]
13. Livingston, G.; Huntley, J.; Sommerlad, A.; Ames, D.; Ballard, C.; Banerjee, S.; Brayne, C.; Burns, A.; Cohen-Mansfield, J.; Cooper, C.; et al. Dementia prevention, intervention, and care: 2020 report of the Lancet Commission. *Lancet* **2020**, *396*, 413–446. [CrossRef]
14. Stamati, P.; Siokas, V.; Aloizou, A.M.; Karampinis, E.; Arseniou, S.; Rakitskii, V.N.; Tsatsakis, A.; Spandidos, D.A.; Gozes, I.; Mitsias, P.D.; et al. Does SCFD1 rs10139154 polymorphism decrease Alzheimer's disease risk? *J. Mol. Neurosci.* **2019**, *69*, 343–350. [CrossRef] [PubMed]
15. Morris, M.C.; Evans, D.A.; Tangney, C.C.; Bienias, J.L.; Wilson, R.S. Fish consumption and cognitive decline with age in a large community study. *Arch. Neurol.* **2005**, *62*, 1849–1853. [CrossRef]
16. Morris, M.C.; Evans, D.A.; Tangney, C.C.; Bienias, J.L.; Wilson, R.S. Associations of vegetable and fruit consumption with age-related cognitive change. *Neurology* **2006**, *67*, 1370–1376. [CrossRef]
17. Nooyens, A.C.; Bueno-de-Mesquita, H.B.; van Boxtel, M.P.; van Gelder, B.M.; Verhagen, H.; Verschuren, W.M. Fruit and vegetable intake and cognitive decline in middle-aged men and women: The Doetinchem Cohort Study. *Br. J. Nutr.* **2011**, *106*, 752–761. [CrossRef]
18. Martinez-Lapiscina, E.H.; Clavero, P.; Toledo, E.; Estruch, R.; Salas-Salvado, J.; San Julian, B.; Sanchez-Tainta, A.; Ros, E.; Valls-Pedret, C.; Martinez-Gonzalez, M.A. Mediterranean diet improves cognition: The PREDIMED-NAVARRA randomised trial. *J. Neurol. Neurosurg. Psychiatry* **2013**, *84*, 1318–1325. [CrossRef]
19. Morris, M.C.; Tangney, C.C.; Wang, Y.; Sacks, F.M.; Barnes, L.L.; Bennett, D.A.; Aggarwal, N.T. MIND diet slows cognitive decline with aging. *Alzheimers Dement.* **2015**, *11*, 1015–1022. [CrossRef]

20. Smith, P.J.; Blumenthal, J.A.; Babyak, M.A.; Craighead, L.; Welsh-Bohmer, K.A.; Browndyke, J.N.; Strauman, T.A.; Sherwood, A. Effects of the dietary approaches to stop hypertension diet, exercise, and caloric restriction on neurocognition in overweight adults with high blood pressure. *Hypertension* **2010**, *55*, 1331–1338. [CrossRef]

21. Tanaka, T.; Talegawkar, S.A.; Jin, Y.; Colpo, M.; Ferrucci, L.; Bandinelli, S. Adherence to a mediterranean diet protects from cognitive decline in the invecchiare in Chianti study of aging. *Nutrients* **2018**, *10*, 2007. [CrossRef]

22. Berti, V.; Murray, J.; Davies, M.; Spector, N.; Tsui, W.H.; Li, Y.; Williams, S.; Pirraglia, E.; Vallabhajosula, S.; McHugh, P.; et al. Nutrient patterns and brain biomarkers of Alzheimer's disease in cognitively normal individuals. *J. Nutr. Health Aging* **2015**, *19*, 413–423. [CrossRef] [PubMed]

23. Mosconi, L.; Murray, J.; Davies, M.; Williams, S.; Pirraglia, E.; Spector, N.; Tsui, W.H.; Li, Y.; Butler, T.; Osorio, R.S.; et al. Nutrient intake and brain biomarkers of Alzheimer's disease in at-risk cognitively normal individuals: A cross-sectional neuroimaging pilot study. *BMJ Open* **2014**, *4*, e004850. [CrossRef] [PubMed]

24. Adani, G.; Filippini, T.; Garuti, C.; Malavolti, M.; Vinceti, G.; Zamboni, G.; Tondelli, M.; Galli, C.; Costa, M.; Vinceti, M.; et al. Environmental risk factors for early-onset Alzheimer's dementia and frontotemporal dementia: A case-control study in northern Italy. *Int. J. Environ. Res. Public Health* **2020**, *17*, 7941. [CrossRef] [PubMed]

25. Filippini, T.; Fiore, M.; Tesauro, M.; Malagoli, C.; Consonni, M.; Violi, F.; Arcolin, E.; Iacuzio, L.; Oliveri Conti, G.; Cristaldi, A.; et al. Clinical and lifestyle factors and risk of amyotrophic lateral sclerosis: A population-based case-control study. *Int. J. Environ. Res. Public Health* **2020**, *17*, 857. [CrossRef]

26. Pala, V.; Sieri, S.; Palli, D.; Salvini, S.; Berrino, F.; Bellegotti, M.; Frasca, G.; Tumino, R.; Sacerdote, C.; Fiorini, L.; et al. Diet in the Italian EPIC cohorts: Presentation of data and methodological issues. *Tumori* **2003**, *89*, 594–607. [CrossRef]

27. Pasanisi, P.; Berrino, F.; Bellati, C.; Sieri, S.; Krogh, V. Validity of the Italian EPIC questionnaire to assess past diet. *IARC Sci. Publ.* **2002**, *156*, 41–44.

28. Filippini, T.; Malagoli, C.; Wise, L.A.; Malavolti, M.; Pellacani, G.; Vinceti, M. Dietary cadmium intake and risk of cutaneous melanoma: An Italian population-based case-control study. *J. Trace Elem. Med. Biol.* **2019**, *56*, 100–106. [CrossRef]

29. Malavolti, M.; Fairweather-Tait, S.J.; Malagoli, C.; Vescovi, L.; Vinceti, M.; Filippini, T. Lead exposure in an Italian population: Food content, dietary intake and risk assessment. *Food Res. Int.* **2020**, *137*, 109370. [CrossRef]

30. Sieri, S.; Krogh, V.; Saieva, C.; Grobbee, D.E.; Bergmann, M.; Rohrmann, S.; Tjonneland, A.; Ferrari, P.; Chloptsios, Y.; Dilis, V.; et al. Alcohol consumption patterns, diet and body weight in 10 European countries. *Eur. J. Clin. Nutr.* **2009**, *63* (Suppl. 4), S81–S100. [CrossRef]

31. Trichopoulou, A.; Costacou, T.; Bamia, C.; Trichopoulos, D. Adherence to a Mediterranean diet and survival in a Greek population. *N. Engl. J. Med.* **2003**, *348*, 2599–2608. [CrossRef]

32. Appel, L.J.; Moore, T.J.; Obarzanek, E.; Vollmer, W.M.; Svetkey, L.P.; Sacks, F.M.; Bray, G.A.; Vogt, T.M.; Cutler, J.A.; Windhauser, M.M.; et al. A clinical trial of the effects of dietary patterns on blood pressure. DASH Collaborative Research Group. *N. Engl. J. Med.* **1997**, *336*, 1117–1124. [CrossRef] [PubMed]

33. Sacks, F.M.; Svetkey, L.P.; Vollmer, W.M.; Appel, L.J.; Bray, G.A.; Harsha, D.; Obarzanek, E.; Conlin, P.R.; Miller, E.R., 3rd; Simons-Morton, D.G.; et al. Effects on blood pressure of reduced dietary sodium and the Dietary Approaches to Stop Hypertension (DASH) diet. DASH-Sodium Collaborative Research Group. *N. Engl. J. Med.* **2001**, *344*, 3–10. [CrossRef] [PubMed]

34. Malagoli, C.; Malavolti, M.; Agnoli, C.; Crespi, C.M.; Fiorentini, C.; Farnetani, F.; Longo, C.; Ricci, C.; Albertini, G.; Lanzoni, A.; et al. Diet quality and risk of melanoma in an Italian population. *J. Nutr.* **2015**, *145*, 1800–1807. [CrossRef] [PubMed]

35. Morris, M.C.; Tangney, C.C.; Wang, Y.; Sacks, F.M.; Bennett, D.A.; Aggarwal, N.T. MIND diet associated with reduced incidence of Alzheimer's disease. *Alzheimers Dement.* **2015**, *11*, 1007–1014. [CrossRef]

36. Agnoli, C.; Krogh, V.; Grioni, S.; Sieri, S.; Palli, D.; Masala, G.; Sacerdote, C.; Vineis, P.; Tumino, R.; Frasca, G.; et al. A priori-defined dietary patterns are associated with reduced risk of stroke in a large Italian cohort. *J. Nutr.* **2011**, *141*, 1552–1558. [CrossRef]

37. McGrattan, A.M.; McGuinness, B.; McKinley, M.C.; Kee, F.; Passmore, P.; Woodside, J.V.; McEvoy, C.T. Diet and inflammation in cognitive ageing and Alzheimer's disease. *Curr. Nutr. Rep.* **2019**, *8*, 53–65. [CrossRef]

38. Fung, T.T.; Chiuve, S.E.; McCullough, M.L.; Rexrode, K.M.; Logroscino, G.; Hu, F.B. Adherence to a DASH-style diet and risk of coronary heart disease and stroke in women. *Arch. Intern. Med.* **2008**, *168*, 713–720. [CrossRef]

39. Di Marco, L.Y.; Marzo, A.; Munoz-Ruiz, M.; Ikram, M.A.; Kivipelto, M.; Ruefenacht, D.; Venneri, A.; Soininen, H.; Wanke, I.; Ventikos, Y.A.; et al. Modifiable lifestyle factors in dementia: A systematic review of longitudinal observational cohort studies. *J. Alzheimers Dis.* **2014**, *42*, 119–135. [CrossRef]

40. Devore, E.E.; Kang, J.H.; Breteler, M.M.; Grodstein, F. Dietary intakes of berries and flavonoids in relation to cognitive decline. *Ann. Neurol.* **2012**, *72*, 135–143. [CrossRef]

41. Roman, G.C.; Jackson, R.E.; Gadhia, R.; Roman, A.N.; Reis, J. Mediterranean diet: The role of long-chain omega-3 fatty acids in fish; polyphenols in fruits, vegetables, cereals, coffee, tea, cacao and wine; probiotics and vitamins in prevention of stroke, age-related cognitive decline, and Alzheimer disease. *Rev. Neurol.* **2019**, *175*, 724–741. [CrossRef]

42. Zielinska, M.A.; Bialecka, A.; Pietruszka, B.; Hamulka, J. Vegetables and fruit, as a source of bioactive substances, and impact on memory and cognitive function of elderly. *Postepy Hig. Med. Dosw. (Online)* **2017**, *71*, 267–280. [CrossRef] [PubMed]

43. Barberger-Gateau, P.; Raffaitin, C.; Letenneur, L.; Berr, C.; Tzourio, C.; Dartigues, J.F.; Alperovitch, A. Dietary patterns and risk of dementia: The Three-City cohort study. *Neurology* **2007**, *69*, 1921–1930. [CrossRef] [PubMed]

44. Kang, J.H.; Ascherio, A.; Grodstein, F. Fruit and vegetable consumption and cognitive decline in aging women. *Ann. Neurol.* **2005**, *57*, 713–720. [CrossRef] [PubMed]

45. Morris, M.C.; Wang, Y.; Barnes, L.L.; Bennett, D.A.; Dawson-Hughes, B.; Booth, S.L. Nutrients and bioactives in green leafy vegetables and cognitive decline: Prospective study. *Neurology* **2018**, *90*, e214–e222. [CrossRef] [PubMed]

46. Agarwal, P.; Holland, T.M.; Wang, Y.; Bennett, D.A.; Morris, M.C. Association of strawberries and anthocyanidin intake with Alzheimer's dementia risk. *Nutrients* **2019**, *11*, 3060. [CrossRef]

47. Devore, E.E.; Grodstein, F.; van Rooij, F.J.; Hofman, A.; Rosner, B.; Stampfer, M.J.; Witteman, J.C.; Breteler, M.M. Dietary intake of fish and omega-3 fatty acids in relation to long-term dementia risk. *Am. J. Clin. Nutr.* **2009**, *90*, 170–176. [CrossRef]

48. Larrieu, S.; Letenneur, L.; Helmer, C.; Dartigues, J.F.; Barberger-Gateau, P. Nutritional factors and risk of incident dementia in the PAQUID longitudinal cohort. *J. Nutr. Health Aging* **2004**, *8*, 150–154.

49. Morris, M.C.; Evans, D.A.; Bienias, J.L.; Tangney, C.C.; Bennett, D.A.; Wilson, R.S.; Aggarwal, N.; Schneider, J. Consumption of fish and n-3 fatty acids and risk of incident Alzheimer disease. *Arch. Neurol.* **2003**, *60*, 940–946. [CrossRef]

50. Samieri, C.; Morris, M.C.; Bennett, D.A.; Berr, C.; Amouyel, P.; Dartigues, J.F.; Tzourio, C.; Chasman, D.I.; Grodstein, F. Fish intake, genetic predisposition to Alzheimer disease, and decline in global cognition and memory in 5 cohorts of older persons. *Am. J. Epidemiol.* **2018**, *187*, 933–940. [CrossRef]

51. Pappalardo, A.M.; Copat, C.; Ferrito, V.; Grasso, A.; Ferrante, M. Heavy metal content and molecular species identification in canned tuna: Insights into human food safety. *Mol. Med. Rep.* **2017**, *15*, 3430–3437. [CrossRef]

52. Filippini, T.; Cilloni, S.; Malavolti, M.; Violi, F.; Malagoli, C.; Tesauro, M.; Bottecchi, I.; Ferrari, A.; Vescovi, L.; Vinceti, M. Dietary intake of cadmium, chromium, copper, manganese, selenium and zinc in a Northern Italy community. *J. Trace Elem. Med. Biol.* **2018**, *50*, 508–517. [CrossRef] [PubMed]

53. Russo, R.; Lo Voi, A.; De Simone, A.; Serpe, F.P.; Anastasio, A.; Pepe, T.; Cacace, D.; Severino, L. Heavy metals in canned tuna from Italian markets. *J. Food Prot.* **2013**, *76*, 355–359. [CrossRef]

54. Storelli, M.M.; Barone, G.; Cuttone, G.; Giungato, D.; Garofalo, R. Occurrence of toxic metals (Hg, Cd and Pb) in fresh and canned tuna: Public health implications. *Food Chem. Toxicol.* **2010**, *48*, 3167–3170. [CrossRef] [PubMed]

55. Vinceti, M.; Mandrioli, J.; Borella, P.; Michalke, B.; Tsatsakis, A.; Finkelstein, Y. Selenium neurotoxicity in humans: Bridging laboratory and epidemiologic studies. *Toxicol. Lett.* **2014**, *230*, 295–303. [CrossRef] [PubMed]

56. Vinceti, M.; Filippini, T.; Mandrioli, J.; Violi, F.; Bargellini, A.; Weuve, J.; Fini, N.; Grill, P.; Michalke, B. Lead, cadmium and mercury in cerebrospinal fluid and risk of amyotrophic lateral sclerosis: A case-control study. *J. Trace Elem. Med. Biol.* **2017**, *43*, 121–125. [CrossRef]

57. Kesse-Guyot, E.; Assmann, K.E.; Andreeva, V.A.; Ferry, M.; Hercberg, S.; Galan, P. Consumption of dairy products and cognitive functioning: Findings from the SU.VI.MAX 2 study. *J. Nutr. Health Aging* **2016**, *20*, 128–137. [CrossRef] [PubMed]

58. Otsuka, R.; Kato, Y.; Nishita, Y.; Tange, C.; Nakamoto, M.; Tomida, M.; Imai, T.; Ando, F.; Shimokata, H. Cereal intake increases and dairy products decrease risk of cognitive decline among elderly female Japanese. *J. Prev. Alzheimers Dis.* **2014**, *1*, 160–167.

59. Lee, J.; Fu, Z.; Chung, M.; Jang, D.J.; Lee, H.J. Role of milk and dairy intake in cognitive function in older adults: A systematic review and meta-analysis. *Nutr. J.* **2018**, *17*, 82. [CrossRef]

60. Ozawa, M.; Ninomiya, T.; Ohara, T.; Doi, Y.; Uchida, K.; Shirota, T.; Yonemoto, K.; Kitazono, T.; Kiyohara, Y. Dietary patterns and risk of dementia in an elderly Japanese population: The hisayama Study1–3. *Am. J. Clin. Nutr.* **2013**, *97*, 1076–1082. [CrossRef]

61. Rahman, A.; Baker, P.S.; Allman, R.M.; Zamrini, E. Dietary factors and cognitive impairment in community-dwelling elderly. *J. Nutr. Health Aging* **2007**, *11*, 49–54.

62. Ano, Y.; Nakayama, H. Preventive effects of dairy products on dementia and the underlying mechanisms. *Int. J. Mol. Sci.* **2018**, *19*, 1927. [CrossRef] [PubMed]

63. Willett, W.C.; Sacks, F.; Trichopoulou, A.; Drescher, G.; Ferro-Luzzi, A.; Helsing, E.; Trichopoulos, D. Mediterranean diet pyramid: A cultural model for healthy eating. *Am. J. Clin. Nutr.* **1995**, *61*, 1402S–1406S. [CrossRef] [PubMed]

64. Wengreen, H.; Munger, R.G.; Cutler, A.; Quach, A.; Bowles, A.; Corcoran, C.; Tschanz, J.T.; Norton, M.C.; Welsh-Bohmer, K.A. Prospective study of Dietary Approaches to Stop Hypertension- and Mediterranean-style dietary patterns and age-related cognitive change: The cache county study on memory, health and aging. *Am. J. Clin. Nutr.* **2013**, *98*, 1263–1271. [CrossRef]

65. Slavin, J. Whole grains and human health. *Nutr. Res. Rev.* **2004**, *17*, 99–110. [CrossRef] [PubMed]

66. Akbaraly, T.N.; Singh-Manoux, A.; Marmot, M.G.; Brunner, E.J. Education attenuates the association between dietary patterns and cognition. *Dement. Geriatr. Cogn. Disord.* **2009**, *27*, 147–154. [CrossRef] [PubMed]

67. Pilleron, S.; Desport, J.C.; Jesus, P.; Mbelesso, P.; Ndamba-Bandzouzi, B.; Dartigues, J.F.; Clement, J.P.; Preux, P.M.; Guerchet, M. Diet, Alcohol consumption and cognitive disorders in central Africa: A study from the EPIDEMCA program. *J. Nutr. Health Aging* **2015**, *19*, 657–667. [CrossRef] [PubMed]

68. Morris, M.C.; Tangney, C.C. Dietary fat composition and dementia risk. *Neurobiol. Aging* **2014**, *35* (Suppl. 2), S59–S64. [CrossRef]

69. Crichton, G.E.; Elias, M.F.; Alkerwi, A. Chocolate intake is associated with better cognitive function: The maine-syracuse longitudinal study. *Appetite* **2016**, *100*, 126–132. [CrossRef]

70. Moreira, A.; Diogenes, M.J.; de Mendonca, A.; Lunet, N.; Barros, H. Chocolate consumption is associated with a lower risk of cognitive decline. *J. Alzheimers Dis.* **2016**, *53*, 85–93. [CrossRef]

71. Barrera-Reyes, P.K.; de Lara, J.C.; Gonzalez-Soto, M.; Tejero, M.E. Effects of cocoa-derived polyphenols on cognitive function in humans. Systematic review and analysis of methodological aspects. *Plant. Foods Hum. Nutr.* **2020**, *75*, 1–11. [CrossRef]

72. Calabro, R.S.; De Cola, M.C.; Gervasi, G.; Portaro, S.; Naro, A.; Accorinti, M.; Manuli, A.; Marra, A.; De Luca, R.; Bramanti, P. The efficacy of cocoa polyphenols in the treatment of mild cognitive impairment: A retrospective study. *Medicina* **2019**, *55*, 156. [CrossRef] [PubMed]

73. Larsson, S.C.; Orsini, N. Coffee consumption and risk of dementia and Alzheimer's disease: A dose-response meta-analysis of prospective studies. *Nutrients* **2018**, *10*, 1501. [CrossRef] [PubMed]

74. Filippini, T.; Tancredi, S.; Malagoli, C.; Cilloni, S.; Malavolti, M.; Violi, F.; Vescovi, L.; Bargellini, A.; Vinceti, M. Aluminum and tin: Food contamination and dietary intake in an Italian population. *J. Trace Elem. Med. Biol.* **2019**, *52*, 293–301. [CrossRef] [PubMed]

75. Malagoli, C.; Malavolti, M.; Farnetani, F.; Longo, C.; Filippini, T.; Pellacani, G.; Vinceti, M. Food and beverage consumption and melanoma risk: A population-based case-control study in northern Italy. *Nutrients* **2019**, *11*, 2206. [CrossRef]

76. Lao, Y.; Hou, L.; Li, J.; Hui, X.; Yan, P.; Yang, K. Association between alcohol intake, mild cognitive impairment and progression to dementia: A dose-response meta-analysis. *Aging Clin. Exp. Res.* **2020**. [CrossRef]

77. Reale, M.; Costantini, E.; Jagarlapoodi, S.; Khan, H.; Belwal, T.; Cichelli, A. Relationship of wine consumption with Alzheimer's disease. *Nutrients* **2020**, *12*, 206. [CrossRef]

78. Deng, J.; Zhou, D.H.; Li, J.; Wang, Y.J.; Gao, C.; Chen, M. A 2-year follow-up study of alcohol consumption and risk of dementia. *Clin. Neurol. Neurosurg.* **2006**, *108*, 378–383. [CrossRef]

79. Orgogozo, J.M.; Dartigues, J.F.; Lafont, S.; Letenneur, L.; Commenges, D.; Salamon, R.; Renaud, S.; Breteler, M.B. Wine consumption and dementia in the elderly: A prospective community study in the Bordeaux area. *Rev. Neurol.* **1997**, *153*, 185–192.

80. Xu, W.; Wang, H.; Wan, Y.; Tan, C.; Li, J.; Tan, L.; Yu, J.T. Alcohol consumption and dementia risk: A dose-response meta-analysis of prospective studies. *Eur. J. Epidemiol.* **2017**, *32*, 31–42. [CrossRef]

81. Berendsen, A.M.; Kang, J.H.; Feskens, E.J.M.; de Groot, C.; Grodstein, F.; van de Rest, O. Association of long-term adherence to the MIND diet with cognitive function and cognitive decline in American women. *J. Nutr. Health Aging* **2018**, *22*, 222–229. [CrossRef]

82. Feart, C.; Samieri, C.; Rondeau, V.; Amieva, H.; Portet, F.; Dartigues, J.F.; Scarmeas, N.; Barberger-Gateau, P. Adherence to a Mediterranean diet, cognitive decline, and risk of dementia. *JAMA* **2009**, *302*, 638–648. [CrossRef] [PubMed]

83. Munoz-Garcia, M.I.; Toledo, E.; Razquin, C.; Dominguez, L.J.; Maragarone, D.; Martinez-Gonzalez, J.; Martinez-Gonzalez, M.A. "A priori" dietary patterns and cognitive function in the SUN project. *Neuroepidemiology* **2020**, *54*, 45–57. [CrossRef] [PubMed]

84. Scarmeas, N.; Stern, Y.; Tang, M.X.; Mayeux, R.; Luchsinger, J.A. Mediterranean diet and risk for Alzheimer's disease. *Ann. Neurol.* **2006**, *59*, 912–921. [CrossRef]

85. Tangney, C.; Hong, L.; Barnes, L.L.; Schneider, J.; Bennett, D.; Morris, M. O1–05–03: Accordance to Dietary Approaches to Stop Hypertension (DASH) is associated with slower cognitive decline. *Alzheimers Dement.* **2013**, *9*, P135. [CrossRef]

86. Tangney, C.C.; Li, H.; Wang, Y.; Barnes, L.; Schneider, J.A.; Bennett, D.A.; Morris, M.C. Relation of DASH- and Mediterranean-like dietary patterns to cognitive decline in older persons. *Neurology* **2014**, *83*, 1410–1416. [CrossRef] [PubMed]

87. Hosking, D.E.; Eramudugolla, R.; Cherbuin, N.; Anstey, K.J. MIND not Mediterranean diet related to 12-year incidence of cognitive impairment in an Australian longitudinal cohort study. *Alzheimers Dement.* **2019**, *15*, 581–589. [CrossRef]

88. Morris, M.C.; Tangney, C.C.; Wang, Y.; Barnes, L.L.; Bennett, D.; Aggarwal, N. MIND diet score more predictive than DASH or Mediterranean Diet scores. *Alzheimer's Dement. J. Alzheimer's Assoc.* **2014**, *10*, P166. [CrossRef]

89. Agarwal, P.; Wang, Y.; Buchman, A.S.; Holland, T.M.; Bennett, D.A.; Morris, M.C. MIND diet associated with reduced incidence and delayed progression of parkinsonism in old age. *J. Nutr Health Aging* **2018**, *22*, 1211–1215. [CrossRef]

90. Cherian, L.; Wang, Y.; Fakuda, K.; Leurgans, S.; Aggarwal, N.; Morris, M. Mediterranean-Dash Intervention for Neurodegenerative Delay (MIND) diet slows cognitive decline after stroke. *J. Prev. Alzheimers Dis.* **2019**, *6*, 267–273.

91. Cherian, L.; Wang, Y.; Holland, T.; Agarwal, P.; Aggarwal, N.; Morris, M.C. DASH and Mediterranean-Dash Intervention for Neurodegenerative Delay (MIND) diets are associated with fewer depressive symptoms over time. *J. Gerontol. A Biol. Sci. Med. Sci.* **2020**. [CrossRef]

92. Morris, M.C. MIND Diet Intervention and Cognitive Decline (MIND). 2018. Available online: https://mind-diet-trial.org/meet-the-researchers/; https://clinicaltrials.gov/ct2/show/NCT02817074; (accessed on 15 November 2020).

93. Morris, M.C. Nutrition and risk of dementia: Overview and methodological issues. *Ann. N. Y. Acad. Sci.* **2016**, *1367*, 31–37. [CrossRef] [PubMed]

94. Biazus-Sehn, L.F.; Schuch, F.B.; Firth, J.; Stigger, F.S. Effects of physical exercise on cognitive function of older adults with mild cognitive impairment: A systematic review and meta-analysis. *Arch. Gerontol. Geriatr.* **2020**, *89*, 104048. [CrossRef] [PubMed]

95. Whitty, E.; Mansour, H.; Aguirre, E.; Palomo, M.; Charlesworth, G.; Ramjee, S.; Poppe, M.; Brodaty, H.; Kales, H.C.; Morgan-Trimmer, S.; et al. Efficacy of lifestyle and psychosocial interventions in reducing cognitive decline in older people: Systematic review. *Ageing Res. Rev.* **2020**, *62*, 101113. [CrossRef] [PubMed]

96. Benedetti, I.; Biggeri, L.; Laureti, T.; Secondi, L. Exploring the Italians' food habits and tendency towards a sustainable diet: The Mediterranean eating pattern. *Agric. Agric. Sci. Procedia* **2016**, *8*, 433–440. [CrossRef]

Publisher's Note: MDPI stays neutral with regard to jurisdictional claims in published maps and institutional affiliations.

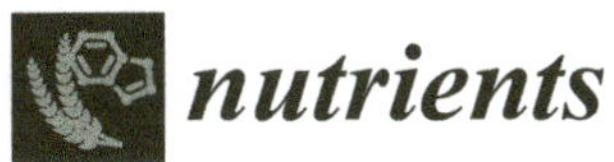

nutrients

Article

Deteriorated Dietary Patterns with Regards to Health and Environmental Sustainability among Hungarian Roma Are Not Differentiated from Those of the General Population

Erand Llanaj [1,2], Ferenc Vincze [1,2], Zsigmond Kósa [3], Helga Bárdos [1], Judit Diószegi [1,4], János Sándor [1] and Róza Ádány [1,4,*]

[1]   Department of Public Health and Epidemiology, Faculty of Medicine, University of Debrecen, Kassai street 26/B, H-4028 Debrecen, Hungary; erand.llanaj@med.unideb.hu (E.L.); vincze.ferenc@med.unideb.hu (F.V.); bardos.helga@med.unideb.hu (H.B.); dioszegi.judit@med.unideb.hu (J.D.); sandor.janos@med.unideb.hu (J.S.)
[2]   Doctoral School of Health Sciences, University of Debrecen, Kassai street 26/B, H-4028 Debrecen, Hungary
[3]   Department of Methodology for Health Visitors and Public Health, Faculty of Health, University of Debrecen, Sóstói street 2-4, H-4400 Nyíregyháza, Hungary; kosa.zsigmond@foh.unideb.hu
[4]   MTA-DE Public Health Research Group, University of Debrecen, Kassai street 26/B, H-4028 Debrecen, Hungary
*   Correspondence: adany.roza@med.unideb.hu; Tel.: +36-52-512-765/77408

Citation: Llanaj, E.; Vincze, F.; Kósa, Z.; Bárdos, H.; Diószegi, J.; Sándor, J.; Ádány, R. Deteriorated Dietary Patterns with Regards to Health and Environmental Sustainability among Hungarian Roma Are Not Differentiated from Those of the General Population. *Nutrients* **2021**, *13*, 721. https://doi.org/10.3390/nu13030721

Academic Editor: Lourdes Varela

Received: 14 January 2021
Accepted: 20 February 2021
Published: 24 February 2021

Publisher's Note: MDPI stays neutral with regard to jurisdictional claims in published maps and institutional affiliations.

Abstract: Nutritional epidemiology studies on Roma people are scarce and, to date, their nutrient-based dietary patterns with regards to both healthy and sustainable dietary considerations have never been reported. We report, for the first time, adherence to healthy and sustainable dietary patterns using scoring and regression models, based on recommendations defined by the World Health Organization, in the Dietary Approaches to Stop Hypertension (DASH) study and the EAT-Lancet report, as well as dietary quality based on Dietary Inflammatory Index (DII) among the Hungarian Roma (HR) population living in North East Hungary, with Hungarian general (HG) adults as reference. Data were obtained from a complex, comparative health survey involving dietary assessment, structured questionnaire-based interview, physical and laboratory examinations on 359 HG and 344 HR subjects in Northeast Hungary. Poisson regressions were fit to models that included DASH, EAT, DII and Healthy Diet Indicator as dependent variables to assess the influence of ethnicity on healthy and sustainable nutrient-based patterns. Adjusted models controlled for all relevant covariates using the residual method indicated poor dietary quality with regards to the selected dietary patterns. These associations were not ethnicity-sensitive, except for DII, where Roma ethnicity was linked to a decrease of DII score ($\beta = -0.455$, 95%CI: -0.720; -0.191, $p < 0.05$). Currently, HR dietary patterns appear to be relatively unhealthy and unsustainable, rendering them vulnerable to elevated risk of ill-health. Nevertheless, their dietary patterns did not strongly differ from HG, which may contribute to Hungarians being one of the most obese and malnourished nations in Europe. Further prospective research on the potential public and environmental health effects of these findings is warranted.

Keywords: nutrition; Roma; Hungary; health; dietary patterns; dietary indicators; sustainability; dietary recall

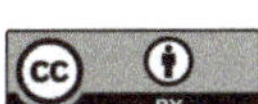

1. Introduction

Ethnicity-based health disparities have been central to the public health discourse in the past decades [1–3] and have remained so, particularly amid the current COVID-19 pandemic [4–7]. Major risk factors for hospitalization, severity and mortality of COVID-19 include diet-related conditions, such as obesity, hypertension and type 2 diabetes, which have been shown to disproportionally affect the most vulnerable [8–10].

Mounting evidence has consistently shown a strong link between ethnic and socio-economic disparities with dietary and nutrient patterns [11–13]. Such inequities exist in many forms, including in diet composition, nutritional behaviors, intake patterns, etc. often resulting in substandard dietary quality, poorer health outcomes and disproportionate burden of disease [14,15]. Along with the growing burden of diet-related noncommunicable diseases (NCDs), there is also a growing interest in characterizing their association with dietary and nutrient patterns in specific, particularly among disadvantaged minority population groups.

In Europe, the Roma population constitutes the largest ethnic minority (estimated to be between 10–12 million) [16] and has been a target of ethnicity-based studies over the past decade [17,18]. Results from different European countries, characterizing dietary aspects of Roma, have revealed inadequate presence of fruits, vegetables [19–32] and dairy products [23,25–27,33] in their diet, frequent fast-foods consumption [34–37], as well as high intake of animal fats [28,31,35,38], sugar-sweetened beverages [22,23,28,37] and sweets [28]. In our previous work, we reported a suboptimal dietary profile and nutritional status of Hungarian Roma (HR) living in segregated colonies in northeastern Hungary, with inadequate nutrient composition and anthropometric status estimates, not strongly different than Hungarian general (HG) population, but occasionally worse among HR. Our findings indicated small differences in meeting nutrient-based dietary recommendations between the two populations, with Roma being less likely to comply with health-promoting nutrient targets [39]. Such information is very useful in informing public health nutrition preventive interventions among Roma, i.e., identifying effective ways of intervening to reduce health inequalities. However, further information on dietary patterns is necessary, in order to gain a higher-resolution and deeper understanding on the current dietary situation and its relation, not only with health, but sustainability considerations as well. What we are eating and how we are producing food is also exerting huge environmental pressures, besides health and nutritional concerns [40]. Diet has emerged as one of the most promising levers to improve health and environmental sustainability, particularly on the demand side of the challenge [41]. It has been demonstrated how health-promoting dietary patterns often have lower environmental impacts, suggesting that dietary shifts that might reduce the risk of NCDs, have the potential to also support attainment of environmental sustainability targets [42,43]. To address the needs emerging from a growing global population, a healthy diet from sustainable food systems was defined by the EAT-Lancet report, a universal reference diet which aims to promote both human health and environmental sustainability [43].

It is reasonable to suppose that diversity and inclusion is key to unlocking sustainability and in creating the kind of development which meets the needs of current generations without compromising the ability of future generations to meet their own needs. Therefore, it is timely and highly relevant to address malnutrition in all its forms and its implications not only with regards to health, but environmental sustainability considerations as well, among underserved groups. With that in mind, we attempt to elucidate the association of Roma ethnicity with regards to dietary patterns shown to strongly influence health (i.e., Healthy Diet Indicator (HDI) and Dietary Inflammatory Index (DII)) and environmental sustainability (i.e., Dietary Approaches to Stop Hypertension (DASH), EAT-Lancet), while considering HG population as reference. To the best of our knowledge, this is the first study among Roma, to date, addressing the relevance of diet for human and planetary health.

2. Materials and Methods

2.1. Study Design

For this report, we analyzed data obtained from a three-pillar (questionnaire-based, physical examination and laboratory examination) complex (health behavior and examination) survey. Details of sampling and data collection and management are thoroughly described elsewhere [44]. In brief, individuals aged 20 to 64 years, were selected randomly, to be representative of the adult HR population living in segregated colonies of northeast Hungary (Hajdú-Bihar and Szabolcs-Szatmár-Bereg counties), where a great proportion of the HR population resides, as well as that of the HG population living in the same counties.

In addition to the demographic, anthropometric, health behavior, physical and laboratory data collection, two 24 h recalls were also obtained to quantify dietary intake. The intended sample size was 500 participants for both study groups, but the final study sample, with full recall data, included 797 participants, of whom 410 subjects were of the HG and 387 individuals of the HR population. The current analysis included 703 participants (359 HG and 344 HR). Detailed information on design, sampling, piloting and validation of the dietary instrument are described elsewhere [39]. In brief, dietary intake data were collected in the case of each participant through a double (one non-consecutive weekday and a weekend day), interviewer-assisted, multiple-pass 24 h dietary recall protocol developed and validated in our previous study [45].

2.2. Dietary Patterns Indexes

In this analysis we used four different nutrient-based dietary quality indexes: HDI, DII, the EAT-Lancet and DASH. EAT-Lancet and DASH are considered environmentally sustainable dietary regimes, in addition to being beneficial to health [46]. The World Health Organization (WHO) guidelines for the prevention of chronic diseases [47] and the 2020 updated healthy diet fact sheet [48] were used to construct a modified version of the HDI originally introduced by Huijbregts et al. [49]. Our HDI used seven nutrient standards and a dichotomous variable was generated for each nutrient according to supplementary Table S1 coding criteria. Further, individual scores were summed and participants received a maximum HDI score of 7 points, if all HDI targets were met, and a minimum of 0 points if none was met. Categories of adherence were created based on the total score (i.e., very low HDI (0–1 points), low HDI (2,3), moderate HDI (4,5), high HDI (6,7)).

Our DASH diet index, used previously by Mellen et al. [50], was an entirely nutrient-based version, constructed on the basis of target nutrient values from the DASH diet used in 2 clinical trials [51,52]. The nine nutrients were those expected to be higher (protein, fiber, magnesium, calcium, and potassium) or lower (total fat, saturated fatty acids (SFAs), sodium, and cholesterol). Individual dietary data were compared against each of the nine dietary component goals. Meeting a dietary component goal received 1 point, while meeting an intermediate goal (defined as the midpoint between the DASH diet goal and the nutrient content of the DASH control diet [51]) received 0.5 point, and meeting neither goal received 0 points. The total score was generated by summing all nine nutrient targets score for a minimum of 0 and a maximum of 9 points (see supplementary Table S2). Further, a categorical outcome was evaluated to estimate the number of individuals achieving modest accordance with the DASH dietary approach. Individuals meeting at least half of the DASH targets (DASH score $\geq$4.5) were considered DASH accordant and the rest, DASH non-accordant.

In 2019, the EAT-Lancet Commission on Healthy Diets from the Sustainable Food Systems report, defined a universal reference diet to promote human and planetary health [43]. To evaluate the adherence of our subjects to this diet, we constructed a novel, nutrient-based EAT index (NB-EAT), based on the nutrient composition of the original EAT-Lancet reference diet. Our NB-EAT included twelve nutrient reference intakes (i.e., α-linolenic acid, carbohydrates, cholesterol, dietary fibers, mono- and poly-unsaturated fats, proteins, saturated fats, total fat, calcium, added sugar, magnesium and potassium) [43].

The individual NB-EAT score was calculated as the sum of nutrient targets met: a value of 1 was given if the participant achieved an EAT-Lancet target for a nutrient and a value of zero was given if target was not met (with a score range from 0 to 12). Categories of adherence were coded based on the achieved score and three categories were created, i.e., low (0–4), moderate (5–8) and high (>8) adherence (supplementary Table S3).

Calculations of dietary inflammatory index (DII) were based on a protocol described by Shivappa et al. [53], while considering methodological aspects for its use and utility [54]. Briefly, nutrient data obtained by 2-day 24 h dietary recall were first linked to the regionally representative world database that was created at the University of South Carolina and provided a robust estimate of a mean and standard deviation for each parameter [53].

These became the multipliers used to express an individual's exposure, relative to the "standard global mean" as a z-score. This was achieved by subtracting the "standard mean" from the amount reported and then dividing this value by the "standard deviation". To minimize the effect of "right skewing", this value was converted to a centered percentile score. The centered percentile score for each food parameter was then multiplied by the respective food parameter effect score. This was derived from the structured review and scoring of 1943 qualifying research articles, to obtain a food parameter-specific DII score for the individual. All of the food parameter–specific DII scores were then summed to create the overall DII score for every participant in the study [53]. Out of 45 possible parameters, a total of 27 nutrients were available to calculate the DII for our study population. The overall index obtained by summing the 27 dietary parameters (i.e., total energy, carbohydrate, protein, total fat, alcohol, fiber, cholesterol, SFAs, caffeine, monounsaturated fatty acids (MUFAs), polyunsaturated fatty acids (PUFAs), omega-3 and omega-6 fatty acids, niacin, thiamine, riboflavin, vitamin B12, vitamin B6, iron, magnesium, zinc, vitamin A, vitamin C, vitamin D, vitamin E, folic acid and beta-carotene), ranged from a minimum of -4.60 (most anti-inflammatory) to a maximum of 3.12 points, with a median value of -1.33. Since there is no current consensus on the optimal DII score values, we addressed this challenge by creating tertiles of the DII score, i.e., statistically dividing our DII score distribution into three parts (=three quantiles).

2.3. Data Analyses

Descriptive univariate analysis with chi-square test were used to evaluate the association between DASH, HDI, DII and NB-EAT scores, as well as socio-demographic and anthropometric factors such as age, sex, and BMI. We considered negative binomial and Poisson regressions for exploring differences between the HG and HR populations with regards to nutrient patterns. Negative binomial regression was chosen if data showed over-dispersion. All sociodemographic and nutritional covariates (age, sex, education, marital status, perceived financial situation, economic activity, BMI and energy intake) were included in the models in a block manner to determine the Roma ethnicity effect, independently from sociodemographic and anthropometric data. Initially, regression models were fit with DASH, HDI, DII and NB-EAT scores as outcome variables and Roma ethnicity controlled for anthropometric data. Secondly, demographic variables were added to each model. Finally, the regression models were fitted with demographic, anthropometric and socioeconomic factors together. Complete regression analysis results and models are provided in supplementary Tables S4–S7. Statistical analyses were carried out using SPSS 26.0 (SPSS, version 26.0; IBM Corp., Armonk, NY, USA) software and R Statistics/R Studio. This work has reported results in accordance with STROBE (STrengthening the Reporting of OBservational studies in Epidemiology) extension for nutrition and dietary assessment [55].

2.4. Research Ethics

Approval for the research protocols and methodology was provided by the Ethical Committee of the Hungarian Scientific Council on Health (61327-2017/EKU). Participants gave their written informed consent in both study populations in accordance with the Declaration of Helsinki and the Science Ethics Code of The Hungarian Academy of Sciences.

3. Results

Table 1 shows relevant basic and nutritional characteristics of our samples. There were no strong statistical differences between the two groups, in terms of basic characteristics and energy intake. Regarding nutrient intake there were significant differences for sodium and cholesterol, both which were higher among HG. Sugar and total carbohydrate (both as percentage of total energy) intakes were significantly higher among HR. Significant associations were observed between ethnicity and economic activity, educational level and perceived financial wellbeing, but there was no association between ethnicity and marital status.

Table 1. Characteristics of study samples.

	Characteristics	Variable [†]	Hungarian General (*n* = 344)	Hungarian Roma (*n* = 359)	*p* [‡]
Basic characteristics	Demographics	Age (years)—mean (std. dev.)	44 (12)	43 (12)	NS
		Females—*n* (%)	188 (52.4)	**248 (72.1)**	***
	Education	Elementary—*n* (%)	76 (21.2)	**292 (84.9)**	
		Secondary/Vocational education—*n* (%)	230 (64.1)	**52 (15.1)**	***
		University degree or higher—*n* (%)	53 (14.8)	**0 (0)**	
	Economic activity	Some type of full-/part-time employment—*n* (%)	296 (82.5)	**256 (74.4)**	
		Student—*n* (%)	8 (2.2)	**0 (0)**	**
		Unable to work/Retired—*n* (%)	40 (11.1)	**32 (9.3)**	
		Unemployed—*n* (%)	15 (4.2)	**56 (16.3)**	
	Marital status	Unmarried/Divorced/Widowed—*n* (%)	136 (37.9)	113 (32.8)	NS
		Married—*n* (%)	223 (62.1)	231 (67.2)	
	Perceived financial wellbeing	Good or very good—*n* (%)	115 (32.8)	**51 (15.0)**	
		Fair—*n* (%)	190 (54.1)	**186 (54.7)**	***
		Challenging or very challenging—*n* (%)	46 (13.1)	**103 (30.3)**	
Nutritional characteristics	Energy intake	Energy (kJ/day)	9146.9 (8824.7; 9469.1)	8836.9 (8537.0; 9136.8)	NS
		Energy (kcal/day)	2188.3 (2111.2; 2265.3)	2114.1 (2042.4; 2185.8)	NS
	Anthropometrics	BMI (kg/m^2)	27.26 (26.7; 27.8)	27.66 (27.0; 28.4)	NS
	Macronutrient intake	Fiber (%E)	3.9 (3.7; 4.0)	4.0 (3.8; 4.2)	NS
		Fiber (g/1000 kcal)	9.7 (9.2; 10.1)	9.9 (9.4; 10.4)	NS
		Protein (%E)	**15.6 (15.2; 15.9)**	15.1 (14.7; 15.4)	*
		Fat (%E)	37.2 (36.3; 38.0)	36.1 (35.2; 37.0)	NS
		SFA (%E)	10.7 (10.3; 11.1)	10.66 (10.3; 11.0)	NS
		Carbohydrates (%E)	46.2 (45.3; 47.1)	**48.2 (47.2; 49.2)**	**
		Sugar (g)	96.3 (89.0; 103.5)	101.5 (94.1; 108.8)	NS
		Sugar (%E)	17.0 (16.0; 18.0)	**18.8 (17.7; 19.8)**	*
		UFA (g)	**20.9 (20.4; 21.4)**	19.7 (19.1; 20.2)	**
		Cholesterol (mg/1000 kcal)	**172.9 (164.7; 181.0)**	159.5 (152.2; 166.8)	*
	Micronutrient intake	Magnesium (mg/1000 kcal)	193.1 (166.0; 220.2)	181.6 (173.8; 189.5)	NS
		Calcium (mg/1000 kcal)	248.5 (233.51; 263.49)	248.0 (234.4; 261.7)	NS
		Potassium (mg/1000 kcal)	1391.1 (1311.4; 1470.8)	1435.3 (1353.3; 1517.4)	NS
		Sodium (mg/1000 kcal)	**2628.1 (2522.8; 2733.4)**	2458.3 (2365.7; 2550.8)	*

[†] All variable values are given with their respective 95% CI, unless otherwise indicated. [‡] * $p \leq 0.05$, ** $p \leq 0.01$, *** $p \leq 0.001$: T-test or Mann–Whitney for differences and Chi-square for associations. Significantly higher values are bolded where appropriate. SFA: saturated fatty acids; UFA: unsaturated fatty acids; (%E): intake as percentage of total energy; IQR: interquartile range. Note: For "Perceived financial wellbeing" some responses were missing.

Dietary Pattern Scores and Quality

Further, when accounting for dietary patterns quality, results showed a high representation of participants with poorer adherence levels for DASH, HDI and NB-EAT, independently of the dietary index used, ethnicity or sex (Table 2). DII tertile and score distribution also showed a considerable representation in the two upper tertiles. Additionally, there was no observed statistical association between sex/ethnicity and the selected dietary indexes, with regards to score differences.

Table 2. Distribution of the dietary indicators among Hungarian general and Roma by sex.

Dietary Indicator		Hungarian General			Hungarian Roma		
		Both Sexes (A)	Females (C)	Males (E)	Both Sexes (B)	Females (D)	Males (F)
HDI	Very low	27 (7.5)	13 (6.9)	14 (8.2)	23 (6.7)	18 (7.3)	5 (5.2)
	Low	172 (47.9)	91 (48.6)	81 (47.4)	152 (44.2)	113 (45.6)	39 (40.6)
	Moderate	140 (39.0)	75 (39.9)	65 (37.0)	158 (45.9)	111 (44.7)	47 (48.9)
	High	20 (5.6)	9 (4.6)	11 (6.4)	11 (3.2)	6 (2.4)	5 (5.2)
DASH	Non-accordant	341 (95.0)	177 (94.1)	164 (95.9)	330 (95.9)	240 (96.8)	90 (93.8)
	Accordant	18 (5.0)	11 (5.9)	7 (4.1)	14 (4.1)	8 (3.2)	6 (6.2)
NB-EAT	Low	324 (90.3)	171 (91.0)	153 (89.5)	305 (88.7)	223 (89.9)	82 (85.4)
	Moderate	35 (9.7)	17 (9.0)	18 (10.5)	39 (11.3)	25 (10.1)	14 (14.6)
	High	0 (0.0)	0 (0.0)	0 (0.0)	0 (0.0)	0 (0.0)	0 (0.0)
DII	Tertile 1	119 (33.1)	66 (35.1)	53 (31.0)	115 (33.5)	84 (33.9)	31 (32.3)
	Tertile 2	109 (30.4)	50 (26.6)	59 (34.5)	126 (36.6)	90 (36.3)	36 (37.5)
	Tertile 3	131 (36.5)	72 (38.3)	59 (34.5)	103 (29.9)	74 (29.8)	29 (30.2)
DASH score (0–9): median (IQR)		1.5 (1.5; 2.0)	1.5 (1.5; 2.0)	1.5 (1.5; 2.0)	1.5 (1.5; 2.0)	1.5 (1.5; 2.0)	1.5 (1.5; 2.0)
NB-EAT score (0–12): median (IQR)		2.0 (2.0; 3.0)	2.0 (2.0; 3.0)	2.0 (2.0; 3.0)	2.0 (2.0; 3.0)	2.0 (2.0; 3.0)	3.0 (3.0; 4.0)
HDI score (0–7): median (IQR)		3.0 (3.0; 4.0)	3.0 (3.0; 4.0)	3.0 (3.0; 4.0)	3.0 (3.0; 4.0)	3.0 (3.0; 4.0)	4.0 (4.0; 5.0)
DII score (−4.60–3.12): median (IQR)		−1.26 (−1.49; −1.06)	−1.31 (−1.80; −0.92)	−1.26 (−1.45; −1.02)	−1.40 (−1.65; −1.23)	−1.34 (−1.64; −1.12)	−1.59 (−1.92; −1.27)

All data are given as n (%) unless otherwise indicated. IQR: Interquartile Range.

Multivariable regression models (Table 3), both adjusted and unadjusted for the indicated and relevant covariates, showed no significant effect of Roma ethnicity on DASH, NB-EAT and HDI scores. On the other hand, DII score was significantly and inversely associated with Roma ethnicity in the adjusted models.

Table 3. Effect of Roma ethnicity on nutrient-based dietary patterns *.

Dietary Score	MODEL 1 (β [95%CI])	MODEL 2 (β [95%CI])	MODEL 3 (β [95%CI])
DASH [†]	−0.023 [−0.176; 0.129]	−0.084 [−0.286; 0.117]	−0.049 [−0.254; 0.156]
HDI [†]	0.038 [−0.131; 0.207]	−0.003 [−0.229; 0.223]	−0.001 [−0.231; 0.230]
DII [‡]	−0.147 [−0.344; 0.049]	**−0.450 [−0.709; −0.191]**	**−0.455 [−0.720; −0.191]**
NB-EAT [†]	0.021 [−0.073; 0.114]	−0.024 [−0.183; 0.136]	−0.017 [−0.179; 0.144]

[†] Poisson regression model; [‡] Multiple linear regression model; * Hungarian general population sample is taken as a reference in these models. Model 1: effect adjusted only for BMI and energy intake; Model 2: effect adjusted for BMI, age, education level, energy intake and sex; Model 3: effect adjusted for BMI, age, education level, energy intake, sex, financial status, marital status and economic activity (see supplementary Tables S4–S7 for more information). Significant effect sizes are bolded. DASH: The Dietary Approaches to Stopping Hypertension; HDI: Healthy Diet Indicator; DII: The Dietary Inflammatory Index; EAT: Nutrient-based EAT-Lancet score; β [95%CI]: beta coefficient of the regression model, accompanied by its corresponding 95% confidence interval.

4. Discussion

Our results indicate substandard adherence to established healthy and sustainable dietary guidelines, as accounted by the nutrient-based dietary indexes used in this work. Ethnicity did not have a strong influence on adherence to selected dietary guidelines. However, being Roma was associated with a lower DII score, i.e., lower dietary inflammatory potential. These findings are in line with our previous results and reinforce the fact that currently the Hungarian population is not close to meeting healthy diet targets, regardless of ethnic background. The cause of such a substandard quality of diet is highly likely to be multifactorial. A relevant contributor may be the lack of adequate dietary guidance/interventions, as nutrition services have not yet been mainstreamed into the Hungarian health care system.

As a result, dietary patterns such as DASH, EAT-Lancet or dietary evaluation based on DII and HDI approach have not been widely promoted in Hungary. At present, provision of general preventive services in primary health care in Hungary is challenging and not based on evidence-informed dietary guidance, i.e., trained dieticians, nutritional experts, etc. [56].

General practitioners (GPs) constitute a significant component of the Hungarian primary healthcare system and are in regular contact with both the healthy and ailing people. According to our data and previous research, lifestyle counselling is the kind of service that patients need most and one of the leading drivers of medical litigation [57]. Coverage and quality of nutritional counselling services, within primary healthcare settings are limited and primarily focused on those suffering from diet-related NCDs, particularly among type 2 diabetes patients [58,59]. People suffering from other diet-related NCDs (e.g., Crohn's disease, gluten sensitivity, etc.) are provided with some dietary advice, only within the context of outpatient care, with no targeted or tailored preventive dietary counselling yet. Additionally, dietary assessment is not common in the routine GP's practice and it is provided only for small proportion of patients (i.e., 24% and mainly hypertonic and diabetic), with almost no monitoring on compliance or providing further counselling and/or follow-up [60].

Dietary services, currently available only in the outpatient and inpatient care, appear to target only those who are already suffering from diet-related NCDs, hence not as a preventive approach. On the other hand, there is a limited number of private dietary and nutritional services, available only in the largest cities, relatively pricy and not clear whether they are effective or not. However, it is crucial to recognize that optimal health and well-being is a human right and not a privilege of only those who can afford to pay. Integrating dietary services within health systems has the potential to generate substantial health gains, while simultaneously being cost-effective [61].

Another aspect of the inadequate access and/or availability of evidence-based nutritional services that merits attention, is the need to raise the profile of nutrition at national level, while aligning resource allocation accordingly. Currently, there is a demand for such services, particularly among high-income, highly-educated Hungarians [62], that seem to have recognized the value of nutritional guidance and interventions (e.g., balanced nutrition, blood glucose lowering and healthy weight control, etc.), among other lifestyle changes.

Currently, nutrition services are not widely supported by the Hungarian national health budget and are typically not delivered by qualified nutrition professionals, since other professions (e.g., personal trainers, self-proclaimed dietitians, etc.) are currently attempting to fill the demand gap [63]. The latter phenomenon has been recognized and there is data showing that such guidance is inadequate and not in line with established guidelines [63,64]. Consequently, despite efforts to improve nutrition [65], Hungarians appear to have a limited exposure to professional and evidence-informed dietary and nutritional preventive services, something which may contribute to our "no difference" findings with regards to nutrient-based dietary patterns.

Additionally, there was a considerable representation of subjects in the upper tertile of the DII in our sample, hinting an elevated inflammatory potential of current dietary patterns. Chronic inflammation plays an important role in the development of several chronic diseases [66].

Since various nutrients and foods have been shown to modulate inflammation, dietary patterns play an important role in the regulation of chronic inflammation [67]. Although the link between diet and disease outcomes needs additional studies to further confirm the health potential of current dietary patterns, longitudinal epidemiological data have already linked poor adherence to healthy dietary patterns to many NCDs and claiming an attributable global death toll of 11 million from diet-related NCDs [68].

Therefore, there is a compelling case for urgently considering the inclusion of nutrition and dietary services as an integral component of primary healthcare [69]. The Hungarian healthcare system has for decades focused on the clinical, pharmacological-oriented model of disease that may ignore fundamental modifiable causes, such as diet and lifestyle. The consequences of this approach can be observed in the poor dietary patterns reported here, with the potential to contribute to an elevated risk of diet-related NCDs. This is further supported by data showing a very high prevalence of metabolic syndrome in both HG and HR populations (i.e., 39.8% and 44.0%, respectively), with no significant difference between the two groups in either females or males [44]. Integrating and mainstreaming nutrition actions into the Hungarian health care system to promote healthier diet, and prevent and treat diet-related NCDs, has the potential to generate substantial health gains and can be highly cost-effective [61].

Furthermore, adherence to sustainable dietary patterns among our participants, can be viewed, not only as a dietary marker, but as one of behavioral commitment towards addressing Climate Change as well. The vast majority of nutrient-based EAT-Lancet reference diet targets were not attained and none of the participants was in the third-upper category of adherence. Considering the detrimental environmental impact of current food systems [70], and concerns raised about their sustainability, there is a pressing need to promote diets that are healthy and have no or low destructive impact on the environment in Hungary and globally. At present, the 'Nutritional recommendations for the adult population in Hungary' (i.e., national food-based dietary guideline [71]) fails to include sustainability criteria, although there is mounting evidence linking overconsumption of, in particular, red and ultra-processed meat products with detrimental human and environmental health outcomes [42,72,73]. Advocating for plant-based diets in Hungary is also timely. Recommending dietary shifts towards plant-based diets may be of great importance in achieving health and sustainability goals [74], as from a food systems point of view, down-right adoption of plant-based diets has the potential to simultaneously optimize food supply, improve health, increase environmental sustainability and advance social justice outcomes [75,76].

Apart from the established health benefits [77–79] DASH diet is also considered an environmental-friendly dietary pattern [46,80]. Our results indicate an extremely high "non-accordance" to DASH pattern (95%), independently of ethnicity. This may be an epidemiological signature, which may signify increased risk for diet-related NCDs, as well as a low potential of the current diet to contribute in improving climate targets. Thus, our findings provide novel insights into dietary situation among HR and HG, as well as key dietary recommendations, which might require special attention during nutrition/public health education campaigns. Moreover, we advocate for nutrition education and research to be extensively integrated in health sciences-related academic programs, with an overarching emphasis and regular reinforcement of the importance of higher fiber, fruit, vegetable and wholegrain intake and substitution of fat sources with beneficial ones, in an energy balanced manner.

In addition to the above-mentioned challenges, the actual nutrition situation is clearly neither a mere consequence of inappropriate quantity/quality of foods in the Hungarian diet, nor as a lack of willpower from the individual [81], but as a consequence of a fundamental global challenge: food systems that have failed in providing healthy, safe, affordable and sustainable diets [82].

The economic, social and environmental implications of further inaction can impact the growth and development of individuals and societies for decades to come [83,84]. As the Lancet Series on the "Double Burden of Malnutrition" has shown, the intricate biological and social pathways of all forms of malnutrition cannot be disrupted through siloed interventions, therefore requiring society-wide and scalable behavioral shifts that can be sustained over time [85,86]. Our findings also point towards the need for triple-duty actions, as described by Swinburn et al. [41] as The Lancet Commission report. Such policy actions have the potential to re-orient major systems of food and agriculture, transport, urban design, and land use that drive this Syndemic—the three co-existing pandemics: obesity, undernutrition and climate change. Such actions need to occur locally, nationally and within a global framework. Implementation of such actions to address these deeper drivers is politically more difficult to achieve and their outcomes are more uncertain compared to downstream actions such as health promotion programs or healthcare service provision. However, their implementation is essential for transformative, systemic changes. More studies are warranted to determine the food system determinants, social drivers of poor dietary intake in Hungary, as well as trials investigating how dietary interventions may effectively influence the current dietary patterns, particularly among Roma.

Finally, the current COVID-19 pandemic has cast a spotlight on longstanding costly and life-threatening inequities that exist in our global society. Those living in economically challenged communities, such as ethnic minorities, are bearing the heaviest burden of COVID-19 infections. It is now accepted that poor metabolic health is one of the most important immunity-impairing factors underlying cardiovascular disease, type 2 diabetes and obesity-related cancers, rendering many people vulnerable to COVID-19 severity and mortality [87]. However, while diet-related NCDs may increase vulnerability to the virus, limited attention has been paid in improving access to healthy and sustainable diets, that can both sustain metabolic health, support a vigorous immune system and contribute to lessening the effect of our footprint on the planet. After this pandemic subsides, a lot more attention needs to be given to the power that our diets have to ward off, not only future medical, economic and social calamities from whatever pathogen next comes down the pike, but to address the bigger "pandemic" as well: climate change.

As governments embark on economic recovery plans in the wake of COVID-19, a great opportunity exists, within the framework of the UN Decade of Action on Nutrition (2016–2025), to invest in a green recovery plan that can tackle the health equity and environmental crises together, to ensure the most effective response to each. Addressing these issues and building forward better starts with our "plates".

Limitations, Strengths and Future Outlooks

There are some potential limitations to our observations that should be recognized. This analysis is based on a double 24 h dietary recall, hence findings need to be interpreted with caution, as long-term dietary patterns of the population under investigation may not be fully captured by this approach. Further, the current findings, although insightful, are relatively incomplete, as linking them with health outcome data (e.g., metabolic syndrome) is crucial in order to better characterize the current situation, and link health effects of an environmentally sustainable diet and further confirm these findings. Although diet is, no doubt, an important modulator of inflammation, it is by no means the only one. Other indexes, including physical activity and stress, should be derived using similar methods. If these could be integrated with the DII, then this could validate and confirm the inflammatory potential of the diet in the current population under investigation. It should be taken also into consideration that, in our study, the representation of females among HR was higher than among HG.

This has also been the case in our previous surveys conducted among segregated Roma colonies in Hungary [88] and also in Roma surveys in other countries [89]. Other potential limitations related to the composition of our sample are described in detail in our previous work [39]. Although this is the first attempt, to the best of our knowledge, to present a nutrient-based index for healthy and sustainable diets based on the rigorous EAT-Lancet reference diet, we recognize that it may need further validation. The EAT-Lancet commission's "healthy and sustainable reference diet" provides values of nutrient composition, as well as intakes for food groups, with the latter being more informative. In our attempt to describe dietary sustainability, NB-EAT's use was chosen due to the inability to obtain dietary intake data at the level of individual food items or food group data—something which we acknowledge that can provide more tangible details on the healthiness and sustainability aspects of the diet. Nevertheless, it was shown that there is a poor adherence to healthy and sustainable dietary targets, independently of the dietary pattern and population group.

Further work on drivers of poor dietary patterns should go beyond measuring the effect of prescribed (but often not followed) dietary guidelines on population-averaged cohorts, towards quantifying the efficiency of dietary and lifestyle advice as well. Even the best dietary advice in the world may be indistinguishable from the worst, when individuals do not or cannot adhere to it due to specific circumstances, e.g., place of residence, access to healthy foods, employment conditions and income. Despite the abovementioned challenges, our findings offer new nutritional insights on dietary aspects that require particular attention during potential interventions and monitoring their effects, when attempting to improve the overall quality of the diet among young adults in Hungary. Decision-makers and experts should approach this issue from a food system's perspective, in order to address and transform the complex web of activities involving the production, processing, transport and consumption of unhealthy diets.

5. Conclusions

Potential nutritional interventions in Hungary, addressing healthy and sustainable nutrition, are not only necessary among Hungarian Roma population, but on a population-wide level as well. Unhealthy nutrient-based dietary patterns appear generally indiscriminate of ethnic background according to our analyses, with both populations (HG and HR) poorly adhering to healthy and sustainable dietary patterns, with no strong mediation by any included factor in this analysis. Identifying dietary patterns that are nutrient-rich, affordable, healthy and sustainable for Hungarians should be a top public health research priority, as well as an opportunity to discern and address social inequalities in nutrition and health. Our cross-sectional analysis also indicates that current nutritional trajectory may not be in line with achieving the sustainable development goals in respect to multiple dietary targets for public health and environmental sustainability. Research and policy action therefore need to be integrated between disciplines and domains, starting with the formulation of integrated national nutrition guidelines, through a sustainability lens and an outlook of long-term challenges to the food system, as well as an agenda to achieve the relevant behavioral change. Further research is warranted to elucidate drivers and ascertain food-based dietary patterns, with sustainability considerations in mind.

Supplementary Materials: The following are available online at https://www.mdpi.com/2072-6643/13//721/s1, Table S1. Healthy diet indicator components used in the current study and their coding criteria based on the World Health Organization's dietary guidelines. Table S2. Nutrient Targets for DASH Score. Table S3. Diet indicator components used in the current study and their coding criteria based on the EAT-Lancet reference diet. Table S4. Regression models for DASH score among Hungarian general and Roma populations. Table S5. Regression models for HDI score among Hungarian general and Roma subjects. Table S6. Regression models for DII score among Hungarian general and Roma subjects. Table S7. Regression models for nutrient-based EAT-Lancet score among Hungarian general and Roma subjects.

Author Contributions: Conceptualization, E.L., R.Á.; Data curation, E.L., F.V.; Formal analysis, E.L.; F.V.; Investigation, E.L., F.V., Z.K., J.D.; Writing original draft, E.L.; Review & editing, R.Á., J.D., F.V., H.B.; Funding acquisition, R.Á.; Methodology, E.L., F.V., H.B.; Resources, R.Á., Z.K., J.S.; Supervision, R.Á. All authors have read and agreed to the published version of the manuscript.

Funding: This work was supported by the GINOP-2.3.2-15-2016-00005 project. The project is co-financed by the European Union under the European Social Fund and European Regional Development Fund, as well as by the Hungarian Academy of Sciences (TK2016-78). Project no. 135784 has also been implemented with the support provided from the National Research, Development and Innovation Fund of Hungary, financed under the K_20 funding scheme.

Institutional Review Board Statement: Approval for the research protocols and methodology was provided by the Ethical Committee of the Hungarian Scientific Council on Health (61327-2017/EKU). Participants gave their written informed consent in both study populations in accordance with the Declaration of Helsinki and the Science Ethics Code of The Hungarian Academy of Sciences.

Informed Consent Statement: Informed consent was obtained from all subjects involved in the study.

Data Availability Statement: All relevant data that support the findings of this study are within the paper and its Supplementary materials. Additional data are available from the corresponding author, upon reasonable request.

Acknowledgments: This work is a contribution of the authors to the United Nations Decade of Action on Nutrition (2016–2025) (https://www.un.org/nutrition/; accessed on 14 January 2021) and UN Nutrition (https://www.unnutrition.org/; accessed on 14 January 2021). We would like to thank Teuta Muhollari for her invaluable help during the design of the visual abstract.

Conflicts of Interest: The authors declare that they have no conflict of interest.

References

1. Arora, V.S.; Kühlbrandt, C.; McKee, M. An examination of unmet health needs as perceived by Roma in Central and Eastern Europe. *Eur. J. Public Health* **2016**, *26*, 737–742. [CrossRef] [PubMed]
2. Ádány, R. Roma health is global ill health. *Eur. J. Public Health* **2014**, *24*, 702–703. [CrossRef]
3. Cook, B.; Wayne, G.F.; Valentine, A.; Lessios, A.; Yeh, E. Revisiting the evidence on health and health care disparities among the Roma: A systematic review 2003–2012. *Int. J. Public Health* **2013**, *58*, 885–911. [CrossRef] [PubMed]
4. Muñoz-Price, L.S.; Nattinger, A.B.; Rivera, F.; Hanson, R.; Gmehlin, C.G.; Perez, A.; Singh, S.; Buchan, B.W.; Ledeboer, N.A.; Pezzin, L.E. Racial Disparities in Incidence and Outcomes Among Patients With COVID-19. *JAMA Netw. Open* **2020**, *3*, e2021892. [CrossRef] [PubMed]
5. Kabarriti, R.; Brodin, N.P.; Maron, M.I.; Guha, C.; Kalnicki, S.; Garg, M.K.; Racine, A.D. Association of Race and Ethnicity With Comorbidities and Survival Among Patients With COVID-19 at an Urban Medical Center in New York. *JAMA Netw. Open* **2020**, *3*, e2019795. [CrossRef]
6. Khazanchi, R.; Evans, C.T.; Marcelin, J.R. Racism, Not Race, Drives Inequity Across the COVID-19 Continuum. *JAMA Netw. Open* **2020**, *3*, e2019933. [CrossRef] [PubMed]
7. Chowkwanyun, M.; Reed, A.L. Racial Health Disparities and Covid-19—Caution and Context. *N. Engl. J. Med.* **2020**, *383*, 201–203. [CrossRef] [PubMed]
8. Richardson, S.; Hirsch, J.S.; Narasimhan, M.; Crawford, J.M.; McGinn, T.; Davidson, K.W.; Northwell, C.-R.C. Presenting Characteristics, Comorbidities, and Outcomes Among 5700 Patients Hospitalized With COVID-19 in the New York City Area. *JAMA* **2020**, *323*, 2052–2059. [CrossRef]
9. EpiCentro. Report sulle Caratteristiche dei Pazienti Deceduti Positivia COVID-19 in Itali all Presente Report è Basato sui Dati Aggiornati al 17 Marzo 2020. Available online: https://www.epicentro.iss.it/coronavirus/bollettino/Report-COVID-2019_17_marzo-v2.pdf (accessed on 11 January 2020).
10. Ryan, D.H.; Ravussin, E.; Heymsfield, S. COVID 19 and the Patient with Obesity—The Editors Speak Out. *Obesity* **2020**, *28*, 847. [CrossRef]
11. Beydoun, M.A.; Gary, T.L.; Caballero, B.H.; Lawrence, R.S.; Cheskin, L.J.; Wang, Y. Ethnic differences in dairy and related nutrient consumption among US adults and their association with obesity, central obesity, and the metabolic syndrome. *Am. J. Clin. Nutr.* **2008**, *87*, 1914–1925. [CrossRef]
12. Dubowitz, T.; Heron, M.; Bird, C.E.; Lurie, N.; Finch, B.K.; Basurto-Dávila, R.; Hale, L.; Escarce, J.J. Neighborhood socioeconomic status and fruit and vegetable intake among whites, blacks, and Mexican Americans in the United States. *Am. J. Clin. Nutr.* **2008**, *87*, 1883–1891. [CrossRef]
13. Kant, A.K.; Graubard, B.I.; Kumanyika, S.K. Trends in black-white differentials in dietary intakes of U.S. adults, 1971-2002. *Am. J. Prev. Med.* **2007**, *32*, 264–272. [CrossRef]
14. Satia, J.A. Diet-related disparities: Understanding the problem and accelerating solutions. *J. Am. Diet. Assoc.* **2009**, *109*, 610–615. [CrossRef]
15. Miranda, J.J.; Barrientos-Gutiérrez, T.; Corvalan, C.; Hyder, A.A.; Lazo-Porras, M.; Oni, T.; Wells, J.C.K. Understanding the rise of cardiometabolic diseases in low- and middle-income countries. *Nat. Med.* **2019**, *25*, 1667–1679. [CrossRef] [PubMed]
16. European Commission. Estimates and Official Numbers of Roma in Europe. Available online: https://rm.coe.int/CoERMPublicCommonSearchServices/DisplayDCTMContent?documentId=0900001680088ea9 (accessed on 29 June 2020).
17. Brüggemann, C.; Friedman, E. The Decade of Roma Inclusion: Origins, Actors, and Legacies. *Eur. Educ.* **2017**, *49*, 1–9. [CrossRef]
18. Sándor, J.; Kósa, Z.; Boruzs, K.; Boros, J.; Tokaji, I.; McKee, M.; Ádány, R. The decade of Roma Inclusion: Did it make a difference to health and use of health care services? *Int. J. Public Health* **2017**, *62*, 803–815. [CrossRef] [PubMed]
19. Valachovicova, M.; Krajcovicova-Kudlackova, M.; Ginter, E.; Paukova, V. Antioxidant vitamins levels–nutrition and smoking. *Bratisl. Med. J.* **2003**, *104*, 411–414.

20. Davidová, E. Zp ůsob života a kultura: Změny ve hmotné kultuře Rom ů—Bydlení, strava. In *Černobílý Život*; Černá, M., Ed.; Gallery: Prague, Czech Republic, 2000; pp. 80–89.
21. Stávková, J.; Brázdová, D.Z. Konzumace ovoce a zeleniny a jiné stravovací zvyklosti Romské populace. *Hygiena* **2014**, *59*, 179–183. [CrossRef]
22. Olišarová, V.; Tóthová, V.; Bártlová, S.; Dolák, F.; Kajanová, A.; Nováková, D.; Prokešová, R.; Šedová, L. Cultural Features Influencing Eating, Overweight, and Obesity in the Roma People of South Bohemia. *Nutrients* **2018**, *10*, 838. [CrossRef] [PubMed]
23. Hijova, E.; Madarasova Geckova, A.; Babinska, I. Do Eating Habits of the Population Living in Roma Settlements Differ from Those of the Majority Population in Slovakia? *Cent. Eur. J. Public Health* **2014**, *22*, S65–S68. [CrossRef]
24. Fundación Secretariado Gitano. Health and the Roma Community: Analysis of the Situation in Europe. Available online: https://www.gitanos.org/upload/07/81/memoria_gral_fin.pdf (accessed on 29 June 2020).
25. Ostrihoňová, T.; Bérešová, J. Occurrence of metabolic syndrome and its risk factors amongst a selected group of Roma inhabitants. *Hygiena* **2010**, *55*, 7–14.
26. Hoxha, A.; Dervishi, G.; Bici, E.; Naum, A.; Seferi, J.; Risilia, K.; Tresa, E. Assessment of nutritional status and dietary patterns of the adult Roma community in Albania. *Alban Med. J.* **2013**, *3*, 32–38.
27. Ciaian, P.; Cupák, A.; Pokrivčák, J.; Rizov, M. Food consumption and diet quality choices of Roma in Romania: A counterfactual analysis. *Food Sec.* **2018**, *10*, 437–456. [CrossRef]
28. Bartosovic, I.; Hegyi, L.; Krcméry, V.; Hanobik, F.; Vasilj, V.; Rothova, P. Poverty & poor eating habits are two of the essential factors that affect the health condition of marginalized Roma population. *CSW* **2014**, *15*. [CrossRef]
29. Sedova, L.; Tothova, V.; Novakova, D.; Olisarova, V.; Bartlova, S.; Dolak, F.; Kajanova, A.; Prokesova, R.; Adamkova, V. Qualification of Food Intake by the Roma Population in the Region of South Bohemia. *Int. J. Environ. Res. Public Health* **2018**, *15*, 386. [CrossRef] [PubMed]
30. Dirección General de Salud Pública Calidad e Innovación. Segunda Encuesta Nacional de Salud a Población Gitana. 2014. Available online: https://www.mscbs.gob.es/en/profesionales/saludPublica/prevPromocion/promocion/desigualdadSalud/docs/ENS2014PG.pdf (accessed on 29 June 2020).
31. Lakatos, S.; Angyal, M.; Solymosy, J.; Bonifácz, S.; Kármán, J.; Csépe, P.; ForraiI, J.; Lökkös, A. Egyenlőség, Egészség és Roma/Cigány Közösség. Available online: http://ec.europa.eu/health/ph_projects/2004/action3/docs/2004_3_01_manuals_hu.pdf (accessed on 26 June 2020).
32. Diószegi, J.; Pikó, P.; Kósa, Z.; Sándor, J.; Llanaj, E.; Ádány, R. Taste and Food Preferences of the Hungarian Roma Population. *Front. Public Health* **2020**, *8*, 359. [CrossRef] [PubMed]
33. Balázs, P.; Rákóczi, I.; Fogarasi-Grenczer, A.; Foley, K.L. Birth-weight differences of Roma and non-Roma neonates–public health implications from a population-based study in Hungary. *Cent. Eur. J. Public Health* **2014**, *22*, 24–28. [CrossRef]
34. Álvarez, M.V.; González, M.M.; San Fabián, J.L. *La Situación de la Infancia Gitana en Asturias. Consejería de Bienestar Social y Vivienda*; Gobierno del Principado de Asturias, Ed.; Instituto Asturiano de Atención Social a la Infancia, Familias y Adolescencia para el Observatorio de la Infancia y la Adolescencia del Principado de Asturias: Oviedo, Spain, 2011; p. 398.
35. Observatorio de Salud Pública de Cantabria. Estudio Sobre Determinantes de la Salud de la Población Gitana Cántabra. Available online: https://www.ospc.es/ficheros/esp/ProyectosFicheros/9F9A2FBE-7DAC-6F48-1AC6-45C6340346CB.pdf/ (accessed on 29 June 2020).
36. Pérez, F.J.; Arias-Gundín, O. La alimentación en un centro educativo donde las minorías son mayoría. *Int. J. Behav. Dev.* **2009**, *2*, 181–189.
37. Velcheva, M.B. Research on the eating habits of pregnant Romani women and mothers of newborns in Bulgaria in 2015: Hristina Velcheva. *Eur. J. Public Health* **2016**, *26*, ckw174.015. [CrossRef]
38. Szabóné Kármán, J. (Ed.) A magyarországi cigány/roma népesség kultúrantropológiai és orvosantropológiai megközelítésben. In *Romológiai Füzetek*; Debreceni Református Hittudományi Egyetem: Debrecen, Hungary, 2018; ISBN 978-615-5853-03-6. ISSN 2560-2209.
39. Llanaj, E.; Vincze, F.; Kósa, Z.; Sándor, J.; Diószegi, J.; Ádány, R. Dietary Profile and Nutritional Status of the Roma Population Living in Segregated Colonies in Northeast Hungary. *Nutrients* **2020**, *12*, 2836. [CrossRef] [PubMed]
40. Poore, J.; Nemecek, T. Reducing food's environmental impacts through producers and consumers. *Science* **2018**, *360*, 987. [CrossRef] [PubMed]
41. Swinburn, B.A.; Kraak, V.I.; Allender, S.; Atkins, V.J.; Baker, P.I.; Bogard, J.R.; Brinsden, H.; Calvillo, A.; De Schutter, O.; Devarajan, R.; et al. The Global Syndemic of Obesity, Undernutrition, and Climate Change: The Lancet Commission report. *Lancet* **2019**, *393*, 791–846. [CrossRef]
42. Clark, M.A.; Springmann, M.; Hill, J.; Tilman, D. Multiple health and environmental impacts of foods. *Proc. Natl. Acad. Sci. USA* **2019**, *116*, 23357–23362. [CrossRef]
43. Willett, W.; Rockström, J.; Loken, B.; Springmann, M.; Lang, T.; Vermeulen, S.; Garnett, T.; Tilman, D.; DeClerck, F.; Wood, A.; et al. Food in the Anthropocene: The EAT-Lancet Commission on healthy diets from sustainable food systems. *Lancet* **2019**, *393*, 447–492. [CrossRef]
44. Ádány, R.; Pikó, P.; Fiatal, S.; Kósa, Z.; Sándor, J.; Bíró, É.; Kósa, K.; Paragh, G.; Bácsné Bába, É.; Veres-Balajti, I. Prevalence of Insulin Resistance in the Hungarian General and Roma Populations as Defined by Using Data Generated in a Complex Health (Interview and Examination) Survey. *Int. J. Environ. Res. Public Health* **2020**, *17*, 4833. [CrossRef] [PubMed]

45. Llanaj, E.; Ádány, R.; Lachat, C.; D'Haese, M. Examining food intake and eating out of home patterns among university students. *PLoS ONE* **2018**, *13*, e0197874. [CrossRef]

46. Llanaj, E.; Hanley-Cook, G.T. Adherence to Healthy and Sustainable Diets Is Not Differentiated by Cost, But Rather Source of Foods among Young Adults in Albania. *Br. J. Nutr.* **2020**, 1–23. [CrossRef] [PubMed]

47. Nishida, C.; Uauy, R.; Kumanyika, S.; Shetty, P. The joint WHO/FAO expert consultation on diet, nutrition and the prevention of chronic diseases: Process, product and policy implications. *Public Health Nutr.* **2004**, *7*, 245–250. [CrossRef] [PubMed]

48. World Health Organization. Healthy Diet: Key Facts (29 April 2020 Update). Available online: https://www.who.int/news-room/fact-sheets/detail/healthy-diet (accessed on 22 December 2020).

49. Huijbregts, P.; Feskens, E.; Räsänen, L.; Fidanza, F.; Nissinen, A.; Menotti, A.; Kromhout, D. Dietary pattern and 20 year mortality in elderly men in Finland, Italy, and the Netherlands: Longitudinal cohort study. *BMJ* **1997**, *315*, 13. [CrossRef] [PubMed]

50. Mellen, P.B.; Gao, S.K.; Vitolins, M.Z.; Goff, D.C., Jr. Deteriorating Dietary Habits Among Adults With Hypertension: DASH Dietary Accordance, NHANES 1988-1994 and 1999-2004. *JAMA Intern. Med.* **2008**, *168*, 308–314. [CrossRef] [PubMed]

51. Appel, L.J.; Moore, T.J.; Obarzanek, E.; Vollmer, W.M.; Svetkey, L.P.; Sacks, F.M.; Bray, G.A.; Vogt, T.M.; Cutler, J.A.; Windhauser, M.M.; et al. A Clinical Trial of the Effects of Dietary Patterns on Blood Pressure. *N. Engl. J. Med.* **1997**, *336*, 1117–1124. [CrossRef] [PubMed]

52. Sacks, F.M.; Svetkey, L.P.; Vollmer, W.M.; Appel, L.J.; Bray, G.A.; Harsha, D.; Obarzanek, E.; Conlin, P.R.; Miller, E.R.; Simons-Morton, D.G.; et al. Effects on Blood Pressure of Reduced Dietary Sodium and the Dietary Approaches to Stop Hypertension (DASH) Diet. *N. Engl. J. Med.* **2001**, *344*, 3–10. [CrossRef]

53. Shivappa, N.; Steck, S.E.; Hurley, T.G.; Hussey, J.R.; Hébert, J.R. Designing and developing a literature-derived, population-based dietary inflammatory index. *Public Health Nutr.* **2014**, *17*, 1689–1696. [CrossRef]

54. Hébert, J.R.; Shivappa, N.; Wirth, M.D.; Hussey, J.R.; Hurley, T.G. Perspective: The Dietary Inflammatory Index (DII)-Lessons Learned, Improvements Made, and Future Directions. *Adv. Nutr.* **2019**, *10*, 185–195. [CrossRef]

55. Lachat, C.; Hawwash, D.; Ocké, M.C.; Berg, C.; Forsum, E.; Hörnell, A.; Larsson, C.; Sonestedt, E.; Wirfält, E.; Åkesson, A.; et al. Strengthening the Reporting of Observational Studies in Epidemiology—Nutritional Epidemiology (STROBE-nut): An Extension of the STROBE Statement. *PLoS Med.* **2016**, *13*, e1002036. [CrossRef] [PubMed]

56. Sándor, J.; Kósa, K.; Papp, M.; Fürjes, G.; Kőrösi, L.; Jakovljevic, M.; Ádány, R. Capitation-Based Financing Hampers the Provision of Preventive Services in Primary Health Care. *Front. Public Health* **2016**, *4*, 200. [CrossRef]

57. Kósa, K.; Sándor, J.; Dobos, É.; Papp, M.; Fürjes, G.; Ádány, R. Human resources development for the operation of general practitioners' cluster. *Eur. J. Public Health* **2013**, *23*, 532–533. [CrossRef] [PubMed]

58. Sándor, J.; Nagy, A.; Jenei, T.; Földvári, A.; Szabó, E.; Csenteri, O.; Vincze, F.; Sipos, V.; Kovács, N.; Pálinkás, A.; et al. Influence of patient characteristics on preventive service delivery and general practitioners' preventive performance indicators: A study in patients with hypertension or diabetes mellitus from Hungary. *Eur. J. Gen. Pract.* **2018**, *24*, 183–191. [CrossRef] [PubMed]

59. Rurik, I.; Ruzsinkó, K.; Jancsó, Z.; Antal, M. Nutritional Counseling for Diabetic Patients: A Pilot Study in Hungarian Primary Care. *Ann. Nutr. Metab.* **2010**, *57*, 18–22. [CrossRef] [PubMed]

60. Sándor, J.; Kósa, K.; Fürjes, G.; Papp, M.; Csordás, Á.; Rurik, I.; Ádány, R. Public health services provided in the framework of general practitioners' clusters. *Eur. J. Public Health* **2013**, *23*, 530–532. [CrossRef] [PubMed]

61. Lee, Y.; Mozaffarian, D.; Sy, S.; Huang, Y.; Liu, J.; Wilde, P.E.; Abrahams-Gessel, S.; Jardim, T.S.V.; Gaziano, T.A.; Micha, R. Cost-effectiveness of financial incentives for improving diet and health through Medicare and Medicaid: A microsimulation study. *PLoS Med.* **2019**, *16*, e1002761. [CrossRef] [PubMed]

62. Gódor, A. The major trends of food consumption in Hungary. *Deturope* **2016**, *8*, 202–211.

63. Kiss, A.; Pfeiffer, L.; Popp, J.; Oláh, J.; Lakner, Z. A Blind Man Leads a Blind Man? Personalised Nutrition-Related Attitudes, Knowledge and Behaviours of Fitness Trainers in Hungary. *Nutrients* **2020**, *12*, 663. [CrossRef]

64. Stacey, D.; Hopkins, M.; Adamo, K.B.; Shorr, R.; Prud'homme, D. Knowledge translation to fitness trainers: A systematic review. *Implement. Sci.* **2010**, *5*, 28. [CrossRef]

65. European Commission. Healthy Lifestyles and Healthy Nutrition. Available online: https://eacea.ec.europa.eu/national-policies/en/content/youthwiki/74-healthy-lifestyles-and-healthy-nutrition-hungary (accessed on 23 November 2020).

66. Minihane, A.M.; Vinoy, S.; Russell, W.R.; Baka, A.; Roche, H.M.; Tuohy, K.M.; Teeling, J.L.; Blaak, E.E.; Fenech, M.; Vauzour, D.; et al. Low-grade inflammation, diet composition and health: Current research evidence and its translation. *Br. J. Nutr.* **2015**, *114*, 999–1012. [CrossRef] [PubMed]

67. Barbaresko, J.; Koch, M.; Schulze, M.B.; Nöthlings, U. Dietary pattern analysis and biomarkers of low-grade inflammation: A systematic literature review. *Nutr. Rev.* **2013**, *71*, 511–527. [CrossRef]

68. Afshin, A.; Sur, P.J.; Fay, K.A.; Cornaby, L.; Ferrara, G.; Salama, J.S.; Mullany, E.C.; Abate, K.H.; Abbafati, C.; Abebe, Z.; et al. Health effects of dietary risks in 195 countries, 1990–2017: A systematic analysis for the Global Burden of Disease Study 2017. *Lancet* **2019**, *393*, 1958–1972. [CrossRef]

69. 2020 Global Nutrition Report: Action on Equity to End Malnutrition. Available online: https://globalnutritionreport.org/reports/2020-global-nutrition-report/ (accessed on 11 January 2021).

70. Béné, C.; Prager, S.D.; Achicanoy, H.A.E.; Toro, P.A.; Lamotte, L.; Bonilla, C.; Mapes, B.R. Global map and indicators of food system sustainability. *Sci. Data* **2019**, *6*, 279. [CrossRef]

71. Országos Egészségfejlesztési Intézet. Dietary Guidelines for the Adult Population in Hungary (Hungarian: Táplálkozási Ajánlások a Magyarországi Felnőtt Lakosság Számára). Available online: http://www.fao.org/3/a-as6840.pdf (accessed on 3 November 2020).
72. Sinha, R.; Cross, A.J.; Graubard, B.I.; Leitzmann, M.F.; Schatzkin, A. Meat Intake and Mortality: A Prospective Study of Over Half a Million People. *Arch. Intern. Med.* **2009**, *169*, 562–571. [CrossRef]
73. Bellavia, A.; Stilling, F.; Wolk, A. High red meat intake and all-cause cardiovascular and cancer mortality: Is the risk modified by fruit and vegetable intake? *Am. J. Clin. Nutr.* **2016**, *104*, 1137–1143. [CrossRef]
74. Bodirsky, B.L.; Dietrich, J.P.; Martinelli, E.; Stenstad, A.; Pradhan, P.; Gabrysch, S.; Mishra, A.; Weindl, I.; Le Mouël, C.; Rolinski, S.; et al. The ongoing nutrition transition thwarts long-term targets for food security, public health and environmental protection. *Sci. Rep.* **2020**, *10*, 19778. [CrossRef] [PubMed]
75. Sabaté, J.; Soret, S. Sustainability of plant-based diets: Back to the future. *Am. J. Clin. Nutr.* **2014**, *100*, 476S–482S. [CrossRef] [PubMed]
76. FAO; WHO. *Strengthening Nutrition Action: A Resource Guide for Countries Based on the Policy Recommendations of the Second International Conference on Nutrition*; WHO: Geneva, Switzerland; FAO: Rome, Italy, 2019.
77. Couch, S.C.; Saelens, B.E.; Khoury, P.R.; Dart, K.B.; Hinn, K.; Mitsnefes, M.M.; Daniels, S.R.; Urbina, E.M. Dietary Approaches to Stop Hypertension Dietary Intervention Improves Blood Pressure and Vascular Health in Youth With Elevated Blood Pressure. *Hypertension* **2020**. [CrossRef]
78. Ali Mohsenpour, M.; Fallah-Moshkani, R.; Ghiasvand, R.; Khosravi-Boroujeni, H.; Mehdi Ahmadi, S.; Brauer, P.; Salehi-Abargouei, A. Adherence to Dietary Approaches to Stop Hypertension (DASH)-Style Diet and the Risk of Cancer: A Systematic Review and Meta-Analysis of Cohort Studies. *J. Am. Coll. Nutr.* **2019**, *38*, 513–525. [CrossRef]
79. Yang, Z.-Q.; Yang, Z.; Duan, M.-L. Dietary approach to stop hypertension diet and risk of coronary artery disease: A meta-analysis of prospective cohort studies. *Int. J. Food Sci. Nutr.* **2019**, *70*, 668–674. [CrossRef] [PubMed]
80. Monsivais, P.; Scarborough, P.; Lloyd, T.; Mizdrak, A.; Luben, R.; Mulligan, A.A.; Wareham, N.J.; Woodcock, J. Greater accordance with the Dietary Approaches to Stop Hypertension dietary pattern is associated with lower diet-related greenhouse gas production but higher dietary costs in the United Kingdom. *Am. J. Clin. Nutr.* **2015**, *102*, 138–145. [CrossRef]
81. Stinson, E.J.; Piaggi, P.; Votruba, S.B.; Venti, C.; Lovato-Morales, B.; Engel, S.; Krakoff, J.; Gluck, M.E. Is Dietary Nonadherence Unique to Obesity and Weight Loss? Results From a Randomized Clinical Trial. *Obesity* **2020**, *28*, 2020–2027. [CrossRef] [PubMed]
82. Branca, F.; Demaio, A.; Udomkesmalee, E.; Baker, P.; Aguayo, V.M.; Barquera, S.; Dain, K.; Keir, L.; Lartey, A.; Mugambi, G.; et al. A new nutrition manifesto for a new nutrition reality. *Lancet* **2020**, *395*, 8–10. [CrossRef]
83. Popkin, B.M.; Corvalan, C.; Grummer-Strawn, L.M. Dynamics of the double burden of malnutrition and the changing nutrition reality. *Lancet* **2019**. [CrossRef]
84. Nugent, R.; Levin, C.; Hale, J.; Hutchinson, B. Economic effects of the double burden of malnutrition. *Lancet* **2020**, *395*, 156–164. [CrossRef]
85. Wells, J.C.; Sawaya, A.L.; Wibaek, R.; Mwangome, M.; Poullas, M.S.; Yajnik, C.S.; Demaio, A. The double burden of malnutrition: Aetiological pathways and consequences for health. *Lancet* **2019**, *395*, 75–88. [CrossRef]
86. Hawkes, C.; Ruel, M.T.; Salm, L.; Sinclair, B.; Branca, F. Double-duty actions: Seizing programme and policy opportunities to address malnutrition in all its forms. *Lancet* **2020**, *395*, 142–155. [CrossRef]
87. Butler, M.J.; Barrientos, R.M. The impact of nutrition on COVID-19 susceptibility and long-term consequences. *Brain Behav. Immun.* **2020**, *87*, 53–54. [CrossRef] [PubMed]
88. Kósa, Z.; Moravcsik-Kornyicki, Á.; Diószegi, J.; Roberts, B.; Szabó, Z.; Sándor, J.; Ádány, R. Prevalence of metabolic syndrome among Roma: A comparative health examination survey in Hungary. *Eur. J. Public Health* **2014**, *25*, 299–304. [CrossRef] [PubMed]
89. Macejova, Z.; Kristian, P.; Janicko, M.; Halanova, M.; Drazilova, S.; Antolova, D.; Marekova, M.; Pella, D.; Madarasova-Geckova, A.; Jarcuska, P. The Roma Population Living in Segregated Settlements in Eastern Slovakia Has a Higher Prevalence of Metabolic Syndrome, Kidney Disease, Viral Hepatitis B and E, and Some Parasitic Diseases Compared to the Majority Population. *Int. J. Environ. Res. Public Health* **2020**, *17*, 3112. [CrossRef] [PubMed]

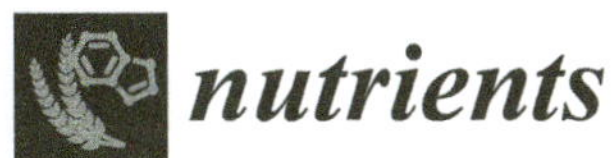

Article

Higher HEI-2015 Score Is Associated with Reduced Risk of Depression: Result from NHANES 2005–2016

Kai Wang [1], Yudi Zhao [2], Jiaqi Nie [1], Haoling Xu [1], Chuanhua Yu [2] and Suqing Wang [1,*]

[1] Department of Nutrition and Food Hygiene, School of Health Science, Wuhan University, 185, Donghu Rd, Wuhan 430071, China; wk1148761305@whu.edu.cn (K.W.); 15502730223@163.com (J.N.); xuhlntl@163.com (H.X.)

[2] Department of Epidemiology and Biostatistics, School of Health Sciences, Wuhan University, 185 Donghu Rd, Wuhan 430071, China; yudi_zhao@whu.edu.cn (Y.Z.); yuchua@whu.edu.cn (C.Y.)

* Correspondence: swang2099@whu.edu.cn

Abstract: Globally, the total estimated number of people living with depression increased by 18.4% between 2005 and 2015, with the prevalence being 4.8% in 2015. Many nutrient and diet patterns are proven to be correlated to depression, so we conducted this analysis to explore whether the Healthy Eating Index 2015 (HEI-2015) score is associated with depression, and possibly to provide dietary measures to reduce the risk of depression. Data came from the National Health and Nutrition Examination Survey (2005–2016), a cross-sectional and nationally representative database. The analytic sample was limited to adults: (1) age ≥20 with complete information of HEI-2015 and depression; (2) no missing data of demographics, BMI, drinking, smoking, and fasting plasma glucose. HEI-2015 was calculated using the Dietary Interview: Total Nutrient Intakes, First Day data file. Depression was assessed using the Patient Health Questionnaire-9 (PHQ-9). Weighted logistic regression models were used to explore the relationship between the HEI-2015 score and depression. The final study sample included 10,349 adults, with 51.4% of them being men, representing a population of about 167.8 million non-institutionalized U.S. adults. After multivariable adjustment, average HEI status (OR: 0.848, 95% CI: 0.846–0.849) and optimal HEI status (OR: 0.455, 95% CI: 0.453–0.456) were associated with reduced odds of depression. Poor diet quality is significantly associated with elevated depressive symptoms in U.S. adults. Aligning with the Dietary Guidelines for Americans reduces the risk of depression.

Keywords: healthy eating index; depression; NHANES; diet pattern; DGA

Citation: Wang, K.; Zhao, Y.; Nie, J.; Xu, H.; Yu, C.; Wang, S. Higher HEI-2015 Score Is Associated with Reduced Risk of Depression: Result from NHANES 2005–2016. *Nutrients* **2021**, *13*, 348. https://doi.org/10.3390/nu13020348

Received: 17 December 2020
Accepted: 19 January 2021
Published: 25 January 2021

Publisher's Note: MDPI stays neutral with regard to jurisdictional claims in published maps and institutional affiliations.

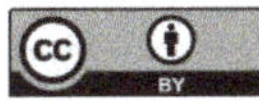

1. Introduction

Depression, clinically characterized by significant and persistent low mood symptoms, is a common and growing globally mental health issue linked with considerably diminished role-functioning and quality of life, medical comorbidity, and mortality [1]. In 2017, about 17.3 million adults aged 18 and over in the US had experienced at least one major depressive episode. The prevalence was about 7.1%, and highest among adults reporting two or more races [2]. According to the Depression and Other Common Mental Disorders: Global Health Estimates published by WHO in 2017, the total number of people living with depression in the world is 322 million. Nearly half of them live in the South-East Asia Region and Western Pacific Region, such as China and India. Meanwhile, the prevalence of depression varies by age, peaking in older adulthood, and was estimated above 7.5% among females aged 55–74 years [3]. A substantial number of researches have shown strong relationships between depression and physical health, including cardiovascular disease [4], Parkinson's disease [5], metabolic disease [6], dementia [7], type 2 diabetes [8], and cancer [9]. Out of the mental and addictive disorders, depressive disorders cause most disability-adjusted life years for both sexes, followed by anxiety disorders in women [10]. In 2015, depressive disorders led to a global total of over 50 million years lived with disability (YLD), more than

80% of which occurred in low- and middle-income countries [4]. Studies in recent decades have shown associations between nutrient intake and the risk of depression, including minerals like zinc, omega-3 fatty acids, and vitamins such as vitamin D [11–14]. Many researchers also found adherence to a specific dietary pattern, such as "dietary approaches to stop hypertension", was correlated with lower depression risk [15–17]. While most of them focused on specific diet pattern or food intake, some research explored the relationship from a macroscopic view. To explore the effect of diet quality in a more macroscopic way, we adopted the latest edition of the Healthy Eating Index (HEI) to determine whether diet quality is related to depression. Through this research, we want to answer whether aligning with the Dietary Guidelines for Americans (DGA) reduces the risk of depression.

2. Materials and Methods

2.1. Sample

Data came from the six continuous National Health and Nutrition Examination Survey (NHANES) cycles from 2005–2016 (https://wwwn.cdc.gov/nchs/nhanes/ContinuousNhanes/Default.aspx?BeginYear=2005). NHANES is a nationally representative, population-based survey for assessing adult and child health and nutritional status in the US. This survey combined health interviews conducted in respondents' homes with health measurements (e.g., DPQ_I, objective physical measures) performed at mobile exam centers (MECs). The examination components consisted of medical, dental, and physiological measurements, and laboratory tests supervised by trained medical personnel. Furthermore, the adoption of various modern equipment enabled the NHANES to collect reliable, high-quality data. Moreover, compensation and a report of medical findings were given to each participant, which increased the compliance of participants [18]. The total sample size of adults from the 2005–2016 assessments was N = 10,349. Additional details of the study design, sampling, and exclusion criteria are described in Figure 1. Only publicly available data was used in the analysis, and no ethical approval was needed in this study.

2.2. Measures

Diet quality: The Healthy Eating Index (HEI) is a measure for assessing dietary quality, precisely, the degree to which a set of foods aligns with the Dietary Guidelines for Americans [19]. The HEI-2015 components were the same as in the HEI-2010, except saturated fat and added sugars replaced empty calories, with the result being 13 components [20]. HEI-2015 scores ranged from 0–100, with higher HEI scores reflecting better diet quality. We utilized the total nutrient intakes on the first day (DR1TOT) to calculate the 13 components of HEI-2015. For further weighted Scott–Rao chi-square test and weighted logistic regressions, an HEI-2015 score less than 50, between 50 and 70, and more than 70 was categorized as inadequate, average and optimal, respectively [21].

Depression: Current depressive symptoms were measured by the Patient Health Questionnaire-9 (PHQ-9). The PHQ-9 is a well-validated (Cronbach's $\alpha = 0.89$) self-report instrument that assesses depression symptoms (i.e., sadness, trouble sleeping, fatigue, problems concentrating) in the past two weeks, and has moderate concordance with clinical psychiatric interviews. The PHQ-9 questionnaire contains nine items, with each item being assessed on a four-point Likert scale, ranging from 0 = not at all to 3 = nearly every day, and summing up a total scale range of 0 to 27. A dichotomous variable indicating no depression (PHQ-9 score <10) or elevated depressive symptoms (PHQ-9 score $\geq$10) was created using a threshold score of 10 [22].

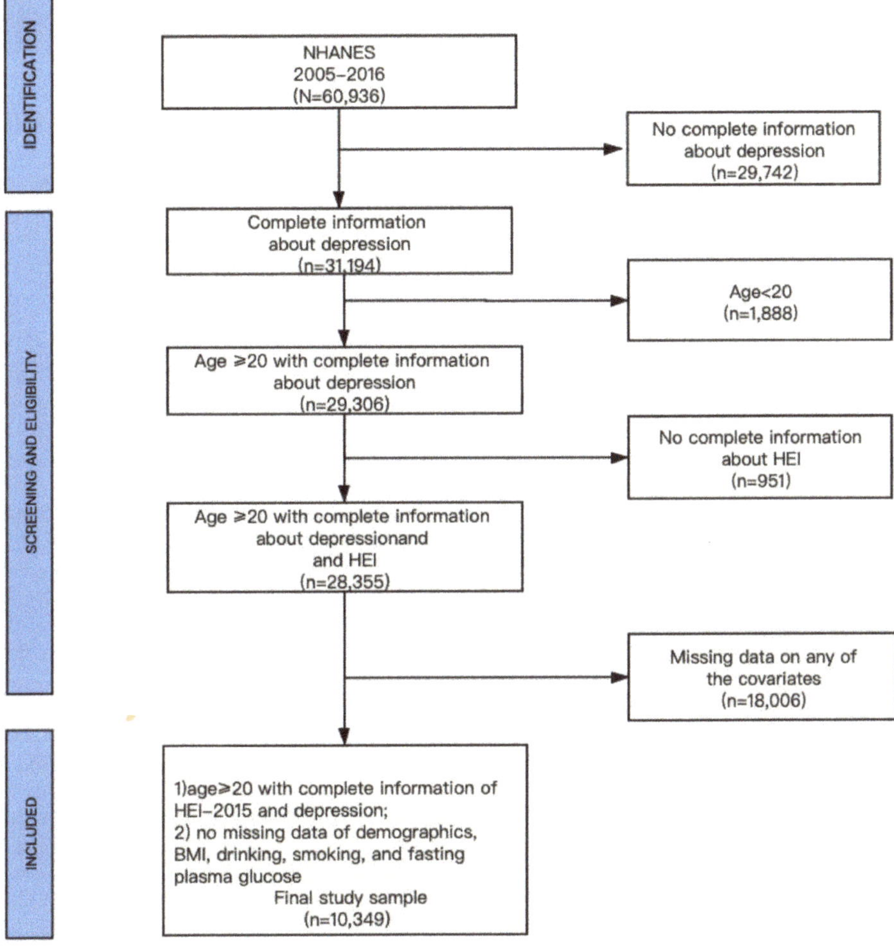

Figure 1. Flowchart of the study population.

Covariates

Each covariant was categorized into a reference group, and other groups. When analyzing, all other groups were compared to this reference group to estimate the relative odds ratio.

Sex: Sex was categorized as male (reference group) and female.

Age: Age was categorized as 20 to 25 years (reference group), 26 to 49 years, and 50+ years [4].

Race: Race was categorized as non-Hispanic white (reference group), non-Hispanic black, Mexican American, and other races [23].

Education level: Education level was categorized as less than a high school diploma (reference group), high school graduate/GED, some college/AA degree, and college graduate or more [24].

Household income: Household income was categorized as ≤130% (reference group), >130% to 350%, and >350% by the ratio of family income to poverty (FPL) [25].

BMI status: body mass index was calculated from measured height and weight as weight/height^2 (kg/m^2), and then categorized into $\leq$25 (reference group), >25 to 30, and >30 [26].

Smoking status: smoking behavior was measured in the "smoking: cigarette use" questionnaire. In the "smoking: cigarette use" questionnaire, respondents were asked if s/he had smoked at least 100 cigarettes in their life, and smoked cigarettes when being questioned. If the respondent had smoked less than 100 cigarettes in their life, s/he was classified as a never smoker. If the respondent had smoked at least 100 cigarettes in his/her life and still smoked when s/he answered the questionnaire, s/he was classified as a current smoker. The respondent was classified as a former smoker if s/he had smoked at least 100 cigarettes in his/her life, and had quit smoking when s/he answered the questionnaire. Smoking status was categorized into never smoker (reference group), former smoker, and current smoker [27].

Drinking status: drinking behavior was measured in the "alcohol use" questionnaire. In the "alcohol use" questionnaire, each respondent was asked how often s/he had drunk alcoholic drinks in the past 12 months, and the average drinks on those days that s/he drank alcoholic beverages. According to these questions, the average number of alcoholic drinks consumed per week in the past 12 months could be calculated. Then it was categorized into four strata (0, <1, 1–<8, and $\geq$8 drinks per week) and defined as none (reference group), light, moderate, and heavy alcohol consumption, respectively. A "drink" was defined as a 12-ounce beer, a 5-ounce glass of wine, or one-and-half ounces of liquor [28].

Diabetes: plasma glucose data were obtained from the plasma fasting glucose laboratory data. Respondents whose fasting plasma glucose was $\geq$6.0 mmol/L were thought to be a diabetic, consistent with American Diabetes Association guidelines [29]. Thus, respondents were categorized into adults with normoglycemia (reference group), and adults with diabetes.

2.3. Statistical Analysis

Initially, the trends of depression and other characteristics in the six continuous cycles were estimated with the Cochran–Armitage trend test. Then, the baseline characteristics of different groups were compared using the weighted Scott–Rao chi-square test [30]. HEI scores were described with a median (P25, P75). Finally, a series of weighted steps forward (likelihood ratio) binary logistic regression models were fit to assess the relationship between diet quality and depression. Estimates were weighted to be representative of the general adult population. All *p* values refer to two-tailed tests. Statistical analyses were conducted using the SPSS statistical package (Version 23.0; SPSS Inc., Chicago, IL, USA).

3. Results

Figure 1 described the study design, sampling, and exclusion; and 18,006 participants were excluded because of missing data on any of the covariates. Among them, 2361, 12, 219, 12, 3594, and 11,808 individuals were excluded because of missing data on income, education, BMI, smoking, drinking, and diabetes, respectively. Our final sample included 10,349 NHANES participants, representing a population of about 167.8 million non-institutionalized U.S. adults, with 48.6% being female and 72.0% being non-Hispanic White.

Table 1 described the prevalence of depression and associated characteristics in six continuous NHANES cycles, in which the trend tests were also conducted. The prevalence of depression grew with time, from 4.8% in 2005–2006 to 7.4% in 2015–2016. In addition, there are other points worth noting. For example, the proportion of women and adults aged over fifty years old increased with time. The proportion of adults with normal or low weight decreased with time, indicating the urgency of body shape management. The prevalence of diabetes increased with time, which reminds adults of the significance of blood glucose control. The proportion of adults with inadequate HEI status decreased with time, showing the improving diet quality in the six cycles.

Table 1. US trends in characteristics among adults aged 20 years or older.

Characteristics	2005–2006 (n = 1595)	2007–2008 (n = 1839)	2009–2010 (n = 1913)	2011–2012 (n = 1619)	2013–2014 (n = 1778)	2015–2016 (n = 1605)	*p* Trend
No. with depressive symptoms	84	157	166	131	159	139	
The prevalence of depression (Weighted %)	4.8	6.8	7.0	7.4	8.0	7.4	<0.001
Sex (No. Weighted %)							<0.001
Male	856 (51.2)	993 (52.7)	983 (51.4)	891 (52.0)	710 (50.7)	856 (50.6)	
Female	739 (48.8)	846 (47.3)	930 (48.7)	728 (48.0)	868 (49.3)	749 (49.4)	
Age group (No. Weighted %)							<0.001
20–24 y	151 (8.9)	136 (9.1)	175 (9.3)	171 (9.6)	143 (9.5)	115 (7.2)	
25–49 y	746 (51.5)	775 (51.0)	809 (47.6)	709 (46.3)	764 (45.4)	670 (44.8)	
50+ y	698 (39.6)	928 (39.9)	929 (43.1)	739 (44.1)	871 (45.0)	820 (45.8)	
Race (No. Weighted %)							<0.001
Non-Hispanic White	865 (75.2)	932 (72.6)	1023 (73.9)	728 (71.9)	868 (70.2)	646 (68.7)	
Non-Hispanic Black	334 (9.7)	364 (10.4)	298 (9.8)	366 (10.1)	339 (10.7)	321 (10.1)	
Mexican American	281 (7.2)	304 (8.0)	331 (7.3)	159 (6.6)	224 (8.3)	240 (7.1)	
Other races	115 (7.9)	239 (9.0)	261 (9.0)	366 (11.4)	347 (10.8)	398 (14.1)	
Education level (No. Weighted %)							<0.001
<High school	373 (14.8)	509 (17.5)	475 (16.2)	323 (14.0)	345 (14.2)	306 (11.9)	
High school/GED	400 (26.2)	453 (23.8)	434 (22.7)	340 (18.7)	384 (20.1)	374 (22.3)	
Some college/AA degree	483 (32.8)	478 (29.4)	567 (30.6)	500 (33.1)	557 (33.2)	506 (32.6)	
College or more	339 (26.1)	399 (29.4)	437 (31.4)	456 (34.2)	492 (32.5)	419 (33.1)	
Household income (No. Weighted %)							<0.001
0–130% FPL	352 (13.3)	503 (17.3)	598 (20.5)	540 (21.8)	574 (23.1)	463 (18.2)	
>130–350% FPL	652 (39.1)	718 (33.6)	711 (36.0)	576 (36.6)	610 (34.3)	665 (37.9)	
>350% FPL	591 (47.6)	618 (49.1)	604 (43.4)	503 (41.9)	594 (42.6)	477 (43.3)	
BMI status (No. Weighted %)							<0.001
Normal or low weight	479 (32.0)	538 (31.6)	540 (31.0)	503 (31.2)	535 (30.0)	422 (26.1)	
Overweight	537 (31.9)	653 (36.1)	665 (34.0)	528 (33.6)	589 (33.2)	534 (32.5)	
Obese	579 (36.2)	648 (32.3)	708 (34.9)	588 (35.2)	654 (36.9)	649 (41.4)	
Smoking status (No. Weighted %)							<0.001
Never	721 (44.6)	863 (50.1)	950 (51.4)	853 (54.1)	911 (53.2)	767 (48.1)	
Former	482 (28.5)	528 (26.7)	531 (28.0)	413 (25.5)	481 (26.8)	469 (31.1)	
Current	392 (27.2)	448 (23.1)	432 (20.6)	353 (20.5)	386 (20.0)	369 (20.8)	
Drinking status (No, Weighted %)							<0.001
None	394 (19.0)	434 (18.5)	385 (16.1)	315 (15.3)	362 (15.6)	307 (15.7)	
Light	516 (33.4)	620 (33.9)	682 (34.0)	591 (34.9)	656 (36.5)	606 (36.0)	
Moderate	457 (30.7)	514 (32.1)	546 (33.3)	453 (31.2)	522 (33.3)	483 (34.3)	
Heavy	228 (16.8)	271 (15.5)	300 (16.7)	238 (18.6)	238 (14.6)	209 (13.9)	
Diabetes (No. Weighted %)							<0.001
No	1448 (93.0)	1617 (92.6)	1707 (92.3)	1445 (92.5)	1570 (90.2)	1370 (88.7)	
Yes	147 (7.0)	222 (7.4)	206 (7.7)	174 (7.5)	208 (9.8)	235 (11.3)	
HEI status (No. Weighted %)							<0.001
Inadequate	889 (57.2)	959 (55.2)	958 (49.3)	825 (49.7)	895 (50.9)	758 (47.3)	
Average	594 (36.4)	751 (38.6)	789 (41.3)	652 (39.8)	704 (40.1)	720 (45.1)	
Optimal	112 (6.4)	129 (6.1)	166 (9.4)	142 (10.5)	179 (9.1)	127 (7.5)	

Values are survey-weighted percentages. FPL = family income to poverty. HEI = healthy eating index.

Table 2 describes the characteristics of participants with the weighted Scott–Rao chi-square test. Adults with depression were more likely to be female, non-Hispanic Black, obese, over 50 years old, current smokers, diabetic, alcoholic, have less than high school education, have low household income, and have inadequate HEI scores.

Table 2. Characteristics among adults aged 20 years or older by depression.

Characteristics	Adults without Depression	Adults with Depression	*p*-Value
No. (Weighted %)	9513 (93.1)	836 (6.9)	
Sex			<0.001
Male	5159 (52.4)	330 (38.1)	
Female	4354 (47.6)	506 (61.9)	
Age group			<0.001
20–24 y	4129 (9.5)	326 (7.4)	
25–49 y	3212 (47.9)	368 (45.6)	
50+ y	2172 (42.6)	142 (47.1)	
Race			<0.001
Non-Hispanic White	4654 (72.3)	408 (69.1)	
Non-Hispanic Black	1846 (9.9)	176 (13.5)	
Mexican American	1430 (7.5)	109 (6.2)	
Other races	1583 (10.3)	143 (11.2)	
Education level			<0.001
<High school	2052 (14.0)	279 (24.9)	
High school/GED	2176 (21.8)	209 (26.3)	
Some college/AA degree	2841 (31.8)	250 (34.4)	
College or more	2444 (32.4)	98 (14.5)	
Household income			<0.001
0–130% FPL	2574 (17.4)	456 (42.3)	
>130–350% FPL	3667 (36.2)	265 (35.7)	
>350% FPL	3272 (46.4)	115 (22.0)	
BMI status			<0.001
Normal or low weight	2795 (30.4)	222 (28.7)	
Overweight	3293 (34.2)	213 (24.8)	
Obese	3425 (35.4)	401 (46.5)	
Smoking status			<0.001
Never	4787 (51.6)	278 (31.8)	
Former	2695 (28.0)	209 (24.3)	
Current	2031 (20.3)	349 (44.0)	
Drinking status			<0.001
None	1979 (16.2)	218 (23.0)	
Light	3336 (34.6)	335 (37.9)	
Moderate	2833 (33.4)	142 (20.6)	
Heavy	1365 (15.8)	141 (18.5)	
Diabetes			<0.001
No	8463 (92.0)	694 (85.6)	
YES	1050 (8.0)	142 (14.4)	
HEI status			<0.001
Inadequate	4783 (50.8)	501 (62.4)	
Average	3908 (40.7)	302 (34.3)	
Optimal	822 (8.5)	33 (3.2)	

Values are survey-weighted percentages. FPL = family income to poverty.

Table 3 shows the results of three weighted logistic regression models. Model 1 was adjusted for demographics characteristics (i.e., sex, age group, race, income, and education). Model 2 was adjusted for all Model 1 covariates and BMI, smoking, and drinking status. Moreover, Model 3 was adjusted for all Model 2 covariates and diabetes. After adjusting for demographic characteristics, optimal HEI status was associated with 0.378 times lower odds (95% CI, 0.377–0.379) of current depression, relative to inadequate HEI status. Additional adjustment for BMI, smoking, drinking, and diabetes status did not substantially attenuate these relationships. After multivariable adjustment, adults with average HEI status (OR: 0.848, 95% CI: 0.846–0.849) and optimal HEI status (OR: 0.455, 95% CI: 0.453–0.456) were associated with reduced odds of depression. Adults with diabetes were more likely to suffer from depression, with the odds ratio being 1.637 (95% CI: 1.634–1.640).

Table 3. Relationship between HEI and Depression among Adults aged 20 years or older.

Variable	OR (95% CI)		
	Model 1	**Model 2**	**Model 3**
Sex (reference, Male)			
Female	1.799 (1.787, 1.791)	1.850 (1.847, 1.852)	1.889 (1.887, 1.892)
Age group (reference, 20–24 y)			
25–49 y	1.669 (1.665, 1.673)	1.495 (1.491, 1.499)	1.472 (1.468, 1.476)
50+ y	2.128 (2.123, 2.133)	1.968 (1.963, 1.973)	1.827 (1.822, 1.832)
Race (reference, Non-Hispanic White)			
Non-Hispanic Black	0.963 (0.961, 0.965)	0.958 (0.956, 0.960)	0.958 (0.956, 0.960)
Mexican American	0.535 (0.534, 0.537)	0.670 (0.668, 0.672)	0.656 (0.655, 0.658)
Other races	0.976 (0.974, 0.978)	1.062 (1.060, 1.064)	1.048 (1.046, 1.050)
Education level (reference, <High school)			
High school/GED	0.812 (0.810, 0.813)	0.848 (0.846, 0.849)	0.852 (0.850, 0.853)
Some college/AA degree	0.835 (0.833, 0.836)	0.952 (0.950, 0.953)	0.962 (0.961, 0.964)
College or more	0.479 (0.478, 0.480)	0.647 (0.646, 0.649)	0.655 (0.653, 0.656)
Household income (reference, 0–130% FPL)			
>130–350% FPL	0.407 (0.406, 0.407)	0.456 (0.456, 0.457)	0.456 (0.455, 0.457)
>350% FPL	0.230 (0.230, 0.231)	0.274 (0.273, 0.274)	0.277 (0.276, 0.277)
HEI status (reference, Inadequate)			
Average	0.766 (0.765, 0.767)	0.842 (0.841, 0.843)	0.848 (0.846, 0.849)
Optimal	0.378 (0.377, 0.379)	0.448 (0.447, 0.450)	0.455 (0.453, 0.456)
BMI (reference, Normal or low weight)			
Overweight		0.844 (0.843, 0.846)	0.833 (0.832, 0.835)
Obese		1.341 (1.339, 1.343)	1.265 (1.263, 1.267)
Smoking status (reference, Never)			
Former		1.286 (1.284, 1.288)	1.274 (1.272, 1.276)
Current		2.546 (2.542, 2.550)	2.564 (2.560, 2.568)
Drinking status (reference, None)			
Light		0.955 (0.954, 0.957)	0.971 (0.969, 0.973)
Moderate		0.702 (0.701, 0.703)	0.722 (0.720, 0.723)
Heavy		1.141 (1.139, 1.144)	1.181 (1.179, 1.184)
Diabetes (reference, No)			
YES			1.637 (1.634, 1.640)

FPL = family income to poverty; CI = confidence interval; OR = odds ratio. Model 1 = adjusted for demographics characteristics (i.e., sex, age group, race, income, and education); Model 2 = Model 1 covariates + BMI, smoking, and drinking status; Model 3 = Model 2 covariates + diabetes.

Figure 2 shows the trend of the HEI-2015 score in the form of a violin plot. HEI score increased from 47.77 (39.39, 56.51) in 2005–2006, to 50.74 (43.13, 59.13) in 2015–2016. The proportion of adults with inadequate HEI status decreased with time, and that of adults with optimal HEI status increased with time.

Figure 3 shows the results of three weighted logistic regression models in the form of a forest plot. As is shown, average and optimal HEI status are both protective factors for depression, reducing the depression risk by 15.2% and 54.5%. Diabetes is the risk factor of depression, increasing the depression risk by 63.7%. Cigarette smoking and heavy drinking are both behavioral risk factors.

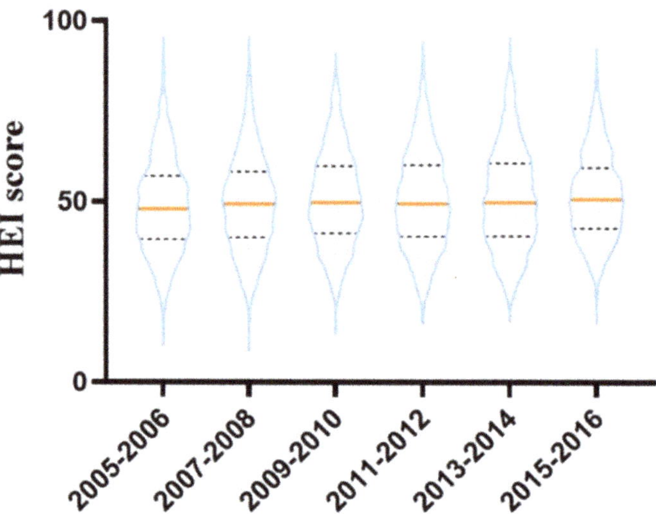

Figure 2. The trends of HEI-2015 score in the six cycles from 2005–2016 in NHANES.

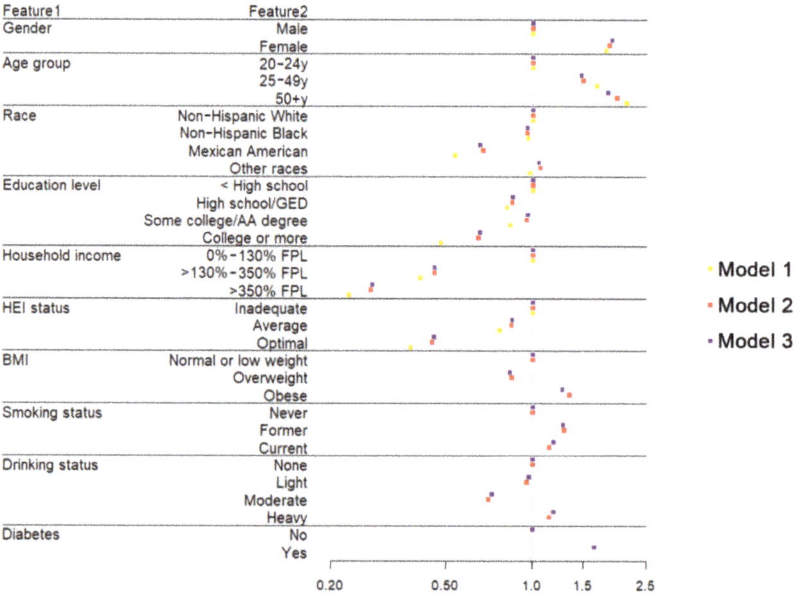

Figure 3. The forest plot shows the odds ratios of analyzing variables in three weighted logistic regression models.

4. Discussion

The results revealed that a higher HEI score was significantly correlated to less elevated depression symptoms, so we concluded that higher diet quality was significantly correlated to a lower risk of depression. Our findings also suggest that Mexican Americans are less likely to suffer from depression, which needs further analyses of genetic factors.

We analyzed the depression status of participants from nine symptomatic questions from the PHQ in 2005–2016 NHANES data, and the results revealed a depression prevalence of 6.9%. Since the sample is generalizable to the non-institutionalized civilian U.S.

population, we assume the prevalence to be credible, similar to the data published by the WHO in 2017.

To our knowledge, many factors are associated with the occurrence of depression, for instance, alcohol consumption and diabetes. Moreover, it has been found by many researchers that women are more susceptible to depression than men [31–33], in accordance with our results (odds ratio, 1.889). Moreover, three logistic regression models were adopted in this analysis to explore a more appropriate model.

Some results have been widely recognized by many researchers. For example, the results of the weighted logistic models revealed that the risk of adults aged over 50 years old suffering from depression was 1.827 times that of adults aged 20–24 years old. The report from the WHO also concluded that the prevalence varies by age, peaking in older adulthood, similar to our results [3]. After multivariable adjustment, the odds ratio for other races changed from less than one, to more than one, which needs more specific classification. Our results revealed higher education level reduced the depression risk, similar to other studies [34–36]. In addition, our results revealed a negative correlation between household income and depression, consistent with other research [37–39]. It is recognized by many experts that a positive association exists between smoking and depression, as in our results [40–42]. Among the results, we found some interesting facts. Compared with normal and low weight participants, overweight adults were less likely to suffer from depression, contrary to our original thoughts. However, we found that Z Ul-Haq got a similar result from a cross-sectional study consisting of 37,272 participants, which revealed that overweight participants had better mental health than the normal-weight group [43]. Generally, overweight and obese adults suffer more ridicule and gossip than normal and low weight adults, which may be a reason for depression. After further analyses, we found that overweight adults accounted for about one third of American adults, so were obese adults. This meant high BMI is typical among American adults, and discrimination in the US is not as high as in China, leading to less psychological pressure in overweight adults. At the same time, overweight adults relieve pressure through diet, and are less susceptible to depression.

Another fact is that light and moderate drinking is a protective factor for depression. A meta-analysis in 2013 concluded that light drinking increased the risk of cancer of the oral cavity and pharynx, esophagus, and female breast [44]. However, many researchers have found that light and moderate drinking also have some health benefits, including reducing the risk of dementia [45], heart failure [46], ischemic stroke [47], type 2 diabetes [48], and all-cause mortality [49]. In a cohort study with ten years of follow up, a J-shaped association was found with increased psychological distress among abstainers and heavy drinkers compared to light or moderate drinkers [50]. Our analysis believes that light and moderate drinking helps people deal with emotional issues and refresh themselves, thus reducing the risk of depression.

Physical activity has been found to be correlated to depression in a substantial number of studies [51–54]. However, three versions of the physical activity questionnaire were adopted in 2005–2016, and no identical and detailed information could be used to conduct an analysis. Therefore, physical activity was not included as a covariant in this analysis.

Diet quality was reported to be correlated to diabetes in many studies, not only in randomized controlled trials, but also in large population-based cohorts [55,56]. The relationship between diabetes and depression was recognized by R J Anderson in 2001 [57], yet whether there is a causal relationship is still under debate.

Thus, we conducted a mediation analysis to figure out whether diet quality influenced depression through diabetes. The HEI-2015 score was the independent variable, and the PHQ-9 score was the dependent variable. The result showed a mediating effect, but the mediating effect's proportion was only 0.14%. For further mechanism analysis, we need to explore more possible factors causing the mediation effect.

The present study has several limitations. The cross-sectional design of the study is the primary limitation, and no causation should be inferred from this study. Second, using self-reported 24-h dietary recall data and the PHQ-9 questionnaire is a limitation, as they are subject to over- or under-reporting. Finally, 18,006 participants were excluded because of missing data on any of the covariates, which may have affected the results. Despite these limitations, our study has several strengths. Using a large, nationally representative database to estimate diet quality is a major strength of the present study. Adopting the latest edition of HEI is another strength. Moreover, data in six cycles were combined to increase the sample size.

Since we found that a higher HEI-2015 score is associated with a lower risk of depression, the next step of our plan is to figure out the pathway by which HEI-2015 influences depression, with structural equation models.

By virtue of this article, we would like to make the public aware of the significance of better diet quality on depression. Since better diet quality is associated with less depression risk, why do we not improve our diet quality to reduce the risk of depression?

5. Conclusions

This study's primary finding is that depression is rapidly growing in prevalence among American adults, from 4.8% in 2005–2006, to 7.4% in 2015–2016. Poor diet quality is significantly associated with elevated depressive symptoms. An optimal HEI-2015 score reduces the risk of suffering from elevated depressive symptoms by 54.5% compared to an inadequate HEI-2015 score.

Author Contributions: Conceptualization, K.W.; methodology, K.W. and C.Y.; software, K.W. and S.W.; validation, K.W. and S.W.; formal analysis, K.W.; investigation, K.W.; resources, S.W.; data curation, K.W.; writing—original draft preparation, K.W.; writing—review and editing, Y.Z.; visualization, K.W. and C.Y.; supervision, J.N.; project administration, H.X. All authors have read and agreed to the published version of the manuscript.

Funding: This research received no external funding.

Institutional Review Board Statement: Not applicable.

Informed Consent Statement: Not applicable.

Data Availability Statement: Publicly available datasets were analyzed in this study. This data can be found here: [https://wwwn.cdc.gov/nchs/nhanes/ContinuousNhanes/Default.aspx?BeginYear=2005].

Conflicts of Interest: The authors declare no conflict of interest.

References

1. Park, L.T.; Zarate, C.A., Jr. Depression in the Primary Care Setting. *N. Engl. J. Med.* **2019**, *380*, 559–568. [CrossRef] [PubMed]
2. Anxiety and Depression Association of America. Available online: https://adaa.org/understanding-anxiety/depression#Types%20of%20Depression (accessed on 17 August 2020).
3. World Health Organization. Available online: https://www.who.int/publications/i/item/depression-global-health-estimates (accessed on 19 July 2020).
4. Carney, R.M.; Freedland, K.E. Depression and coronary heart disease. *Nat. Rev. Cardiol.* **2017**, *14*, 145–155. [CrossRef] [PubMed]
5. Wang, S.; Mao, S.; Xiang, D.; Fang, C. Association between depression and the subsequent risk of Parkinson's disease: A meta-analysis. *Prog. Neuropsychopharmacol. Biol. Psychiatry* **2018**, *86*, 186–192. [CrossRef]
6. Hidese, S.; Asano, S.; Saito, K.; Sasayama, D.; Kunugi, H. Association of depression with body mass index classification, metabolic disease, and lifestyle: A web-based survey involving 11,876 Japanese people. *J. Psychiatr. Res.* **2018**, *102*, 23–28. [CrossRef] [PubMed]
7. Byers, A.L.; Yaffe, K. Depression and risk of developing dementia. *Nat. Rev. Neurol.* **2011**, *7*, 323–331. [CrossRef]
8. Nouwen, A.; Winkley, K.; Twisk, J.; Lloyd, C.E.; Peyrot, M.; Ismail, K.; Pouwer, F.; European Depression in Diabetes (EDID) Research Consortium. Type 2 diabetes mellitus as a risk factor for the onset of depression: A systematic review and meta-analysis. *Diabetologia* **2010**, *53*, 2480–2486. [CrossRef]
9. Wakefield, C.E.; Butow, P.N.; Aaronson, N.A.; Hack, T.F.; Hulbert-Williams, N.J.; Jacobsen, P.B.; International Psycho-Oncology Society Research Committee. Patient-reported depression measures in cancer: A meta-review. *Lancet Psychiatry* **2015**, *2*, 635–647. [CrossRef]
10. Rehm, J.; Shield, K.D. Global Burden of Disease and the Impact of Mental and Addictive Disorders. *Curr. Psychiatry Rep.* **2019**, *21*, 10. [CrossRef]

11. Li, Z.; Wang, W.; Xin, X.; Song, X.; Zhang, D. Association of total zinc, iron, copper and selenium intakes with depression in the US adults. *J. Affect. Disord.* **2018**, *228*, 68–74. [CrossRef] [PubMed]

12. Nakamura, M.; Miura, A.; Nagahata, T.; Shibata, Y.; Okada, E.; Ojima, T. Low Zinc, Copper, and Manganese Intake is Associated with Depression and Anxiety Symptoms in the Japanese Working Population: Findings from the Eating Habit and Well-Being Study. *Nutrients* **2019**, *11*, 847. [CrossRef]

13. Sánchez-Villegas, A.; Álvarez-Pérez, J.; Toledo, E.; Salas-Salvadó, J.; Ortega-Azorín, C.; Zomeño, M.D.; Vioque, J.; Martínez, J.A.; Romaguera, D.; Pérez-López, J.; et al. Seafood Consumption, Omega-3 Fatty Acids Intake, and Life-Time Prevalence of Depression in the PREDIMED-Plus Trial. *Nutrients* **2018**, *10*, 2000. [CrossRef] [PubMed]

14. Anglin, R.E.; Samaan, Z.; Walter, S.D.; McDonald, S.D. Vitamin D deficiency and depression in adults: Systematic review and meta-analysis. *Br. J. Psychiatry* **2013**, *202*, 100–107. [CrossRef] [PubMed]

15. Perez-Cornago, A.; Sanchez-Villegas, A.; Bes-Rastrollo, M.; Gea, A.; Molero, P.; Lahortiga-Ramos, F.; Martinez-Gonzalez, M.Á. Relationship between adherence to Dietary Approaches to Stop Hypertension (DASH) diet indices and incidence of depression during up to 8 years of follow-up. *Public Health Nutr.* **2017**, *20*, 2383–2392. [CrossRef] [PubMed]

16. Cherian, L.; Wang, Y.; Holland, T.; Agarwal, P.; Aggarwal, N.; Morris, M.C. DASH and Mediterranean-Dash Intervention for Neurodegenerative Delay (MIND) Diets are Associated with Fewer Depressive Symptoms Over Time. *J. Gerontol. A Biol. Sci. Med. Sci.* **2020**. [CrossRef]

17. Fresán, U.; Bes-Rastrollo, M.; Segovia-Siapco, G.; Sanchez-Villegas, A.; Lahortiga, F.; de la Rosa, P.A.; Martínez-Gonzalez, M.A. Does the MIND diet decrease depression risk? A comparison with Mediterranean diet in the SUN cohort. *Eur. J. Nutr.* **2019**, *58*, 1271–1282. [CrossRef]

18. National Health and Nutrition Examination Survey. Available online: https://www.cdc.gov/nchs/nhanes/about_nhanes.htm (accessed on 15 June 2020).

19. *Nutrition and Your Health: 2015–2020 Dietary Guidelines for Americans*, 8th ed.; US Government Printing Office: Washington, DC, USA, 2015. Available online: https://health.gov/our-work/food-nutrition/previous-dietary-guidelines/2015 (accessed on 20 May 2020).

20. Krebs-Smith, S.M.; Pannucci, T.E.; Subar, A.F.; Kirkpatrick, S.I.; Lerman, J.L.; Tooze, J.A.; Wilson, M.M.; Reedy, J.; Reedy, J. Update of the Healthy Eating Index: HEI-2015. *J. Am. Acad. Nutr. Diet.* **2018**, *118*, 1591–1602. [CrossRef]

21. Cruz, N.; Shabaneh, O.; Appiah, D. The Association of Ideal Cardiovascular Health and Ocular Diseases among U.S Adults. *Am. J. Med.* **2020**. [CrossRef]

22. Kroenke, K.; Spitzer, R.L.; Williams, J.B. The PHQ-9: Validity of a brief depression severity measure. *J. Gen. Intern. Med.* **2001**, *16*, 606–613. [CrossRef]

23. Tsai, J.; Homa, D.M.; Gentzke, A.S.; Mahoney, M.; Sharapova, S.R.; Sosnoff, C.S.; Caron, K.T.; Wang, L.; Melstrom, P.C.; Trivers, K.F. Exposure to Secondhand Smoke Among Nonsmokers—United States, 1988–2014. *MMWR Morb. Mortal. Wkly. Rep.* **2018**, *67*, 1342–1346. [CrossRef]

24. Scholes, S.; Bann, D. Education-related disparities in reported physical activity during leisure-time, active transportation, and work among US adults: Repeated cross-sectional analysis from the National Health and Nutrition Examination Surveys, 2007 to 2016. *BMC Public Health* **2018**, *18*, 926. [CrossRef]

25. Montgomery, J.; Lu, J.; Ratliff, S.; Mezuk, B. Food Insecurity and Depression among Adults with Diabetes: Results from the National Health and Nutrition Examination Survey (NHANES). *Diabetes Educ.* **2017**, *43*, 260–271. [CrossRef] [PubMed]

26. Dreimüller, N.; Lieb, K.; Tadić, A.; Engelmann, J.; Wollschläger, D.; Wagner, S. Body mass index (BMI) in major depressive disorder and its effects on depressive symptomatology and antidepressant response. *J. Affect. Disord.* **2019**, *256*, 524–531. [CrossRef] [PubMed]

27. ALHarthi, S.S.Y.; Natto, Z.S.; Midle, J.B.; Gyurko, R.; O'Neill, R.; Steffensen, B. Association between time since quitting smoking and periodontitis in former smokers in the National Health and Nutrition Examination Surveys (NHANES) 2009 to 2012. *J. Periodontol.* **2019**, *90*, 16–25. [CrossRef] [PubMed]

28. Gay Isabel, C.; Tran Duong, T.; Paquette David, W. Alcohol intake and periodontitis in adults aged ≥30 years: NHANES 2009–2012. *J. Periodontol.* **2018**, *89*, 625–634.

29. Caspard, H.; Jabbour, S.; Hammar, N.; Fenici, P.; Sheehan, J.J.; Kosiborod, M. Recent trends in the prevalence of type 2 diabetes and the association with abdominal obesity lead to growing health disparities in the USA: An analysis of the NHANES surveys from 1999 to 2014. *Diabetes Obes. Metab.* **2018**, *20*, 667–671. [CrossRef] [PubMed]

30. Rao, J.N.K.; Scott, A.J. On Simple Adjustments to Chi-Square Tests with Sample Survey Data. *Ann. Stat.* **1987**, *15*, 385–397. [CrossRef]

31. Salk, R.H.; Hyde, J.S.; Abramson, L.Y. Gender differences in depression in representative national samples: Meta-analyses of diagnoses and symptoms. *Psychol. Bull.* **2017**, *143*, 783–822. [CrossRef]

32. Culbertson, F.M. Depression and gender. An international review. *Am. Psychol.* **1997**, *52*, 25–31. [CrossRef]

33. Fletcher, J.M. Adolescent depression and educational attainment: Results using sibling fixed effects. *Health Econ.* **2010**, *19*, 855–871. [CrossRef]

34. Korhonen, K.; Remes, H.; Martikainen, P. Education as a social pathway from parental socioeconomic position to depression in late adolescence and early adulthood: A Finnish population-based register study. *Soc. Psychiatry Psychiatr. Epidemiol.* **2017**, *52*, 105–116. [CrossRef]

35. Freeman, A.; Tyrovolas, S.; Koyanagi, A.; Chatterji, S.; Leonardi, M.; Ayuso-Mateos, J.L.; Tobiasz-Adamczyk, B.; Koskinen, S.; Rummel-Kluge, C.; Haro, J.M. The role of socio-economic status in depression: Results from the COURAGE (aging survey in Europe). *BMC Public Health* **2016**, *16*, 1098. [CrossRef] [PubMed]

36. Çakıcı, M.; Gökçe, Ö.; Babayiğit, A.; Çakıcı, E.; Eş, A. Depression: Point-prevalence and risk factors in a North Cyprus household adult cross-sectional study. *BMC Psychiatry* **2017**, *17*, 387. [CrossRef] [PubMed]

37. Gero, K.; Kondo, K.; Kondo, N.; Shirai, K.; Kawachi, I. Associations of relative deprivation and income rank with depressive symptoms among older adults in Japan. *Soc. Sci. Med.* **2017**, *189*, 138–144. [CrossRef] [PubMed]

38. Fukuda, Y.; Hiyoshi, A. Influences of income and employment on psychological distress and depression treatment in Japanese adults. *Environ. Health Prev. Med.* **2012**, *17*, 10–17. [CrossRef]

39. Tomita, A.; Manuel, J.I. Evidence on the Association Between Cigarette Smoking and Incident Depression from the South African National Income Dynamics Study 2008–2015: Mental Health Implications for a Resource-Limited Setting. *Nicotine Tob. Res.* **2020**, *22*, 118–123. [CrossRef]

40. Luger, T.M.; Suls, J.; Vander Weg, M.W. How robust is the association between smoking and depression in adults? A meta-analysis using linear mixed-effects models. *Addict. Behav.* **2014**, *39*, 1418–1429. [CrossRef]

41. Tjora, T.; Hetland, J.; Aarø, L.E.; Wold, B.; Wiium, N.; Øverland, S. The association between smoking and depression from adolescence to adulthood. *Addiction* **2014**, *109*, 1022–1030. [CrossRef]

42. Shafer, K.; Pace, G.T. Gender differences in depression across parental roles. *Soc. Work* **2015**, *60*, 115–125. [CrossRef]

43. Ul-Haq, Z.; Mackay, D.F.; Fenwick, E.; Pell, J.P. Association between body mass index and mental health among Scottish adult population: A cross-sectional study of 37,272 participants. *Psychol. Med.* **2014**, *44*, 2231–2240. [CrossRef]

44. Bagnardi, V.; Rota, M.; Botteri, E.; Tramacere, I.; Islami, F.; Fedirko, V.; Scotti, L.; Jenab, M.; Turati, F.; Pasquali, E.; et al. Light alcohol drinking and cancer: A meta-analysis. *Ann. Oncol.* **2013**, *24*, 301–308. [CrossRef]

45. Xu, W.; Wang, H.; Wan, Y.; Tan, C.; Li, J.; Tan, L.; Yu, J.T. Alcohol consumption and dementia risk: A dose-response meta-analysis of prospective studies. *Eur. J. Epidemiol.* **2017**, *32*, 31–42. [CrossRef] [PubMed]

46. Larsson, S.C.; Wallin, A.; Wolk, A. Alcohol consumption and risk of heart failure: Meta-analysis of 13 prospective studies. *Clin. Nutr.* **2018**, *37*, 1247–1251. [CrossRef] [PubMed]

47. Larsson, S.C.; Wallin, A.; Wolk, A.; Markus, H.S. Differing association of alcohol consumption with different stroke types: A systematic review and meta-analysis. *BMC Med.* **2016**, *14*, 178. [CrossRef] [PubMed]

48. Knott, C.; Bell, S.; Britton, A. Alcohol Consumption and the Risk of Type 2 Diabetes: A Systematic Review and Dose-Response Meta-analysis of More Than 1.9 Million Individuals from 38 Observational Studies. *Diabetes Care* **2015**, *38*, 1804–1812. [CrossRef] [PubMed]

49. Xi, B.; Veeranki, S.P.; Zhao, M.; Ma, C.; Yan, Y.; Mi, J. Relationship of Alcohol Consumption to All-Cause, Cardiovascular, and Cancer-Related Mortality in U.S. Adults. *J. Am. Coll. Cardiol.* **2017**, *70*, 913–922, Erratum in: *J. Am. Coll. Cardiol.* **2017**, *70*, 1542. [CrossRef] [PubMed]

50. Alati, R.; Lawlor, D.A.; Najman, J.M.; Williams, G.M.; Bor, W.; O'Callaghan, M. Is there really a 'J-shaped' curve in the association between alcohol consumption and symptoms of depression and anxiety? Findings from the Mater-University Study of Pregnancy and its outcomes. *Addiction* **2005**, *100*, 643–651. [CrossRef]

51. Korczak, D.J.; Madigan, S.; Colasanto, M. Children's Physical Activity and Depression: A Meta-analysis. *Pediatrics* **2017**, *139*, e20162266. [CrossRef]

52. Kandola, A.; Ashdown-Franks, G.; Hendrikse, J.; Sabiston, C.M.; Stubbs, B. Physical activity and depression: Towards understanding the antidepressant mechanisms of physical activity. *Neurosci. Biobehav. Rev.* **2019**, *107*, 525–539. [CrossRef]

53. Choi, K.W.; Chen, C.Y.; Stein, M.B.; Klimentidis, Y.C.; Wang, M.J.; Koenen, K.C.; Smoller, J.W.; Major Depressive Disorder Working Group of the Psychiatric Genomics Consortium. Assessment of Bidirectional Relationships between Physical Activity and Depression among Adults: A 2-Sample Mendelian Randomization Study. *JAMA Psychiatry* **2019**, *76*, 399–408. [CrossRef]

54. Kvam, S.; Kleppe, C.L.; Nordhus, I.H.; Hovland, A. Exercise as a treatment for depression: A meta-analysis. *J. Affect. Disord.* **2016**, *202*, 67–86. [CrossRef]

55. Ley, S.H.; Hamdy, O.; Mohan, V.; Hu, F.B. Prevention and management of type 2 diabetes: Dietary components and nutritional strategies. *Lancet* **2014**, *383*, 1999–2007. [CrossRef]

56. Ley, S.H.; Pan, A.; Li, Y.; Manson, J.E.; Willett, W.C.; Sun, Q.; Hu, F.B. Changes in Overall Diet Quality and Subsequent Type 2 Diabetes Risk: Three U.S. Prospective Cohorts. *Diabetes Care* **2016**, *39*, 2011–2018. [CrossRef] [PubMed]

57. Anderson, R.J.; Freedland, K.E.; Clouse, R.E.; Lustman, P.J. The prevalence of comorbid depression in adults with diabetes: A meta-analysis. *Diabetes Care* **2001**, *24*, 1069–1078. [CrossRef] [PubMed]

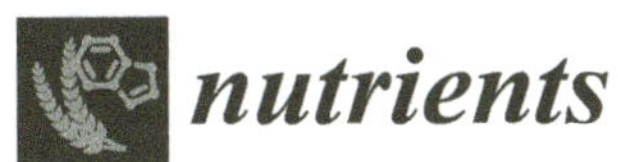 *nutrients* 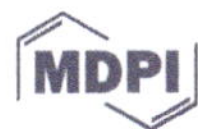

Article

DNA Methylation Profiles of Vegans and Non-Vegetarians in the Adventist Health Study-2 Cohort

Fayth L. Miles [1,2,3,4], Andrew Mashchak [1], Valery Filippov [4], Michael J. Orlich [1,2,5], Penelope Duerksen-Hughes [4], Xin Chen [4,6], Charles Wang [4,6], Kimberly Siegmund [7] and Gary E. Fraser [1,2,5,*]

1   Adventist Health Study, Loma Linda University, Loma Linda, CA 92350, USA; fmiles@llu.edu (F.L.M.); amashchak@llu.edu (A.M.); morlich@llu.edu (M.J.O.)
2   Center for Nutrition, Healthy Lifestyle, and Disease Prevention, School of Public Health, Loma Linda University, Loma Linda, CA 92350, USA
3   Department of Preventive Medicine, School of Medicine, Loma Linda University, Loma Linda, CA 92350, USA
4   Department of Basic Sciences, School of Medicine, Loma Linda University, Loma Linda, CA 92350, USA; vfilippov@llu.edu (V.F.); pdhughes@llu.edu (P.D.-H.); xchen@llu.edu (X.C.); chwang@llu.edu (C.W.)
5   Department of Medicine, School of Medicine, Loma Linda University, Loma Linda, CA 92350, USA
6   Center for Genomics, School of Medicine, Loma Linda University, Loma Linda, CA 92350, USA
7   Department of Preventive Medicine, Keck School of Medicine of the University of Southern California, Los Angeles, CA 90033, USA; kims@usc.edu
*   Correspondence: gfraser@llu.edu; Tel.: +1-(909)-558-4753

Received: 15 October 2020; Accepted: 23 November 2020; Published: 30 November 2020

Abstract: We sought to determine if DNA methylation patterns differed between vegans and non-vegetarians in the Adventist Health Study-2 cohort. Genome-wide DNA methylation derived from buffy coat was profiled in 62 vegans and 142 non-vegetarians. Using linear regression, methylation of CpG sites and genes was categorized or summarized according to various genic/intergenic regions and CpG island-related regions, as well as the promoter. Methylation of genes was measured as the average methylation of available CpG's annotated to the nominated region of the respective gene. A permutation method defining the null distribution adapted from Storey et al. was used to adjust for false discovery. Differences in methylation of several CpG sites and genes were detected at a false discovery rate < 0.05 in region-specific and overall analyses. A vegan diet was associated predominantly with hypomethylation of genes, most notably methyltransferase-like 1 (*METTL1*). Although a limited number of differentially methylated features were detected in the current study, the false discovery method revealed that a much larger proportion of differentially methylated genes and sites exist, and could be detected with a larger sample size. Our findings suggest modest differences in DNA methylation in vegans and non-vegetarians, with a much greater number of detectable significant differences expected with a larger sample.

Keywords: DNA methylation; epigenetics; Adventist Health Study-2; vegetarian diet; linear regression; permutation

1. Introduction

Findings from the Adventist Health Study-2 (AHS-2) cohort have been prominent among epidemiologic studies linking a vegetarian dietary pattern to lower risks of diabetes, metabolic syndrome, and coronary heart disease [1–5] as well as lower risks of gastrointestinal and prostate cancers, among others [6–8]. Besides avoiding meat, vegetarians and particularly vegans in this cohort have markedly higher consumption of plant-based foods including fruits, vegetables, whole grains, soy, and nuts, but lower consumption of sweets, snack foods, refined grains, and caloric beverages [9], and healthier profiles of biomarkers of dietary intake, including phytochemicals or bioactive compounds [10] relative to non-vegetarians. However, there is limited understanding of the underlying molecular mechanisms that could help explain the probable ability of vegetarian dietary patterns to prevent chronic diseases, or to buttress causal interpretations.

DNA methylation involves the chemical addition of a methyl group at the 5′ position of a cytosine residue, and may be influenced by diet, among other lifestyle or environmental factors. Such modifications can potentially alter gene expression and the development of chronic, autoimmune, or aging-related diseases [11,12]. Diet may influence gene-specific or global DNA methylation by (1) providing or modifying the availability of methyl donor compounds or cofactors that regulate one-carbon metabolism [13], (2) regulating enzymes that catalyze or reverse methylation, such as DNA methyl transferases (DNMTs) or ten or eleven translocation (TET) enzymes [14,15], and (3) indirectly regulating inflammation or oxidative stress [16]. Vegetarian or plant-based diets are rich in polyphenols and secondary plant metabolites that could inhibit the activity of DNMT to prevent cancer [14,17,18]. On the other hand, diets high in animal-based and fatty foods may generate pro-inflammatory compounds [19–22] and metabolites [15,23] that alter methylation and increase activity of TET enzymes to promote cancer.

Besides specific dietary components, there is some evidence from animal studies and human intervention trials that dietary conditions such as high fat content or caloric restriction may alter genome-wide and gene-specific DNA methylation [24–30]. However, it is not clear how habitual dietary patterns differing in consumption of plant- and animal-based foods differ in terms of DNA methylation patterns. The aim of the current study was to examine genome-wide DNA methylation patterns in long-term vegan and non-vegetarian participants of the AHS-2 cohort to identify differentially methylated genes. Our approach involved a covariate-adjusted analysis of methylation of individual CpG sites, as well as of CpGs annotated to their respective genes (gene methylation), considering various gene regions, and employing an adapted Storey et al. [31,32] permutation method to correct for false discovery.

2. Materials and Methods

2.1. Study Population

Participants in the current study are members of the larger AHS-2 cohort, established in 2002–2007 as a national study of Seventh-day Adventists, about $\frac{1}{2}$ of whom are vegetarian. In this sub-study, 143 participants were Caucasian, and 61 were African-American or Black. Subjects were selected from the AHS-2 biorepository for DNA methylation analyses conducted at three separate times variably balanced by age, sex, diet group, and/or ethnic group. All subjects were pooled for the analyses performed in the current study. Participants were classified a priori into vegetarian diet groups based on their responses to the food frequency questionnaire (FFQ) completed upon enrollment as follows: vegans never or rarely (less than once per month) consumed eggs, dairy, fish and other meats, and non-vegetarians consumed non-fish meats at least once a month and any meat (including but not only fish) more than once per week.

All investigations were carried out following the rules of the Declaration of Helsinki of 1975, revised in 2013. The project was originally approved by the Loma Linda University institutional review board, protocol: 48134.

2.2. Laboratory Analysis and Data Processing

Fasting blood samples were collected at field clinics held in church halls, as described previously [33]. Buffy coat was removed and diluted to a final volume of 8 mL with phosphate buffered saline, then aliquoted into straws and frozen at −180 °C in nitrogen vapor for storage in the AHS-2 biorepository. Genomic DNA from buffy coat samples was isolated using the Quick-gDNA

MiniPrep kit (Zymo Research, Irvine, CA, USA) according to the manufacturer's protocol. After bisulfite sequencing, genome-wide methylation analysis was performed using the Infinium MethylationEPIC (n = 67) and HumanMethylation450 BeadChip (n = 137) arrays at the University of California, Los Angeles Neuroscience Genomics Core. Raw data were summarized into BeadStudio IDAT files for further analysis.

Methylation data were processed using R version 3.6.1. Initial preprocessing and normalization procedures were conducted using the minfi package in R [34]. Raw data generated from methylation analysis were normalized with the single-sample normal-exponential out-of-band (ssNoob) method as recommended by Fortin (2017) for combined 450 k and EPIC datasets. Probes were excluded that were cross-reactive, within 10 bp of single nucleotide polymorphisms (SNPs) [35,36], or present on X/Y chromosomes. Furthermore, CpG probes with bead counts less than 3 in more than 2% of samples or detection p values above 0.01 in more than 1% samples were excluded. After these normalization and processing steps, 313,206 CpG sites (common to both BeadChip arrays) remained for analysis.

As an additional layer of control and primarily to adjust for unwanted variation including batch, chip, positional, cell heterogeneity, and study effects, a surrogate variable analysis was used from the SmartSVA R package. With this method, influential principal components of residuals from regressions of CpG methylation on dietary groups are converted into surrogate variables, and subsequently included in final regression models, thereby accounting for unwanted variation from other sources of "error" [37].

2.3. Statistical Analyses

DNA methylation β values were obtained from the BeadChip array, representing the methylation frequency within an individual sample (ratio of methylated signal divided by the sum of methylated and unmethylated signals) for each target CpG or gene ranging from 0 (not methylated) to 1 (fully methylated). Subsequently the log2 ratio of the methylated to unmethylated signal was calculated to obtain M values. Using SmartSVA (39), surrogate variables were created from regression residuals conditional on covariates, age (continuous), sex (male, female), ethnic group (Black, Caucasian), and body mass index (BMI; continuous). To examine the association between dietary pattern and DNA methylation, a linear model was then fitted where the response variable was the residual when the M values were regressed on these covariates (except BMI) and the surrogate variables [38]. This represents non-BMI covariate-adjusted methylation levels for individual CpG sites [39], or the average of covariate-adjusted methylation level for CpGs associated with each gene. The independent variable came from residuals when dietary pattern was regressed on these same covariates, this then representing covariate-adjusted dietary pattern. Body mass index was not included as a covariate, given that it may be a mediator in some cases between diet and CpG methylation.

For comparison, separate linear regression models were fitted excluding the SmartSVA method, where models were additionally adjusted for position on the BeadChip (n = 8 rows), the original sub-study (n = 3) along with array (450 K, 800 K), and cell type heterogeneity (CD8T, CD4T, NK, Bcell Mono, Gran) using the approach of Houseman et al. [38].

CpG sites were associated with genes by calculating an unweighted average of covariate-adjusted M values of all CpG sites in the dataset that were annotated to the gene of interest and in the nominated gene region, where applicable. When analyzing a particular region, genes were only included where at least two CpG sites were available in that region. Thus, besides analyzing methylation of all represented sites, or average methylation across a gene, methylation was also analyzed according to 1) genic/intergenic region (200 or 1500 base pairs upstream of the transcription start site (TSS200 and TSS1500, respectively), the 5′ untranslated region (UTR), first exon, gene body, 3′ UTR, and intergenic regions, 2) in relation to CpG islands (CpG island, north shore, south shore, north shelf, south shelf, and open sea regions), and 3) in the promoter, including CpG islands within the promoter.

An adapted permutation-identified null distribution (Storey et al. method, references 31, 32) was used to adjust for multiple comparisons to avoid the risk of severe false discovery. The measure of

DNA methylation differences by diet pattern for each CpG site or gene is the corresponding partial t statistic for each CpG site, and for genes a joint t statistic averaging multivariable-adjusted methylation status across relevant CpGs in a particular gene. The permutation method was used to define the null distribution of the t scores for CpG sites. Then for genes, in separate analyses, all CpG sites in a nominated region relevant to that gene were used in the averaging process, not only the CpG sites that were previously statistically significant. To adjust for covariates when planning a permutation approach, the residual method was used as has been recommended [40], this being applied to both the independent variables aside from diet (the exposure of interest) and the dependent variable as described above. This reduces the independent variables to one for permutation, which already takes account of covariances between the covariates. Covariances between the residualized dependent M values are retained as these dependent variables are not permuted. Recognizing that the real data are a mixture of null and non-null methylation sites/genes, an estimate of the proportion of null features allows a direct estimate of the false discovery rate (FDR) [32], and hence the more useful selection of only those with small FDR. The method also allows an estimate of the number of all differentially methylated sites/genes [31,32]), although only a proportion can be individually identified with acceptable FDR in this relatively small dataset. All statistical analyses were performed with R software.

3. Results

3.1. Methylation Differences in Vegans and Non-Vegetarians

Demographic characteristics of study participants are shown in Table 1. There were no statistically significant differences in the distribution of males and females, or in age, comparing vegans and non-vegetarians. As expected, vegans had lower BMI relative to non-vegetarians (24.3 vs. 28.0; $p < 0.001$). This was viewed as a potentially mediating variable in statistical analyses.

Table 1. Demographic characteristics of study population [1].

	Vegan	**Non-Vegetarian**	*p*
Participants (*n*)	62	142	
Sex (%)			0.57
Male	30 (48.4)	61 (43)	
Female	32 (51.6)	81 (57.0)	
Age (years)	67.3 (9.0)	65.9 (8.4)	0.28
BMI (kg/m^2)	24.3 (4.6)	28 (5.1)	<0.001
Ethnicity (%)			0.50
Caucasian	46 (74.2)	97 (68.3)	
Black	16 (25.8)	45 (31.7)	

[1] Values presented as mean (SD) or as *n* (%) where indicated.

For this study, we compared methylation of individual CpG sites and genes in vegans relative to non-vegetarians, dividing CpG sites into separate categories defined by gene region, namely, genic/intergenic, relation to CpG islands, and promoter regions.

3.1.1. Differential Methylation of Select Regions Associated with Individual Genes

1. Proportions of Differentially Methylated Gene Regions

There were greater proportions of genes with at least two probes in a related CpG island (74%) or TSS1500 (72%) region, followed by those with sites in the gene body (65%) (Table 2). The majority of differentially methylated genes were hypomethylated in vegans. When differential methylation was analyzed after averaging CpG methylation across an entire gene, within each of the 18,627 genes (i.e., labelled "All") represented on the array and in our analytical dataset, a total of 18 genes (4 hypermethylated, 14 hypomethylated) were found to be differentially methylated after adjustment for false discovery (Table 2). When differential methylation was analyzed according to methylation of genic/intergenic regions, 21 genes (including three identified in the analysis of overall gene methylation, "All") showed differential methylation in the gene body, representing the most differentially methylated genes for any region. Identifying a central linear region of a plot of cumulative probabilities of the null vs. actual distributions of t scores (adaptation of methods in references [31,32]) revealed that an estimated 1081 (6%) of the 18,627 genes analyzed are non-null (Table 2 and Appendix A), although the majority of these cannot be specifically identified here. The greatest proportion of estimated non-null genes relative to the respective total number of genes for methylation of a given region were genes defined by methylation of the gene body (9%, see Figure A1 of Appendix A), with relatively high proportions also noted when defined by methylation of the TSS1500 (7%), north shelf (7%), and open sea (7%) regions. As only t-scores of non-null sites will systematically increase (in absolute value) as sample sizes increase, it is possible to estimate the effects of larger sample size on the proportion of differentially methylated genes that could then be identified (Appendix A). With increasing sample size, the number of differentially methylated genes comparing vegans with non-vegetarians steadily increases (Table 3). Fewer differentially methylated genes were observed with exclusion of surrogate variables (SmartSVA) from the analytical approach (Supplementary Table S1), although greater numbers of differentially methylated CpG sites than genes (observed and non-null) were noted in analyses excluding surrogate variables (Supplementary Table S2).

2.   Unique Genes Showing Differential Methylation

Methyltransferase-like 1 (*METTL1*) was significantly and consistently hypomethylated in vegans in both analyses of promoter methylation (62,398 CpG sites distributed among 9131 genes) and overall methylation of all genes present on the array and in our analytical set (313,161 CpG sites distributed among 18,627 genes), this with either the inclusion of SmartSVA (Tables 4 and 5) or the exclusion of surrogate variables from models (Supplementary Tables S3 and S4). Other genes that were significantly hypomethylated in the promoter regions in analyses both with and without surrogate variables included *ribosomal protein L38* (*RPL38*), *snurportin 1* (*SNUPN*), FLVCR heme transporter 2 (*FLVCR2*), and *CKLF-like MARVEL transmembrane domain containing 7* (*CMTM7*). Two genes, *METTL1* and *nei-like DNA glycosylase 2* (*NEIL2*), were significantly hypomethylated in CpG islands within the promoter, in analyses with and without SmartSVA (Table 5 and Supplementary Table S4). Besides *METTL1*, genes showing differential methylation in analyses of both promoter methylation and overall methylation of all genes included *RPL38* (SmartSVA analysis) (Tables 4 and 5), and *FLVCR2* (analysis excluding SmartSVA) (Supplementary Tables S3 and S4). Differential methylation of *D-dopachrome tautomerase-like* (*DDTL*) and *aryl hydrocarbon receptor nuclear translocator 2* (*ARNT2*) was observed in analyses of genes defined by methylation of the gene body, as well as of all genes (SmartSVA analysis, Table 4), and the same was true for *LIM homeobox protein 3* (*LHX3*) in models excluding surrogate variables (Supplementary Table S3). *Glutathione S-transferase theta pseudogene 1* (*GSTTP1*), detected in analysis of the open sea region showed the most marked hypomethylation in vegans (fold change of 0.72 and 0.76 in models with and without SmartSVA, respectively), whereas NACHT and WD repeat domain containing 2 (NWD2), identified in analysis of methylation of the south shore region, showed the greatest increase in gene methylation (fold change, 1.12) (Table 5 and Supplementary Table S4).

Table 2. Estimated non-null and observed differentially methylated genes (false discovery rate < 0.05) summarized according to gene region or in relation to CpG islands comparing vegans with non-vegetarians [1].

Region [2]	Total Genes		Estimated Non-Null		Significantly Hypermethylated		Significantly Hypomethylated	
	n	% of All Genes	n [3]	% of Region-Specific Total	n	Fold Change [4]	n	Fold Change [4]
All	18,627	100	1081	5.8	4	1.02	14	0.97
Genic/intergenic								
TSS200	10,008	53.7	388	3.9	4	1.03	4	0.96
TSS1500	13,373	71.8	954	7.1	2	1.03	7	0.97
3′ UTR	1935	10.4	55	2.8	1	1.04	2	0.98
5′ UTR	7686	41.3	475	6.2	2	1.02	6	
Gene Body	12,072	64.8	1100	9.1	7	1.03	14	0.97
1st Exon	6262	33.6	405	6.5	1	1.07	9	0.97
Intergenic	8049	43.2	449	5.6	1	1.05	7	0.97
Island-related								
CpG Island	13,688	73.5	649	4.7	4	1.03	2	0.97
North Shelf	2562	13.8	180	7.0	2	1.03	2	0.97
North Shore	8315	44.6	424	5.1	1	1.03	7	0.96
South Shelf	2278	12.2	146	6.4	3	1.04	7	0.97
South Shore	7137	38.3	441	6.2	5	1.06	7	0.96
Open Sea	11,884	63.8	798	6.7	2	1.04	14	0.96
Promoter								
All	9131	49.0	459	5.0	2	1.05	9	0.98
CpG Island	7693	41.3	60	0.8	1	1.02	2	0.97

[1] Number of actual differentially methylated genes determined using linear regression with SmartSVA followed by adapted Storey et al. [32] permutation approach to adjust for false discovery. [2] Individual CpGs may have been represented in more than one region when determining gene methylation of a given region. [3] Number of genes estimated to show non-null differences in methylation. [4] Fold change represents ratio of the mean methylation of vegans to that of non-vegetarians for differentially methylated (hypomethylated or hypermethylated) genes in a given region. This is averaged across significant genes.

Table 3. Numbers of genes expected to be detected with FDR < 0.05 as differentially methylated in vegans relative to non-vegetarians [1].

Region	Fold Increase in Sample Size—Hypomethylated Genes						Fold Increase in Sample Size—Hypermethylated Genes					
	1	1.5	2	3	4	5	1	1.5	2	3	4	5
All	14	28	42	66	79	86	4	29	103	266	377	456
Body	14	23	37	58	68	91	7	17	65	159	254	309
TSS1500	7	7	24	31	43	49	2	25	108	254	350	411
TSS200	4	4	4	12	19	19	4	9	44	141	203	254
3′ UTR	2	2	2	2	2	2	1	1	10	30	47	57
5′ UTR	6	6	12	17	26	28	2	15	47	122	172	226
1st Exon	9	10	23	33	37	43	1	10	45	96	142	169
Island	2	2	12	26	27	33	4	27	98	243	336	397
North Shore	7	7	12	23	24	28	1	8	47	144	222	260
South Shore	7	7	16	24	31	36	5	19	60	124	175	229
North Shelf	2	2	2	7	7	7	2	4	17	46	69	83
South Shelf	7	7	7	7	7	7	3	9	21	39	59	71
Promoter Associated	9	9	12	16	17	20	2	12	62	145	214	250
Promoter and CpG Island	2	2	2	5	10	13	1	8	45	112	161	201
Open Sea	14	20	28	44	58	61	2	11	61	144	218	256
Intergenic	7	8	19	30	40	51	1	7	40	101	154	185

[1] Number of differentially methylated genes determined by adapted Storey et al. [32] based on plots of cumulative distributions of p values (derived from t statistics) from real and hypothetical null data.

Table 4. Differential methylation of genic/intergenic regions associated with individual genes at FDR < 0.05 (based on SmartSVA method) [1].

Gene ID	Gene Symbol	Description	Fold Change
TSS200			
341,350	OVCH1 (1)	ovochymase 1	0.93
8499	PPFIA2	PTPRF interacting protein alpha 2	0.96
51,099	ABHD5	abhydrolase domain containing 5, lysophosphatidic acid acyltransferase	0.98
51,205	ACP6	acid phosphatase 6, lysophosphatidic	0.98
9874	TLK1	tousled-like kinase 1	1.02
10,440	TIMM17A	translocase of inner mitochondrial membrane 17A	1.02
1132	CHRM4	cholinergic receptor, muscarinic 4	1.03
9570	GOSR2	lgi SNAP receptor complex member 2	1.03
TSS1500			
151,313	FAHD2B	fumarylacetoacetate hydrolase domain containing 2B	0.95
10,653	SPINT2	serine peptidase inhibitor, Kunitz type 2	0.96
100,302,640	LINC00882	Long Intergenic Non-Protein Coding RNA 882	0.96
84,838	ZNF496 (1)	zinc finger protein 496	0.96
4234	METTL1	methyltransferase-like 1	0.98
9054	NFS1	NFS1 cysteine desulfurase	0.98
1263	PLK3	polo-like kinase 3	0.98
8546	AP3B1	adaptor-related protein complex 3 subunit beta 1	1.02
11,267	SNF8	SNF8 subunit of ESCRT-II	1.04
3′ UTR			
79,960	JADE1	jade family PHD finger 1	0.97
667	DST	dystonin	0.98
54,820	NDE1	nudE neurodevelopment protein 1	1.04
5′ UTR			
252,969	NEIL2	nei-like DNA glycosylase 2	0.96
4147	MATN2	matrilin 2	0.97
5928	RBBP4	RB binding protein 4, chromatin remodeling factor	0.97
3792	KEL	Kell metallo-endopeptidase (Kell blood group)	0.97
9772	TMEM94	transmembrane protein 94	0.98
63,924	CIDEC	cell death-inducing DFFA-like effector c	0.99
51,465	UBE2J1	ubiquitin conjugating enzyme E2 J1	1.02
1374	CPT1A	carnitine palmitoyltransferase 1A	1.03
Body			
100,037,417	DDTL	D-dopachrome decarboxylase-like protein	0.92
154,007	SNRNP48	small nuclear ribonucleoprotein U11/U12 subunit 48	0.95
8120	AP3B2	adaptor-related protein complex 3 subunit beta 2	0.96
89,781	HPS4	HPS4, biogenesis of lysosomal organelles complex 3 subunit 2	0.96
2668	GDNF	glial cell line derived neurotrophic factor	0.96
56,666	PANX2	pannexin 2	0.97
91,010	FMNL3	formin-like 3	0.98
117,246	FTSJ3	FtsJ RNA 2′-O-methyltransferase 3	0.98
11,052	CPSF6	cleavage and polyadenylation-specific factor 6	0.98
149,297	FAM78B	family with sequence similarity 78 member B	0.98
399,671	HEATR4	HEAT repeat containing 4	0.98
285,987	DLX6-AS1	DLX6 antisense RNA 1	0.99
64,784	CRTC3	CREB regulated transcription coactivator 3	0.99
5361	PLXA1	plexin A1	0.99
Body			
9915	ARNT2	aryl hydrocarbon receptor nuclear translocator 2	1.02
5170	PDPK1	3-phosphoinositide dependent protein kinase 1	1.02
10,610	ST6GALNAC2	ST6 N-acetylgalactosaminide alpha-2,6-sialyltransferase 2	1.02
57,459	GATAD2B	GATA zinc finger domain containing 2B	1.03
3694	ITGB6	integrin subunit beta 6	1.04
58	ACTA1	actin alpha 1, skeletal muscle	1.05
9963	SLC23A1	solute carrier family 23 member 2	1.06
First Exon			
2201	FBN2	fibrillin 2	0.96
100,303,453	TSNAX-DISC1	Disrupted in schizophrenia 1 isoform 51	0.96
10,274	STAG1	stromal antigen 1	0.97
252,969	NEIL2	nei-like DNA glycosylase 2	0.97
3489	IGFBP6	insulin-like growth factor binding protein 6	0.97

Table 4. *Cont.*

Gene ID	Gene Symbol	Description	Fold Change
5928	RBBP4	RB binding protein 4, chromatin remodeling factor	0.97
6727	SRP14	signal recognition particle 14	0.97
9167	COX7A2L (1)	cytochrome c oxidase subunit 7A2-like	0.97
1802	DPH2(1)	diphthamide biosynthesis 2	0.98
23,336	SYNM	Synemin	1.07
All			
100,037,417	DDTL	D-dopachrome tautomerase-like	0.95
284,680	SPATA46	spermatogenesis associated 46	0.96
100,113,403	LIN28B-AS1	LIN28B antisense RNA 1	0.96
64,220	STRA6	signaling receptor and transporter of retinol STRA6	0.97
4234	METTL1	methyltransferase-like 1	0.97
27,179	IL36A	interleukin 36 alpha	0.98
90,379	DCAF15	DDB1 and CUL4 associated factor 15	0.98
89,781	HPS4	HPS4, biogenesis of lysosomal organelles complex 3 subunit 2	0.98
136,371	ASB10	ankyrin repeat and SOCS box containing 10	0.98
397	ARHGDIB	Rho GDP dissociation inhibitor beta	0.98
6169	RPL38	ribosomal protein L38	0.98
55,222	LRRC20	leucine rich repeat containing 20	0.99
9491	PSMF1	proteasome inhibitor subunit 1	0.99
154,150	HDGFL1	HDGF-like 1	0.99
9915	ARNT2	aryl hydrocarbon receptor nuclear translocator 2	1.02
219,990	OOSP2	oocyte secreted protein 2	1.02
114,757	CYGB	cytoglobin	1.02
7284	TUFM	Tu translation elongation factor, mitochondrial	1.02
Intergenic			
136,371	ASB10	Ankyrin repeat and SOCS box protein 10	0.95
100,113,403	LIN28B-AS1	LIN28B antisense RNA 1	0.96
23,704	KCNE4	Potassium voltage-gated channel subfamily E member 4	0.97
27,319	BHLHE22	Class E basic helix-loop-helix protein 22	0.97
9935	MAFB	Transcription factor MafB	0.98
7100	TLR5	Toll-like receptor 5	0.98
154,150	HDGFL1	Hepatoma-derived growth factor-like protein 1	0.99
284,889	MIF-AS1	MIF antisense RNA	1.05

[1] Number of differentially methylated CpG sites associated with each gene shown in brackets.

Table 5. Differential methylation of island-related and promoter regions associated with individual genes at FDR < 0.05 (based on SmartSVA method) [1].

Gene ID	Gene Symbol	Description	Fold Change
Island			
80,070	ADAMTS20	ADAM metallopeptidase with thrombospondin type 1 motif 20	0.95
101,409,261	OGFR-AS1	OGFR Antisense RNA 1	0.98
4609	MYC	MYC proto-oncogene	1.01
161,145	TMEM229B	transmembrane protein 229B	1.02
7284	TUFM	Tu translation elongation factor, mitochondrial	1.04
273	AMPH	amphiphysin	1.05
North Shelf			
4000	LMNA	lamin A/C	0.97
123,041	SLC24A4	solute carrier family 24 member 4	0.97
100,534,592	URGCP-MRPS24	URGCP-MRPS24 readthrough	1.02
116,844	LRG1	leucine rich alpha-2-glycoprotein 1	1.04
North Shore			
8022	LHX3	LIM homeobox protein 3	0.92
10,653	SPINT2	serine peptidase inhibitor, Kunitz type 2	0.95
6169	RPL38	ribosomal protein L38	0.96
23,200	ATP11B	Probable phospholipid-transporting ATPase IF	0.96
7707	ZNF148	Zinc finger protein 148	0.97
26,156	RSL1D1	ribosomal L1 domain containing 1	0.97
9379	NRXN2	Neurexin-2	0.98
9480	ONECUT2	one cut homeobox 2	1.03

Table 5. *Cont.*

Gene ID	Gene Symbol	Description	Fold Change
South Shelf			
55,608	ANKRD10	ankyrin repeat domain 10	0.95
26,693	OR2V1	olfactory receptor family 2 subfamily V member 1	0.96
2180	ACSL1	acyl-CoA synthetase long chain family member 1	0.96
399,829	LINC01168	long intergenic non-protein coding RNA 1168	0.97
2774	GNAL	G protein subunit alpha L	0.97
64,319	FBRS	fibrosin	0.97
84,286	TMEM175	transmembrane protein 175	0.97
140,706	CCM2L	cerebral cavernous malformation 2-like	1.04
1112	FOXN3	forkhead box N3	1.04
10,410	IFITM3	interferon-induced transmembrane protein 3	1.04
South Shore			
41	ASIC1	acid-sensing (proton-gated) ion channel 1	0.94
151,313	FAHD2B	fumarylacetoacetate hydrolase domain containing 2B	0.95
84,838	ZNF496 (2)	zinc finger protein 496	0.95
116,988	AGAP3	ArfGAP with GTPase domain, ankyrin repeat and PH domain 3	0.95
9735	KNTC1	kinetochore associated 1	0.96
29,993	PACSIN1	protein kinase C and casein kinase substrate in neurons 1	0.96
85,395	FAM207A	family with sequence similarity 207 member A	0.97
57,186	RALGAPA2	Ral GTPase activating protein catalytic subunit alpha 2	1.03
55,243	KIRREL1	kirre-like nephrin family adhesion molecule 1	1.03
11,267	SNF8	SNF8 subunit of ESCRT-II	1.04
375,061	FAM89A	family with sequence similarity 89, member A	1.06
57,495	NWD2	NACHT and WD repeat domain containing 2	1.12
Open Sea			
25,774	GSTTP1	glutathione S-transferase theta 4	0.72
402,381	SOHLH1	spermatogenesis and oogenesis specific basic helix-loop-helix 1	0.96
3034	HAL	histidine ammonia-lyase	0.96
64,220	STRA6	signaling receptor and transporter of retinol STRA6	0.97
134,510	UBLCP1	ubiquitin-like domain containing CTD phosphatase 1	0.97
1188	CLCNKB	Chloride channel protein ClC-Kb	0.97
1610	DAO	D-amino-acid oxidase	0.98
397	ARHGDIB	Rho GDP-dissociation inhibitor 2	0.98
27,179	IL36A	interleukin 36 alpha	0.98
54,989	ZNF770	zinc finger protein 770	0.98
83,394	PITPNM3	PITPNM family member 3	0.98
79,981	FRMD1	FERM domain containing 1	0.98
55,137	FIGN	fidgetin	0.99
114,879	OSBPL5	oxysterol binding protein-like 5	0.99
219,990	OOSP2	oocyte secreted protein 2	1.02
100,130,673	LOC100130673	phosphoribosyl pyrophosphate synthetase 2 pseudogene	1.06
Promoter			
55,640	FLVCR2	FLVCR heme transporter 2	0.95
79,695	GALNT12	polypeptide N-acetylgalactosaminyltransferase 12	0.96
6169	RPL38	ribosomal protein L38	0.97
4234	METTL1	methyltransferase-like 1	0.97
112,616	CMTM7	CKLF-like MARVEL transmembrane domain containing 7	0.98
10,073	SNUPN	snurportin 1	0.98
80,321	CEP70	centrosomal protein 70	0.98
9167	COX7A2L	cytochrome c oxidase subunit 7A2-like	0.99
100,288,142	NBPF20	NBPF member 20	0.99
8546	AP3B1	adaptor-related protein complex 3, beta 1 subunit	1.01
100,506,334	LINC00649 (1)	long intergenic non-protein coding RNA 649	1.08
Islands in Promoter			
4234	METTL1	methyltransferase-like 1	0.97
252,969	NEIL2	nei-like DNA glycosylase 2	0.97
200,312	RNF215	ring finger protein 215	1.02

[1] Number of differentially methylated CpG sites associated with each gene shown in parentheses.

3.1.2. Differential Methylation of CpG Sites

1. Proportions of Differentially Methylated CpG Sites by Region

Considering CpG sites, the majority of CpG sites are mapped to the gene body (36%), open sea (34%), and island (32%) regions (Table 6). A large proportion of the promoter region (66%) overlapped with CpG islands, and the promoter region also showed overlap with the TSS200 and TSS1500 regions (25% and 24%, respectively) (Supplementary Figure S1). Analysis of individual CpG sites revealed few identifiable differentially methylated sites and roughly a balance of hypo- and hypermethylated sites (SmartSVA method, Table 6). In spite of the relatively low numbers of differentially methylated sites, we estimated that 9% ($n = 27{,}276$) of CpG sites were actually non-null. Out of all CpG sites represented in our analytical dataset ($n = 313{,}161$), 4–9% were estimated to be non-null CpG sites across individual gene regions (Table 6). Relatively fewer numbers of differentially methylated CpG sites were observed in analyses excluding SmartSVA (Supplementary Table S2).

2. Genes Associated with Differentially Methylated CpGs

Individual CpG sites that were differentially methylated were annotated to many of the genes identified as differential in the analysis of gene methylation. cg15613340 in *protocadherin beta 5* (*PCDHB5*) was significantly hypomethylated in vegans in the analysis of methylation of all sites and of the first exon, with a fold change of 0.81 (analyses with SmartSVA), and cg25026992 in *protocadherin beta 7* (*PCDHB7*) was similarly hypomethylated (fold change, 0.81) in analysis of the 3′ UTR region (analyses without SmartSVA), representing the most marked hypomethylation observed among CpG sites. The most marked hypermethylation was that of Cg07967210 in *SNF8 subunit of ESCRT-II* (*SNF8*), identified in the analysis of promoter methylation (fold change, 1.17) (Supplementary Tables S5–S8).

Table 6. Estimated non-null and observed differentially methylated CpG sites (FDR < 0.05) summarized according to genic/intergenic region or in relation to CpG islands comparing vegans with non-vegetarians [1].

Region [2]	Total Genes		Estimated Non-Null		Significantly Hypermethylated		Significantly Hypomethylated	
	n	% of All CpG Sites	*n* [3]	% of Region-Specific Total	*n*	Fold Change [4]	*n*	Fold Change [4]
All	313,161	100	27,276	8.7	6	1.06	8	0.92
Genic/intergenic								
TSS200	40,816	13.0	2355	5.8	5	1.05	3	0.91
TSS1500	57,450	18.3	3950	6.9	5	1.06	8	0.93
3′ UTR	12,840	4.1	633	4.9	3	1.04	6	0.93
5′ UTR	43,313	13.8	3270	7.6	4	1.08	3	0.95
Gene Body	114,095	36.4	9835	8.6	7	1.08	6	0.95
1st Exon	25,662	8.2	2082	8.1	1	1.04	7	0.92
Intergenic	72,524	23.2	5798	8.0	9	1.06	3	0.92
Island-related								
CpG Island	99,350	31.7	7883	7.9	4	1.07	4	0.92
North Shelf	15,106	4.8	923	6.1	7	1.05	6	0.93
North Shore	43,549	13.9	3542	8.1	6	1.06	3	0.94
South Shelf	13,564	4.3	974	7.2	9	1.06	3	0.93
South Shore	33,905	10.8	2652	7.8	5	1.08	7	0.93
Open Sea	107,687	34.4	8266	7.7	5	1.06	5	0.93
Promoter								
All	62,398	19.9	2308	3.7	6	1.08	3	0.95
CpG Island	39,230	12.5	1713	4.4	1	1.07	3	0.96

[1] Number of differentially methylated CpG sites determined using linear regression with SmartSVA, followed by adapted Storey et al. [32] approach to adjust for false discovery. [2] Some CpG sites represented in more than one gene region. [3] Number of CpG sites estimated to show non-null differences in methylation. [4] Fold change represents ratio of the mean methylation of vegans to that of non-vegetarians for differentially methylated (hypomethylated or hypermethylated) sites for a given region. This is averaged across significant sites.

4. Discussion

DNA methylation is one mechanism that links lifestyle with genomic alterations. The goal of this study was to determine if habitual vegan and non-vegetarian dietary patterns differentially influenced DNA methylation. Using a permutation-based adapted Storey et al. [32] approach, and considering various genomic regions, we could detect a modest number of genes that differed significantly in their methylation status between vegans and non-vegetarians, noting that much larger proportions of apparently differentially methylated CpG sites and genes are in fact present, and should be detected with larger samples.

The majority of differentially methylated genes detected were hypomethylated in vegans, both when considering gene methylation overall, as well as in various gene regions. The greatest differences in gene methylation were found when considering the gene body. The region-specific differences in the number of detected differentially methylated genes are in part a reflection of the nonuniformity in the distribution of probes selected for the BeadChip array (i.e., a large number of CpG sites were present in the gene body). However, there were fewer observed and predicted non-null differentially methylated genes defined by the TSS1500 and CpG island regions, in spite of greater total numbers of genes with CpG sites in these regions, relative to the gene body. The gene body may therefore be the most susceptible to diet-induced alterations in methylation. Overall, we have estimated larger proportions of differentially methylated, non-null genes (6% of all genes) and CpG sites (9% of all CpG sites) to be detected with sufficiently large samples, using our adapted Storey approach. It should be noted that results from our permutation-based adapted Storey approach showed strong agreement with results from the simpler Benjamini–Hochberg approach for false discovery.

There is little other published evidence on the influence of plant-based dietary patterns on DNA methylation. Global methylation (LINE1) has been associated with consumption of fruits and vegetables or flavonoids in dietary intervention studies [41,42], as well as with energy restriction in overweight participants [43,44] although the latter has not been consistently observed [45]. It is unclear how a vegan diet impacted global (overall) methylation in the current study, given our array-based approach. However, of the significantly hypermethylated CpG sites, the majority were located in the intergenic region, which houses many transposable elements, including LINE1. Our findings show some consistency with those reported by Perfilyev et al., where high fat feeding (both saturated and polyunsaturated combined) was associated with hypermethylation of genes (>99%) [27]. These findings seem to complement our results as vegans who have lower fat consumption [9] and lower proportions of saturated fatty acids in adipose tissue [10], showed decreased gene methylation overall. However, the differential patterns of methylation between vegans and non-vegetarians in our study was not merely due to differences in fat, as our findings were only slightly attenuated when adjusted for total/saturated fat. Additionally, associations persisted when controlling for BMI, which could also be thought of as a surrogate of long-term energy intake and energy balance.

Many genes differentially methylated in the analysis of overall methylation of all genes have roles in RNA transport or ribosome assembly/regulation of translation (*RPL38, TUFM* [46,47]), as well as lysosome regulation (HPS4 [48]), protein degradation or ubiquitination (*DCAF15, PSMF1* [49,50]), cytokine or B cell receptor signaling (*CMTM7, IL36A* [51,52]), and metabolism (*STRA6, COX7A2L, GALNT12* [53–56]), among other pathways. Alterations in many of these processes impact protein synthesis and may have pathophysiological implications [57,58].

We have highlighted methylation differences in the promoter region particularly, as such alterations may have a greater impact on gene transcription. *METTL1* consistently showed hypomethylation in all relevant analyses—i.e., analyses of methylation of genes defined by CpGs in associated promoter regions, as well as of overall methylation of all genes, this being in analyses including or excluding SmartSVA variables, and after adjustment for false discovery. *METTL1* encodes a methyltransferase that promotes methylguanine methylation of RNA, including miRNAs such as let7, which results in processing of the miRNA [59]. Let-7 miRNA has roles in regulating cell growth and metabolism, and is also considered a tumor suppressor, showing downregulation in a number of cancers [60]. *METTL1* along with *NEIL2*, encoding an enzyme involved in DNA repair [61], were significantly hypomethylated in CpG islands within the promoter independent of SmartSVA variables. Hypermethylation of CpG islands within the promoter is associated with silencing of tumor suppressor genes [62–65]. Thus, hypomethylation and consequent increases in these genes might be associated with sustained expression of tumor suppressors, and thus cancer prevention.

Besides METTL1 and NEIL2, several of the differentially methylated genes identified by analysis of associated promoter methylation, or of all genes, have roles in cancer biology. For example, *LIN28B* regulates let-7 miRNA [66], *CMTM7* is potential tumor suppressor, possibly silenced by promoter methylation [49,67]), and *ARGHDIB*, a regulator of Rho family signaling, can be upregulated in tumors [68]. Interestingly, *GALNT12*, *DDT*, and *ARNT2* have been found to be over-represented in cancer, including colorectal cancer among others [69–72], with ARNT2 showing promoter hypermethylation in hepatoma cells [73]. We have found that vegans and other vegetarians in AHS-2 have lower risk of certain types of cancer and other chronic diseases [2,3,6]. Thus, DNA methylation alterations in genes with relevance to cancer could help explain some of the differences in cancer outcomes between dietary groups in the AHS-2 cohort. However, it is unclear if transcriptional changes are associated with any of the observed methylation alterations.

The observed trend towards hypomethylation of genes in vegans could be explained in part by inhibition of activity of DNMT enzymes by polyphenols and various secondary plant metabolites [14,74]. We have shown that vegetarians in the AHS-2 cohort have significantly increased consumption of plant-based foods including fruits, vegetables, legumes, nuts, and seeds [9], which are high in polyphenols. Furthermore, we recently demonstrated that vegetarians, particularly vegans, have significantly higher levels of bioactive compounds and phytochemicals-enterolactone, isoflavones, carotenoids, as well as total omega-3 fatty acids (attributable to alpha linolenic acid) in plasma, urine, and adipose tissue, many of which could theoretically modulate methylation [75]. Additionally, methyl donor compounds, folate, choline, methionine and cofactors (vitamin B), which are obtained from various foods, may influence both gene-specific and global DNA methylation, as demonstrated through observational and intervention studies; however, activity may be context, dose, or tissue dependent [13,30,76,77]. It is not clear if any of these methyl donor compounds differ between vegans and non-vegetarians in the current study. Thus, gene-specific and genome-wide alterations in methylation may be determined by a complex interplay of methyl donors, micronutrients, polyphenols, macronutrient composition, and inflammatory status, among other possible factors, including physical activity and stress.

Methylation activity of CpGs within the same gene, and particularly the same region, may be coordinated. This correlation of CpG sites could partly explain why our analysis of gene methylation revealed greater differential alterations than analysis of individual CpG sites, although a much greater number of sites are estimated to be non-null and detectable with a larger sample. Findings from our study suggest that methylation alterations associated with dietary patterns (and likely other environmental exposures) may be characterized by coordinated methylation of CpG sites in a specific gene and within select regions of the gene. This approach of analyzing CpGs within select regions after annotation to their respective genes is, in general, similar to the region-centric approach taken by Bacalini et al. involving the grouping together of probes mapping to the same island or gene [78].

The effect size of methylation differences was low overall, with average regional methylation differences in the range of 2–4% for significant genes and 4–9% for significant CpG sites (at FDR < 0.05), though fold changes were much larger for select genes or CpG sites. Effect sizes of low magnitude (≤1–5%) have been previously reported in dietary studies. Besides the high fat feeding study by Perfilyev et al. [27], interventions examining alterations associated with a Mediterranean diet or diet enriched in flavonoids and isothiocyanates also found very subtle but significant changes (~1% methylation difference in LINE1) [41,44]. Smaller changes in methylation tend to be disregarded [79,80], but the physiological relevance of such small effects is unclear. It is possible that such changes over the long-term contribute to sustained, physiologically meaningful epigenetic differences. These "small" changes may translate into permanent changes in gene expression, and consequently phenotype, and be inherited by daughter cells [81]. The location of methylation alterations also holds much relevance, as methylation of one site can contribute to gene silencing if the methylated site blocks binding of a transcription factor [82,83].

This is the first study to our knowledge analyzing differences in DNA methylation between vegans and non-vegetarians. The AHS-2 cohort is unique in its relatively large number of vegans (~9% of cohort), thereby enabling such a study, although it should be noted that AHS-2 non-vegetarians tend to have lower meat consumption relative to the general population. The examination of habitual, long-term dietary patterns is a major strength, as epigenetic marks are more stable, reflecting long-term dietary conditions. We have shown that the majority of cohort members remain in the same diet group from one decade to the next [84]. Because of the habitual, a priori-classified dietary patterns, there was likely minimal measurement error in the classification of diet group. Additionally, our study was strengthened by leveraging multiple analytical approaches, comparing the SmartSVA method which adjusts for surrogate variables and thus unwanted variation, with linear regression models not including these surrogate variables but adjusting for other known technical variations.

Our study has some noteworthy limitations. Methylation alterations are best paralleled with gene expression data. In the absence of such data there are limitations in the interpretation of our findings. As mentioned, it is not clear how other dietary or lifestyle influences (exercise, methyl donors) may have altered results. Furthermore, we do not know how methylation alterations in leukocytes correlate with those in other tissues, although there is evidence that methylation patterns or alterations in blood may be reflective of patterns in other tissues [85–87]. Additionally, the two dietary groups examined were somewhat heterogeneous in terms of consumption of animal- and plant-based foods. For example, it is not clear how methylation patterns differ comparing individuals with very high consumption of red or processed meat with individuals following a diet comprised largely of fruits, vegetables, and whole plant foods.

5. Conclusions

In summary, modest specific differences in methylation of genes and CpG sites were detected, comparing vegans and non-vegetarians, with clear indication that many more such differences exist, but are yet to be specifically identified with larger studies. This study thus lays the foundation for the identification of transcriptional alterations and molecular functions associated with these diet-influenced methylation patterns.

Supplementary Materials: The following are available online at http://www.mdpi.com/2072-6643/12/12/3697/s1. Figure S1: Overlap of promoter with gene- or island-related regions, Table S1: Estimated non-null and observed differentially methylated genes (FDR < 0.05) summarized according to genic/intergenic region or in relation to CpG islands in vegans relative to non-vegetarians (without SmartSVA method), Table S2: Estimated non-null and observed differentially methylated CpG sites (at FDR < 0.05) summarized according to genic/intergenic region or in relation to CpG islands in vegans relative to non-vegetarians (without SmartSVA), Table S3: Genes differentially methylated at FDR < 0.05 according to genic/intergenic region, Table S4: Genes differentially methylated at FDR < 0.05 in island-related and promoter regions, Table S5: CpGs differentially methylated at FDR < 0.05 according to genic/intergenic region (based on SmartSVA method), Table S6: CpGs differentially methylated at FDR < 0.05 in island-related and promoter regions (based on SmartSVA method), Table S7: CpGs differentially methylated at FDR < 0.05 according to genic/intergenic region, Table S8: CpGs differentially methylated at FDR < 0.05 in island-related and promoter regions.

Author Contributions: The authors' responsibilities were as follows: Conceptualization and design, G.E.F., F.L.M., K.S. and P.D.-H.; Methodology, A.M., V.F., G.E.F., F.L.M., C.W., K.S. and X.C.; Data analysis, A.M., G.E.F. and F.L.M.; Writing—Original Draft Preparation, F.L.M. and G.E.F.; Data curation, A.M., G.E.F. and V.F.; Writing—Review and Editing, G.E.F., F.L.M., K.S., M.J.O., P.D.-H., A.M. and C.W. All authors have read and agreed to the published version of the manuscript.

Funding: This research was funded by Ardmore Institute of Health, the National Institute of Health (National Cancer Institute, R01 CA094594, National Institute of Aging, 1R01AG026348, and by Loma Linda University through Grants for Research and Partnerships awards (2120211, 2130279, 2170322).

Conflicts of Interest: The authors declare no conflict of interest. The funders had no role in the design of the study; in the collection, analyses, or interpretation of data; in the writing of the manuscript, or in the decision to publish the results.

Appendix A

A Method of Power Calculations, Estimating Ability to Detect Differentially Methylated Sites with a Given False Discovery Rate

First, in what follows, p values are defined as the cumulative probabilities of the chosen test statistics when the null hypothesis is satisfied, thus ranging from 0 to 1.0. As noted by Storey et al. [32], a plot of the density of p values for a central t distribution (or other distributions) is a uniform plot, when the data conform to the null (the hypothesis that the p value is defined to represent). Then, it is assumed that the observed data to be evaluated (consisting of a large number, say R, independent t statistics), represent a mix from two types of CpG (or gene) populations. Namely, these are a population of true null data, and a second population where the true distribution for each t statistic is non-null (non-central), but not otherwise specified.

In that situation the density plot of p values (estimated, say, from a central t distribution) should devolve into a central uniform portion, at a density less than 1.0, say R_0/R, and tails at either end that slope upward from the uniform region represent an excess of p values in regions more sparsely populated under the null. The total area under the curve must, as usual, equal 1.0, by the definition of density. One can compare this to a plot that would be expected if all values came from a null distribution, which would be a uniform plot at a value of 1.0. It is easy to show that the value R_0/R represents the proportion of the t values in the real data that come from a null distribution. Then $R—R_0$ is the estimated number of t statistics that come from non-null distributions.

To gain some extra stability, we have simply translated this same rationale to cumulative distributions of p values from both observed data and hypothetical null data. In the null situation the cumulative distribution is a diagonal line from lower left to upper right. In the observed data, the central uniform density cumulates to a straight line that can be shown to have slope R_0/R. Relative excess densities at small p values cumulate to push the left end of the curve higher than the diagonal with slopes that exceed 1.0, thus flattening the straight line null portion that begins at the end of this elevated segment. Unless there are no non-null data at the right-hand higher-valued end, the central straight portion necessarily crosses the diagonal. Then later, at the end of the null straight portion, again develops slopes greater than 1.0, representing non-null high-value P statistics, finally meeting the diagonal again when $p = 1.0$. In these plots the slope of the straight line portion estimates the proportion of underlying null distributions, and of course again $(R—R_0)/R$ is the proportion that are non-null.

An example from the DNA methylation data (average of CpG sites in gene body regions) described in this paper is shown as Figure A1. Here, the deviation in slope of the central linear region from the diagonal is relatively small, but important, and in part due to large numbers, is not due to chance ($p < 2 \times 10^{-16}$). The size of the population studies, and the relatively small fold change values (that translate to smaller non-centrality parameters for the non-null t distributions) account for the modest deviation from the diagonal in the figure. Increasing n (the number of subjects) will change this (see Table 4). An example from a metabolomics dataset—also comparing non-vegetarians to vegans—includes t distributions with much greater non-centrality parameters and is shown below for illustrative purposes (Figure A2).

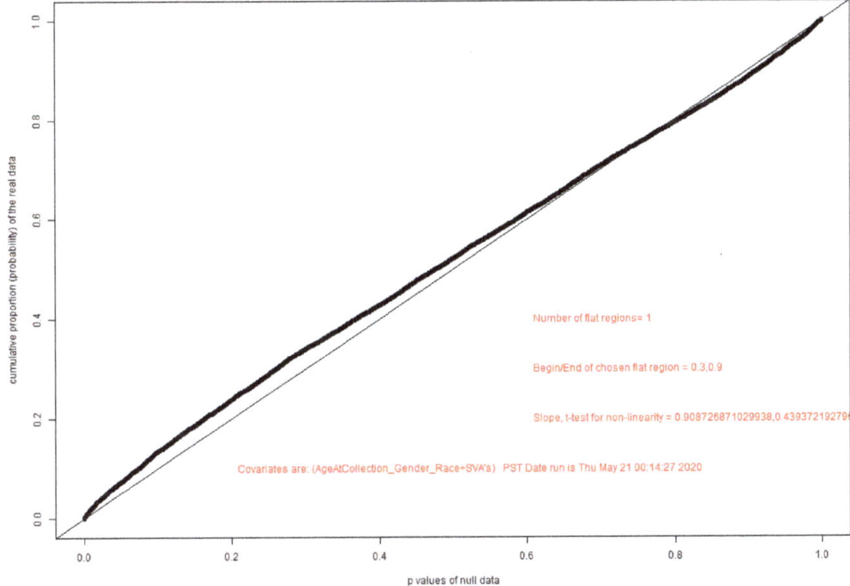

Figure A1. Plot of cumulative *p* values from real data (dark line), and from a hypothetical data where all data are null (fine line). Differential methylation: average of CpG sites in gene body regions, comparing non-vegetarians to vegans.

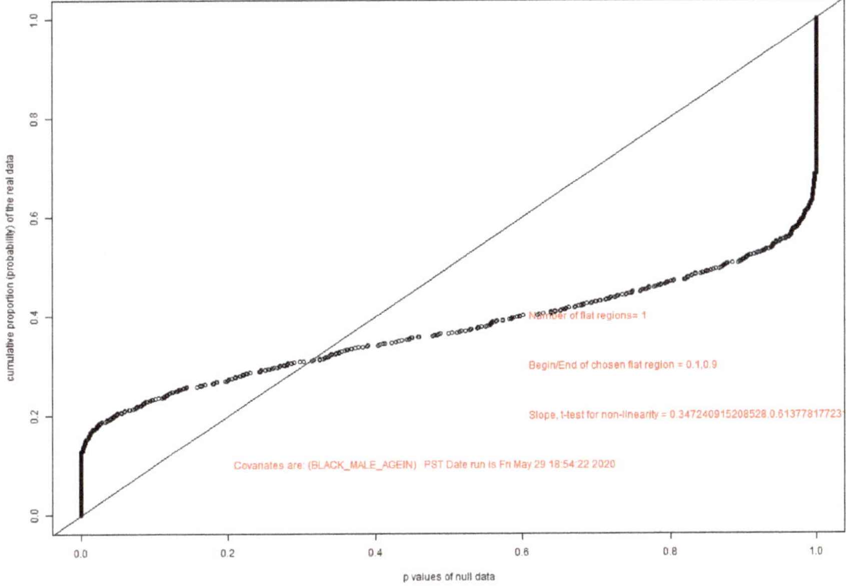

Figure A2. Cumulative *p* plots (real and hypothetical null data) for a metabolomics panel comparing non-vegetarians to vegans.

This situation can be used to estimate power, and how, in a particular dataset, this depends on *n*. Power is here expressed as the false discovery rate (FDR) associated with sample size *n*2, where $n1$ is the size of the observed data, and where critical t statistic values are nominated for exploratory purposes. This is dependent on the observation that as n increases, the distribution of t statistics from null sites does not change. The reason for this is that the numerator of each t value is (mean(non-vegetarians)—mean(vegans)) for that site or gene, and its expectation by definition under the null, is zero. Thus, the underlying random errors in these means will shrink as n increases according to the inverse square root law, decreasing the range of the random differences between the two means (the numerator). The denominator that measures the standard error of this difference between means shrinks by an exactly equivalent amount; however, the ratio t statistic remains unchanged, with other things being equal.

However, the situation for non-null t values is different—the numerators, again by definition, have a non-zero expected value (that differs from methylation site to methylation site). As n increases, this expected value does not change, but the denominator (Standard Error of the difference) shrinks as usual, driving the non-null t statistics to ever more extreme values. This has the most helpful consequence of drawing the non-null results ever more toward the tails of the observed distribution as numbers increase. So, for any nominated critical t value, the tails will contain the usual number of randomly extreme t statistics from null sites, but an increasing number from non-null sites with increasing numbers of subjects, thus improving the FDR.

Specifically, it can be shown that, for the left-hand tail,

$$\text{FDR(n2)} = \frac{\text{FDR(n1).R.cp(Tcl)}}{\left\{ \text{R.cp}\left(\text{Tcl.} \sqrt{(n1/n2)}\right) - R_0.\left[p\left(\text{Tcl.} \sqrt{(n1/n2)}\right) - p(\text{Tcl})\right]\right\}},$$

where Tcl is the nominated critical t value for the left-hand tail; p(Tcl) refers to the cumulative probability under the null corresponding to this t value; cp(Tcl) refers to the cumulative probability of this Tcl value in the observed data.

For the right-hand tail where Tcu is the critical value for significance in the upper tail, the expression is

$$\text{FDR(n2)} = \frac{\text{FDR(n1).R.}(1 - \text{cp(Tcu)})}{\left\{ \text{R.}\left(1 - \text{cp}\left(\text{Tcu.} \sqrt{(n1/n2)}\right)\right) - R_0.\left[p(\text{Tcu}) - p\left(\text{Tcu.} \sqrt{(n1/n2)}\right)\right]\right\}}.$$

References

1. Fraser, G.; Katuli, S.; Anousheh, R.; Knutsen, S.; Herring, P.; Fan, J. Vegetarian diets and cardiovascular risk factors in black members of the Adventist Health Study-2. *Public Health Nutr.* **2015**, *18*, 537–545. [CrossRef] [PubMed]
2. Rizzo, N.S.; Sabate, J.; Jaceldo-Siegl, K.; Fraser, G.E. Vegetarian dietary patterns are associated with a lower risk of metabolic syndrome: The adventist health study 2. *Diabetes Care* **2011**, *34*, 1225–1227. [CrossRef] [PubMed]
3. Tonstad, S.; Stewart, K.; Oda, K.; Batech, M.; Herring, R.P.; Fraser, G.E. Vegetarian diets and incidence of diabetes in the Adventist Health Study-2. *Nutr. Metab. Cardiovasc. Dis.* **2013**, *23*, 292–299. [CrossRef] [PubMed]
4. Tharrey, M.; Mariotti, F.; Mashchak, A.; Barbillon, P.; Delattre, M.; Fraser, G.E. Patterns of plant and animal protein intake are strongly associated with cardiovascular mortality: The Adventist Health Study-2 cohort. *Int. J. Epidemiol.* **2018**, *47*, 1603–1612. [CrossRef] [PubMed]
5. Alshahrani, S.M.; Fraser, G.E.; Sabate, J.; Knutsen, R.; Shavlik, D.; Mashchak, A.; Lloren, J.I.; Orlich, M.J. Red and Processed Meat and Mortality in a Low Meat Intake Population. *Nutrients* **2019**, *11*, 622. [CrossRef] [PubMed]
6. Tantamango-Bartley, Y.; Jaceldo-Siegl, K.; Fan, J.; Fraser, G. Vegetarian diets and the incidence of cancer in a low-risk population. *Cancer Epidemiol. Biomark. Prev.* **2013**, *22*, 286–294. [CrossRef]
7. Orlich, M.J.; Singh, P.N.; Sabate, J.; Fan, J.; Sveen, L.; Bennett, H.; Knutsen, S.F.; Beeson, W.L.; Jaceldo-Siegl, K.; Butler, T.L.; et al. Vegetarian dietary patterns and the risk of colorectal cancers. *JAMA Intern. Med.* **2015**, *175*, 767–776. [CrossRef]

8.	Tantamango-Bartley, Y.; Knutsen, S.F.; Knutsen, R.; Jacobsen, B.K.; Fan, J.; Beeson, W.L.; Sabate, J.; Hadley, D.; Jaceldo-Siegl, K.; Penniecook, J.; et al. Are strict vegetarians protected against prostate cancer? *Am. J. Clin. Nutr.* **2016**, *103*, 153–160. [CrossRef]

9.	Orlich, M.J.; Jaceldo-Siegl, K.; Sabate, J.; Fan, J.; Singh, P.N.; Fraser, G.E. Patterns of food consumption among vegetarians and non-vegetarians. *Br. J. Nutr.* **2014**, *112*, 1644–1653. [CrossRef]

10.	Miles, F.L.; Lloren, J.I.C.; Haddad, E.; Jaceldo-Siegl, K.; Knutsen, S.; Sabate, J.; Fraser, G.E. Plasma, Urine, and Adipose Tissue Biomarkers of Dietary Intake Differ Between Vegetarian and Non-Vegetarian Diet Groups in the Adventist Health Study-2. *J. Nutr.* **2019**, *149*, 667–675. [CrossRef]

11.	Field, A.E.; Robertson, N.A.; Wang, T.; Havas, A.; Ideker, T.; Adams, P.D. DNA Methylation Clocks in Aging: Categories, Causes, and Consequences. *Mol. Cell* **2018**, *71*, 882–895. [CrossRef] [PubMed]

12.	Stylianou, E. Epigenetics of chronic inflammatory diseases. *J. Inflamm. Res.* **2019**, *12*, 1–14. [CrossRef]

13.	Anderson, O.S.; Sant, K.E.; Dolinoy, D.C. Nutrition and epigenetics: An interplay of dietary methyl donors, one-carbon metabolism and DNA methylation. *J. Nutr. Biochem.* **2012**, *23*, 853–859. [CrossRef] [PubMed]

14.	Fang, M.Z.; Chen, D.; Sun, Y.; Jin, Z.; Christman, J.K.; Yang, C.S. Reversal of hypermethylation and reactivation of p16INK4a, RARbeta, and MGMT genes by genistein and other isoflavones from soy. *Clin. Cancer Res.* **2005**, *11*, 7033–7041. [CrossRef] [PubMed]

15.	Figueroa, M.E.; Abdel-Wahab, O.; Lu, C.; Ward, P.S.; Patel, J.; Shih, A.; Li, Y.; Bhagwat, N.; Vasanthakumar, A.; Fernandez, H.F.; et al. Leukemic IDH1 and IDH2 mutations result in a hypermethylation phenotype, disrupt TET2 function, and impair hematopoietic differentiation. *Cancer Cell* **2010**, *18*, 553–567. [CrossRef] [PubMed]

16.	Wu, Q.; Ni, X. ROS-mediated DNA methylation pattern alterations in carcinogenesis. *Curr. Drug Targets* **2015**, *16*, 13–19. [CrossRef] [PubMed]

17.	Yang, C.S.; Fang, M.; Lambert, J.D.; Yan, P.; Huang, T.H. Reversal of hypermethylation and reactivation of genes by dietary polyphenolic compounds. *Nutr. Rev.* **2008**, *66* (Suppl. 1), S18–S20. [CrossRef]

18.	Hsu, A.; Wong, C.P.; Yu, Z.; Williams, D.E.; Dashwood, R.H.; Ho, E. Promoter de-methylation of cyclin D2 by sulforaphane in prostate cancer cells. *Clin. Epigenetics* **2011**, *3*, 3. [CrossRef]

19.	Chai, W.; Morimoto, Y.; Cooney, R.V.; Franke, A.A.; Shvetsov, Y.B.; Le Marchand, L.; Haiman, C.A.; Kolonel, L.N.; Goodman, M.T.; Maskarinec, G. Dietary Red and Processed Meat Intake and Markers of Adiposity and Inflammation: The Multiethnic Cohort Study. *J. Am. Coll. Nutr.* **2017**, *36*, 378–385. [CrossRef]

20.	Jiao, L.; Stolzenberg-Solomon, R.; Zimmerman, T.P.; Duan, Z.; Chen, L.; Kahle, L.; Risch, A.; Subar, A.F.; Cross, A.J.; Hollenbeck, A.; et al. Dietary consumption of advanced glycation end products and pancreatic cancer in the prospective NIH-AARP Diet and Health Study. *Am. J. Clin. Nutr.* **2015**, *101*, 126–134. [CrossRef]

21.	Papuc, C.; Goran, G.V.; Predescu, C.N.; Nicorescu, V. Mechanisms of Oxidative Processes in Meat and Toxicity Induced by Postprandial Degradation Products: A Review. *Compr. Rev. Food Sci. Food Saf.* **2017**, *16*, 96–123. [CrossRef]

22.	Welty, F.K. How do elevated triglycerides and low HDL-cholesterol affect inflammation and atherothrombosis? *Curr. Cardiol. Rep.* **2013**, *15*, 400. [CrossRef] [PubMed]

23.	Hoekstra, A.S.; de Graaff, M.A.; Briaire-de Bruijn, I.H.; Ras, C.; Seifar, R.M.; van Minderhout, I.; Cornelisse, C.J.; Hogendoorn, P.C.; Breuning, M.H.; Suijker, J.; et al. Inactivation of SDH and FH cause loss of 5hmC and increased H3K9me3 in paraganglioma/pheochromocytoma and smooth muscle tumors. *Oncotarget* **2015**, *6*, 38777–38788. [CrossRef] [PubMed]

24.	Keleher, M.R.; Zaidi, R.; Hicks, L.; Shah, S.; Xing, X.; Li, D.; Wang, T.; Cheverud, J.M. A high-fat diet alters genome-wide DNA methylation and gene expression in SM/J mice. *BMC Genom.* **2018**, *19*, 888. [CrossRef]

25.	Keleher, M.R.; Zaidi, R.; Shah, S.; Oakley, M.E.; Pavlatos, C.; El Idrissi, S.; Xing, X.; Li, D.; Wang, T.; Cheverud, J.M. Maternal high-fat diet associated with altered gene expression, DNA methylation, and obesity risk in mouse offspring. *PLoS ONE* **2018**, *13*, e0192606. [CrossRef]

26.	Masuyama, H.; Mitsui, T.; Nobumoto, E.; Hiramatsu, Y. The Effects of High-Fat Diet Exposure in Utero on the Obesogenic and Diabetogenic Traits Through Epigenetic Changes in Adiponectin and Leptin Gene Expression for Multiple Generations in Female Mice. *Endocrinology* **2015**, *156*, 2482–2491. [CrossRef]

27.	Perfilyev, A.; Dahlman, I.; Gillberg, L.; Rosqvist, F.; Iggman, D.; Volkov, P.; Nilsson, E.; Riserus, U.; Ling, C. Impact of polyunsaturated and saturated fat overfeeding on the DNA-methylation pattern in human adipose tissue: A randomized controlled trial. *Am. J. Clin. Nutr.* **2017**, *105*, 991–1000. [CrossRef]

28. Gillberg, L.; Jacobsen, S.C.; Ronn, T.; Brons, C.; Vaag, A. PPARGC1A DNA methylation in subcutaneous adipose tissue in low birth weight subjects–impact of 5 days of high-fat overfeeding. *Metabolism* **2014**, *63*, 263–271. [CrossRef]

29. Brons, C.; Jacobsen, S.; Nilsson, E.; Ronn, T.; Jensen, C.B.; Storgaard, H.; Poulsen, P.; Groop, L.; Ling, C.; Astrup, A.; et al. Deoxyribonucleic acid methylation and gene expression of PPARGC1A in human muscle is influenced by high-fat overfeeding in a birth-weight-dependent manner. *J. Clin. Endocrinol. Metab.* **2010**, *95*, 3048–3056. [CrossRef]

30. ElGendy, K.; Malcomson, F.C.; Lara, J.G.; Bradburn, D.M.; Mathers, J.C. Effects of dietary interventions on DNA methylation in adult humans: Systematic review and meta-analysis. *Br. J. Nutr.* **2018**, *120*, 961–976. [CrossRef]

31. Hastie, T.T.R.; Friedman, J. The elements of statistical learning. In *Data Mining, Inference, and Prediction*, 2nd ed.; Springer: Berlin/Heidelberg, Germany, 2009; pp. 687–692.

32. Storey, J.D.; Tibshirani, R. Statistical significance for genomewide studies. *Proc. Natl. Acad. Sci. USA* **2003**, *100*, 9440–9445. [CrossRef] [PubMed]

33. Chan, J.; Knutsen, S.F.; Sabate, J.; Haddad, E.; Yan, R.; Fraser, G.E. Feasibility of running clinics to collect biological specimens in a nationwide cohort study–Adventist Health Study-2. *Ann. Epidemiol.* **2007**, *17*, 454–457. [CrossRef] [PubMed]

34. Aryee, M.J.; Jaffe, A.E.; Corrada-Bravo, H.; Ladd-Acosta, C.; Feinberg, A.P.; Hansen, K.D.; Irizarry, R.A. Minfi: A flexible and comprehensive Bioconductor package for the analysis of Infinium DNA methylation microarrays. *Bioinformatics* **2014**, *30*, 1363–1369. [CrossRef] [PubMed]

35. Chen, Y.A.; Lemire, M.; Choufani, S.; Butcher, D.T.; Grafodatskaya, D.; Zanke, B.W.; Gallinger, S.; Hudson, T.J.; Weksberg, R. Discovery of cross-reactive probes and polymorphic CpGs in the Illumina Infinium HumanMethylation450 microarray. *Epigenetics* **2013**, *8*, 203–209. [CrossRef] [PubMed]

36. Pidsley, R.; Zotenko, E.; Peters, T.J.; Lawrence, M.G.; Risbridger, G.P.; Molloy, P.; Van Djik, S.; Muhlhausler, B.; Stirzaker, C.; Clark, S.J. Critical evaluation of the Illumina MethylationEPIC BeadChip microarray for whole-genome DNA methylation profiling. *Genome Biol.* **2016**, *17*, 208. [CrossRef]

37. Chen, J.; Behnam, E.; Huang, J.; Moffatt, M.F.; Schaid, D.J.; Liang, L.; Lin, X. Fast and robust adjustment of cell mixtures in epigenome-wide association studies with SmartSVA. *BMC Genom.* **2017**, *18*, 413. [CrossRef]

38. Houseman, E.A.; Accomando, W.P.; Koestler, D.C.; Christensen, B.C.; Marsit, C.J.; Nelson, H.H.; Wiencke, J.K.; Kelsey, K.T. DNA methylation arrays as surrogate measures of cell mixture distribution. *BMC Bioinform.* **2012**, *13*, 86. [CrossRef]

39. Seber, G.A.F. Analysis of covariance and missing observations. In *Linear Regression Analyses*; John Wiley and Sons: New York, NY, USA, 1977.

40. Freedman, D.; Lane, D. A Nonstochastic Interpretation of Reported Significance Levels. *J. Bus. Econ. Stat.* **1983**, *1*, 292–298. [CrossRef]

41. Scoccianti, C.; Ricceri, F.; Ferrari, P.; Cuenin, C.; Sacerdote, C.; Polidoro, S.; Jenab, M.; Hainaut, P.; Vineis, P.; Herceg, Z. Methylation patterns in sentinel genes in peripheral blood cells of heavy smokers: Influence of cruciferous vegetables in an intervention study. *Epigenetics* **2011**, *6*, 1114–1119. [CrossRef]

42. Greenlee, H.; Ogden Gaffney, A.; Aycinena, A.C.; Koch, P.; Contento, I.; Karmally, W.; Richardson, J.M.; Shi, Z.; Lim, E.; Tsai, W.Y.; et al. Long-term Diet and Biomarker Changes after a Short-term Intervention among Hispanic Breast Cancer Survivors: The inverted exclamation markCocinar Para Su Salud! Randomized Controlled Trial. *Cancer Epidemiol. Biomark. Prev.* **2016**, *25*, 1491–1502. [CrossRef]

43. Delgado-Cruzata, L.; Zhang, W.; McDonald, J.A.; Tsai, W.Y.; Valdovinos, C.; Falci, L.; Wang, Q.; Crew, K.D.; Santella, R.M.; Hershman, D.L.; et al. Dietary modifications, weight loss, and changes in metabolic markers affect global DNA methylation in Hispanic, African American, and Afro-Caribbean breast cancer survivors. *J. Nutr.* **2015**, *145*, 783–790. [CrossRef] [PubMed]

44. Martin-Nunez, G.M.; Cabrera-Mulero, R.; Rubio-Martin, E.; Rojo-Martinez, G.; Olveira, G.; Valdes, S.; Soriguer, F.; Castano, L.; Morcillo, S. Methylation levels of the SCD1 gene promoter and LINE-1 repeat region are associated with weight change: An intervention study. *Mol. Nutr. Food Res.* **2014**, *58*, 1528–1536. [CrossRef] [PubMed]

45. Duggan, C.; Xiao, L.; Terry, M.B.; McTiernan, A. No effect of weight loss on LINE-1 methylation levels in peripheral blood leukocytes from postmenopausal overweight women. *Obesity* **2014**, *22*, 2091–2096. [CrossRef] [PubMed]

46. Kondrashov, N.; Pusic, A.; Stumpf, C.R.; Shimizu, K.; Hsieh, A.C.; Ishijima, J.; Shiroishi, T.; Barna, M. Ribosome-mediated specificity in Hox mRNA translation and vertebrate tissue patterning. *Cell* **2011**, *145*, 383–397. [CrossRef]

47. Travers, A.A.; Kamen, R.I.; Schleif, R.F. Factor necessary for ribosomal RNA synthesis. *Nature* **1970**, *228*, 748–751. [CrossRef]

48. Nazarian, R.; Falcon-Perez, J.M.; Dell'Angelica, E.C. Biogenesis of lysosome-related organelles complex 3 (BLOC-3): A complex containing the Hermansky-Pudlak syndrome (HPS) proteins HPS1 and HPS4. *Proc. Natl. Acad. Sci. USA* **2003**, *100*, 8770–8775. [CrossRef]

49. Li, H.; Li, J.; Su, Y.; Fan, Y.; Guo, X.; Li, L.; Su, X.; Rong, R.; Ying, J.; Mo, X.; et al. A novel 3p22.3 gene CMTM7 represses oncogenic EGFR signaling and inhibits cancer cell growth. *Oncogene* **2014**, *33*, 3109–3118. [CrossRef]

50. Uehara, T.; Minoshima, Y.; Sagane, K.; Sugi, N.H.; Mitsuhashi, K.O.; Yamamoto, N.; Kamiyama, H.; Takahashi, K.; Kotake, Y.; Uesugi, M.; et al. Selective degradation of splicing factor CAPERalpha by anticancer sulfonamides. *Nat. Chem. Biol.* **2017**, *13*, 675–680. [CrossRef]

51. Russell, S.E.; Horan, R.M.; Stefanska, A.M.; Carey, A.; Leon, G.; Aguilera, M.; Statovci, D.; Moran, T.; Fallon, P.G.; Shanahan, F.; et al. IL-36alpha expression is elevated in ulcerative colitis and promotes colonic inflammation. *Mucosal Immunol.* **2016**, *9*, 1193–1204. [CrossRef]

52. Zhang, Y.F.; Wang, J.Y.; Han, W.L. A role for CMTM7 in BCR expression and survival in B-1a but not B-2 cells. *Int. Immunol.* **2014**, *26*, 47–57. [CrossRef]

53. Bennett, E.P.; Mandel, U.; Clausen, H.; Gerken, T.A.; Fritz, T.A.; Tabak, L.A. Control of mucin-type O-glycosylation: A classification of the polypeptide GalNAc-transferase gene family. *Glycobiology* **2012**, *22*, 736–756. [CrossRef] [PubMed]

54. Cogan, U.; Kopelman, M.; Mokady, S.; Shinitzky, M. Binding Affinities of Retinol and Related Compounds to Retinol Binding-Proteins. *Eur. J. Biochem.* **1976**, *65*, 71–78. [CrossRef] [PubMed]

55. Kawaguchi, R.; Zhong, M.; Kassai, M.; Ter-Stepanian, M.; Sun, H. STRA6-Catalyzed Vitamin A Influx, Efflux, and Exchange. *J. Membr. Biol.* **2012**, *245*, 731–745. [CrossRef]

56. Lapuente-Brun, E.; Moreno-Loshuertos, R.; Acin-Perez, R.; Latorre-Pellicer, A.; Colas, C.; Balsa, E.; Perales-Clemente, E.; Quiros, P.M.; Calvo, E.; Rodriguez-Hernandez, M.A.; et al. Supercomplex assembly determines electron flux in the mitochondrial electron transport chain. *Science* **2013**, *340*, 1567–1570. [CrossRef]

57. Drummond, D.A.; Wilke, C.O. Mistranslation-induced protein misfolding as a dominant constraint on coding-sequence evolution. *Cell* **2008**, *134*, 341–352. [CrossRef]

58. Roy, H.; Ibba, M. Molecular biology: Sticky end in protein synthesis. *Nature* **2006**, *443*, 41–42. [CrossRef]

59. Pandolfini, L.; Barbieri, I.; Bannister, A.J.; Hendrick, A.; Andrews, B.; Webster, N.; Murat, P.; Mach, P.; Brandi, R.; Robson, S.C.; et al. METTL1 Promotes let-7 MicroRNA Processing via m7G Methylation. *Mol. Cell* **2019**, *74*, 1278–1290.e9. [CrossRef]

60. Wang, T.; Wang, G.; Hao, D.; Liu, X.; Wang, D.; Ning, N.; Li, X. Aberrant regulation of the LIN28A/LIN28B and let-7 loop in human malignant tumors and its effects on the hallmarks of cancer. *Mol. Cancer* **2015**, *14*, 125. [CrossRef]

61. Chakraborty, A.; Wakamiya, M.; Venkova-Canova, T.; Pandita, R.K.; Aguilera-Aguirre, L.; Sarker, A.H.; Singh, D.K.; Hosoki, K.; Wood, T.G.; Sharma, G.; et al. Neil2-null Mice Accumulate Oxidized DNA Bases in the Transcriptionally Active Sequences of the Genome and Are Susceptible to Innate Inflammation. *J. Biol. Chem.* **2015**, *290*, 24636–24648. [CrossRef]

62. Feinberg, A.P.; Ohlsson, R.; Henikoff, S. The epigenetic progenitor origin of human cancer. *Nat. Rev. Genet.* **2006**, *7*, 21–33. [CrossRef]

63. Robert, M.F.; Morin, S.; Beaulieu, N.; Gauthier, F.; Chute, I.C.; Barsalou, A.; MacLeod, A.R. DNMT1 is required to maintain CpG methylation and aberrant gene silencing in human cancer cells. *Nat. Genet.* **2003**, *33*, 61–65. [CrossRef] [PubMed]

64. Grewal, S.I.; Moazed, D. Heterochromatin and epigenetic control of gene expression. *Science* **2003**, *301*, 798–802. [CrossRef] [PubMed]

65. Stirzaker, C.; Taberlay, P.C.; Statham, A.L.; Clark, S.J. Mining cancer methylomes: Prospects and challenges. *Trends Genet.* **2014**, *30*, 75–84. [CrossRef] [PubMed]

66. Ustianenko, D.; Chiu, H.S.; Treiber, T.; Weyn-Vanhentenryck, S.M.; Treiber, N.; Meister, G.; Sumazin, P.; Zhang, C. LIN28 Selectively Modulates a Subclass of Let-7 MicroRNAs. *Mol. Cell* **2018**, *71*, 271–283.e275. [CrossRef]

67. Liu, B.; Su, Y.; Li, T.; Yuan, W.; Mo, X.; Li, H.; He, Q.; Ma, D.; Han, W. CMTM7 knockdown increases tumorigenicity of human non-small cell lung cancer cells and EGFR-AKT signaling by reducing Rab5 activation. *Oncotarget* **2015**, *6*, 41092–41107. [CrossRef] [PubMed]

68. Garcia-Mata, R.; Boulter, E.; Burridge, K. The 'invisible hand': Regulation of RHO GTPases by RHOGDIs. *Nat. Rev. Mol. Cell Biol.* **2011**, *12*, 493–504. [CrossRef] [PubMed]

69. Coleman, A.M.; Rendon, B.E.; Zhao, M.; Qian, M.W.; Bucala, R.; Xin, D.; Mitchell, R.A. Cooperative regulation of non-small cell lung carcinoma angiogenic potential by macrophage migration inhibitory factor and its homolog, D-dopachrome tautomerase. *J. Immunol.* **2008**, *181*, 2330–2337. [CrossRef]

70. Liang, Y.; Li, W.W.; Yang, B.W.; Tao, Z.H.; Sun, H.C.; Wang, L.; Xia, J.L.; Qin, L.X.; Tang, Z.Y.; Fan, J.; et al. Aryl hydrocarbon receptor nuclear translocator is associated with tumor growth and progression of hepatocellular carcinoma. *Int. J. Cancer* **2012**, *130*, 1745–1754. [CrossRef] [PubMed]

71. Pasupuleti, V.; Du, W.; Gupta, Y.; Yeh, I.J.; Montano, M.; Magi-Galuzzi, C.; Welford, S.M. Dysregulated D-dopachrome tautomerase, a hypoxia-inducible factor-dependent gene, cooperates with macrophage migration inhibitory factor in renal tumorigenesis. *J. Biol. Chem.* **2014**, *289*, 3713–3723. [CrossRef]

72. Shi, S.L.; Yoon, D.Y.; Hodge-Bell, K.C.; Bebenek, I.G.; Whitekus, M.J.; Zhang, R.X.; Cochran, A.J.; Huerta-Yepez, S.; Yim, S.H.; Gonzalez, F.J.; et al. The aryl hydrocarbon receptor nuclear translocator (Arnt) is required for tumor initiation by benzo[a]pyrene. *Carcinogenesis* **2009**, *30*, 1957–1961. [CrossRef]

73. Hao, N.; Bhakti, V.L.; Peet, D.J.; Whitelaw, M.L. Reciprocal regulation of the basic helix-loop-helix/Per-Arnt-Sim partner proteins, Arnt and Arnt2, during neuronal differentiation. *Nucleic Acids Res.* **2013**, *41*, 5626–5638. [CrossRef] [PubMed]

74. Bishop, K.S.; Ferguson, L.R. The interaction between epigenetics, nutrition and the development of cancer. *Nutrients* **2015**, *7*, 922–947. [CrossRef] [PubMed]

75. Van Dijk, S.J.; Zhou, J.; Peters, T.J.; Buckley, M.; Sutcliffe, B.; Oytam, Y.; Gibson, R.A.; McPhee, A.; Yelland, L.N.; Makrides, M.; et al. Effect of prenatal DHA supplementation on the infant epigenome: Results from a randomized controlled trial. *Clin. Epigenetics* **2016**, *8*, 114. [CrossRef] [PubMed]

76. Mahmoud, A.M.; Ali, M.M. Methyl Donor Micronutrients that Modify DNA Methylation and Cancer Outcome. *Nutrients* **2019**, *11*, 608. [CrossRef]

77. Crider, K.S.; Yang, T.P.; Berry, R.J.; Bailey, L.B. Folate and DNA methylation: A review of molecular mechanisms and the evidence for folate's role. *Adv. Nutr.* **2012**, *3*, 21–38. [CrossRef]

78. Bacalini, M.G.; Boattini, A.; Gentilini, D.; Giampieri, E.; Pirazzini, C.; Giuliani, C.; Fontanesi, E.; Remondini, D.; Capri, M.; Del Rio, A.; et al. A meta-analysis on age-associated changes in blood DNA methylation: Results from an original analysis pipeline for Infinium 450k data. *Aging* **2015**, *7*, 97–109. [CrossRef]

79. Bouchard, L.; Rabasa-Lhoret, R.; Faraj, M.; Lavoie, M.E.; Mill, J.; Perusse, L.; Vohl, M.C. Differential epigenomic and transcriptomic responses in subcutaneous adipose tissue between low and high responders to caloric restriction. *Am. J. Clin. Nutr.* **2010**, *91*, 309–320. [CrossRef]

80. Milagro, F.I.; Campion, J.; Cordero, P.; Goyenechea, E.; Gomez-Uriz, A.M.; Abete, I.; Zulet, M.A.; Martinez, J.A. A dual epigenomic approach for the search of obesity biomarkers: DNA methylation in relation to diet-induced weight loss. *FASEB J.* **2011**, *25*, 1378–1389. [CrossRef]

81. Breton, C.V.; Marsit, C.J.; Faustman, E.; Nadeau, K.; Goodrich, J.M.; Dolinoy, D.C.; Herbstman, J.; Holland, N.; LaSalle, J.M.; Schmidt, R.; et al. Small-Magnitude Effect Sizes in Epigenetic End Points are Important in Children's Environmental Health Studies: The Children's Environmental Health and Disease Prevention Research Center's Epigenetics Working Group. *Environ. Health Perspect.* **2017**, *125*, 511–526. [CrossRef]

82. Li, Y.; Liu, L.; Tollefsbol, T.O. Glucose restriction can extend normal cell lifespan and impair precancerous cell growth through epigenetic control of hTERT and p16 expression. *FASEB J.* **2010**, *24*, 1442–1453. [CrossRef]

83. Tate, P.H.; Bird, A.P. Effects of DNA methylation on DNA-binding proteins and gene expression. *Curr. Opin. Genet. Dev.* **1993**, *3*, 226–231. [CrossRef]

84. Martins, M.C.T.; Jaceldo-Siegl, K.; Orlich, M.; Fan, J.; Mashchak, A.; Fraser, G.E. A New Approach to Assess Lifetime Dietary Patterns Finds Lower Consumption of Animal Foods with Aging in a Longitudinal Analysis of a Health-Oriented Adventist Population. *Nutrients* **2017**, *9*, 1118. [CrossRef] [PubMed]

85. Byun, H.M.; Siegmund, K.D.; Pan, F.; Weisenberger, D.J.; Kanel, G.; Laird, P.W.; Yang, A.S. Epigenetic profiling of somatic tissues from human autopsy specimens identifies tissue- and individual-specific DNA methylation patterns. *Hum. Mol. Genet.* **2009**, *18*, 4808–4817. [CrossRef] [PubMed]
86. Crujeiras, A.B.; Diaz-Lagares, A.; Sandoval, J.; Milagro, F.I.; Navas-Carretero, S.; Carreira, M.C.; Gomez, A.; Hervas, D.; Monteiro, M.P.; Casanueva, F.F.; et al. DNA methylation map in circulating leukocytes mirrors subcutaneous adipose tissue methylation pattern: A genome-wide analysis from non-obese and obese patients. *Sci. Rep.* **2017**, *7*, 41903. [CrossRef]
87. Wu, H.C.; Wang, Q.; Yang, H.I.; Tsai, W.Y.; Chen, C.J.; Santella, R.M. Global DNA methylation levels in white blood cells as a biomarker for hepatocellular carcinoma risk: A nested case-control study. *Carcinogenesis* **2012**, *33*, 1340–1345. [CrossRef]

Publisher's Note: MDPI stays neutral with regard to jurisdictional claims in published maps and institutional affiliations.

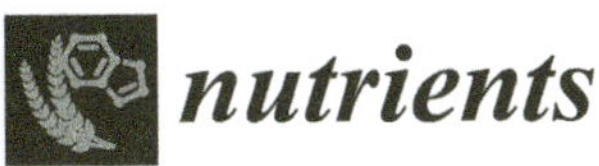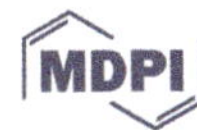

Article

The Association between Daily Total Dietary Nutrient Intake and Recent Glycemic Control States of Non-Pregnant Adults 20+ Years Old from NHANES 1999–2018 (Except for 2003–2004)

Yin Bai [1], Hao Zhang [2], Jie Yang [3] and Lei Peng [4],*

[1]   Department of Marketing, College of Management and Economics, Tianjin University, Tianjin 300072, China; baiyin@tju.edu.cn
[2]   Department of Social Medicine and Health Education, School of Public Health, Peking University, Beijing 100000, China; 2011210118@stu.pku.edu.cn
[3]   Public Health Clinical Center of Chengdu, Chengdu 610066, China; yangjieHJ@gmail.com
[4]   Department of Epidemiology, School of Clinical Oncology, Peking University, Beijing 100143, China
*   Correspondence: 2011210593@stu.pku.edu.cn; Tel.: +86-138-0828-2849

Abstract: Background: Although daily total dietary nutrient intakes were potentially important factors in maintaining glycemic balance, their overall effect on glycemic control was still unclear among American adults. Objectives: We aimed to examine the association between daily total dietary nutrient intake and recent glycemic control status (RGCS). Methods: This cohort was composed of 41,302 individuals from the National Health and Nutrition Examination Survey (NHANES). The daily total intake of dietary nutrients and RGCS were independent and dependent variables, respectively. To evaluate their association, we carried out binary logistic regression, model fitting, linear discriminant analysis, and the receiver operator characteristic (ROC) analysis. Results: The result of robust check model showed that only the daily total dietary vitamin B6 intake (adjusted OR = 0.848; 95% CI: 0.738, 0.973; *p*-value = 0.019) was significantly negatively correlated with RGCS. When daily total dietary vitamin B6 intake and glycosylated hemoglobin (HbA1c) were used as independent variables and dependent variables, respectively, to fit the curves and lines, the established robust check model could distinguish American adults with different RGCS well. Moreover, the robust check model results of ROC analysis indicated that daily total dietary vitamin B6 intake might be a potential predictor for RGCS (AUC = 0.977; 95% CI: 0.974, 0.980; *p*-value < 0.001). Conclusions: This study showed that only daily total dietary vitamin B6 intake was a beneficial factor in RGCS, but it might need further multicenter or prospective studies to verify whether vitamin B6 had biological implications and public health meaning for glycemic control among American adults (specifically referred to non-pregnant participants over 20 years old).

Keywords: daily total intake of dietary nutrients; RGCS; HbA1c; NHANES; odds ratio

Citation: Bai, Y.; Zhang, H.; Yang, J.; Peng, L. The Association between Daily Total Dietary Nutrient Intake and Recent Glycemic Control States of Non-Pregnant Adults 20+ Years Old from NHANES 1999–2018 (Except for 2003–2004). *Nutrients* **2021**, *13*, 4168. https://doi.org/10.3390/nu13114168

Academic Editor: Lourdes Varela

Received: 18 September 2021
Accepted: 19 November 2021
Published: 21 November 2021

1. Introduction

Dietary nutrients play an important role in maintaining the balance of blood glucose as a necessary substance to regulate the normal physiological function of the body, being roughly divided into macronutrients [1–3], dietary fiber (as an independent factor that distinguishes carbohydrates, included in this study) [4–6], minerals [7–9], and vitamins [10–13]. Many studies have shown that there was a positive correlation between recent glycemic control status (RGCS) and serum chromium, zinc, and magnesium levels [7,14–20]. Glycosylated hemoglobin (HbA1c), an irreversible product of blood glucose and hemoglobin, could provide information for long-term glycemic control [21]. Moreover, after the relationship between RGCS and HbA1c concentration was widely confirmed, the serum index was applied to diabetes diagnosis and glycemic monitoring practice [21,22]. Therefore, it was appropriate to use HbA1c as a predictor for RGCS among American adults (specifically referred to non-pregnant participants over 20 years old).

At present, most of the research conclusions on the association between daily total nutrient intake and RGCS have been one-sided. They did not analyze the overall effect of various nutrients on RGCS but analyzed minerals, vitamins, and macronutrients separately, which was not complete and systematic, and might have even led to obtaining inconsistent conclusions [23,24]. Although findings on the association between daily total dietary nutrient intake and RGCS were inconsistent and not enough to prove the relationship, these results, to a certain extent, could supply research hypotheses for future large-scale prospective or multi-center verification. Therefore, if we further explored the association between the adults' RGCS and daily total dietary nutrient intakes, it was necessary to construct a holistic and optimal model to combine the macronutrients, minerals, and vitamins of daily total nutrient intake, as well as demographic characteristics, in order to draw a reliable conclusion.

In addition, most studies on dietary factors affecting glycemic control have been conducted on diabetes patients [5,11,25–27], and therefore these conclusions could not be suitable for American adults to control blood glucose. Moreover, it is worth noting that insufficient sample size might also lead to biased conclusions, for instance, in the study of Intra et al. [26], the sample size of cases group was very small (cases group, n = 84; controls group, n = 2745), and therefore the results of this study might have a larger systematic bias. Therefore, we conducted the follow-up sampling survey study to estimate the association between daily total nutrient intake and RGCS among non-pregnant adults 20+ years old using a large-scale database from National Health and Nutrition Examination Survey (NHANES 1999–2018, except for 2003–2004).

2. Methods

2.1. Database and Study Population

We used the NHANES database, a nationally representative survey database collected biennially by the National Center for Health Statistics (NCHS), and employed a complex, multistage, probabilistic sampling design [28]. The database was publicly available on the Internet and can be downloaded by researchers around the world. All details about the database could be efficiently acquired at http://www.cdc.gov/nchs/nhanes/ (accessed on 27 May 2021), including relevant information such as strict quality control measures for the questionnaire data undertaken by NHANES. The 24 h dietary recall data from non-pregnant adults 20+ years of age participating in NHANES 1999–2002 and 2005–2018 surveys were followed biennially for all analyses. The database for analysis consisted of five parts: demographics data, dietary data, examination data, laboratory data, and questionnaire data.

During the 1999–2018 NHANES survey cohorts, 101,316 preliminary participants were included in the study. Individuals without physical examination data (n = 2096), under 20 years of age (n = 47,208), pregnant (n = 2527), without an unusual diet compared food consumed yesterday and without reliable data (n = 6431), and 2003–2004 survey cycle data with the missing outcome variable (n = 1752) were excluded. Those with complete or reliable 24 h recall data (only day 1 data used) as judged by the United States Department of Agriculture's (USDA) Food Surveys Research Group staff were included in the analyses. In addition, of the 41302 participants, 58 of the dietary survey data contained some missing indices (such as the intake of dietary fiber and folic acid), and we used the median to fill them. Finally, 41,302 subjects (20,458 males and 20,844 females, 50.0 ± 17.9 years for males and 50.2 ± 17.8 years for females) were certainly included in this study (Figure S1). All serum samples were collected under fasting condition. HCHS obtained the written informed consent from all participants and the ethical review committee approved all NHANES protocols.

2.2. Variables

In this study, the independent variables were daily total dietary nutrient intakes, containing protein, carbohydrate, total fat, dietary fiber, vitamin B1, vitamin B2, vitamin

B6, total folate, vitamin B12, vitamin E, calcium, magnesium, iron, zinc, and copper. It is worth mentioning that the dietary energy value different from the category of dietary nutrients was also included in the follow-up analysis as an independent important parameter. The dependent variable was RGCS (HbA1c < 6.5% represents good RGCS, and HbA1c ≥ 6.5% represents poor RGCS). All variables involved in this study were divided into continuous variables and categorical variables. Continuous variables included energy, protein, carbohydrate, dietary fiber, total fat, total folate, vitamin B1, vitamin B2, vitamin B6, vitamin B12, vitamin E, calcium, magnesium, iron, zinc, copper, poverty income ratio (PIR), insulin, glucose, and hemoglobin. Categorical variables included gender, age, race, education level, body mass index (BMI), moderate or severe physical activity, hypertension, the doctor informing them they had diabetes, having at least 12 cups of alcoholic drink per year, consuming over 100 cigarettes in their lifetime, and adult food security. Details of all variable acquisition procedures can be found at http://www.cdc.gov/nchs/nhanes/.

2.3. Statistical Analysis

The results of normality test showed that it could not be considered that all continuous variables obeyed normal distribution. Therefore, in the stages of statistical description and single variable analysis, all continuous variables and categorical variables were expressed as median (25% percentile–75% percentile) and percentage (proportion), respectively. We used a nonparametric test (Mann–Whitney U test) for all continuous variables that did not obey normal distribution, as well as Pearson's chi-squared test for all categorical variables. Then, in the multivariate analysis stage, we controlled different confounders and established four binary logistic regression models with the RGCS as the dependent variable to adjust the potential bias. Eventually, we performed model fitting with the HbA1c index as the dependent variable, and receiver operator characteristic (ROC) analysis was performed to calculate the area under the curve (AUC). The result of the collinearity diagnosis showed that there was no collinearity (variance inflation factor, VIF < 10) among the independent variables studied. Statistical significance was considered when p-value was below 0.05 (two-tailed). Data processing, statistical analysis, and graphic drawing were carried out with Stata version 13.1, IBM SPSS version 26.0, GraphPad Prism version 7.00, R version 4.0.2 (http://www.R-project.org, The R Foundation), and EmpowerStats software version 2.1 (http://www.empowerstats.com, X&Y Solutions, Inc., Boston, MA, USA).

3. Result

3.1. Baseline Characteristics

The description of demographic and medical characteristics is shown in Table 1. Among the participants, 49.5% (n = 20,458) were male, 44.6% (n = 18,404) were non-Hispanic White, 20.5% (n = 8458) were non-Hispanic Black, and 17.3% (n = 7153) were Mexican American. In addition, the statistical description of daily dietary nutrient intakes in our study showed that their distribution fluctuated over time (Figure 1). Therefore, the time effect was often a potential confusion factor, which should be placed in subsequent analysis.

Table 1. Characteristics by RGCS of non-pregnant adults 20+ years old from NHANES 1999–2018 (except for 2003–2004).

Characteristics	Good RGCS (HbA1 < 6.5%) [#] n = 36,594	Poor RGCS (HbA1 ≥ 6.5%) [#] n = 4708	χ^2/Z Value	p-Value
Gender (%)			21.006	<0.001
Male	17,978 (87.9)	2480 (12.1)		
Female	18,616 (89.3)	2228 (10.7)		
Age (%)			2119.291	<0.001
≥60 years old	11,414 (80.1)	2843 (19.9)		
40–59 years old	12,125 (88.6)	1554 (11.4)		
<40 years old	13,055 (97.7)	311 (2.3)		

Table 1. *Cont.*

Characteristics	Good RGCS (HbA1 < 6.5%) [#] n = 36,594	Poor RGCS (HbA1 ≥ 6.5%) [#] n = 4708	χ^2/Z Value	*p*-Value
Race (%)			322.688	<0.001
Non-Hispanic White	16,857 (91.6)	1547 (8.4)		
Non-Hispanic Black	7201 (85.1)	1257 (14.9)		
Mexican American	6140 (85.8)	1013 (14.2)		
Other Races	6396 (87.8)	891 (12.2)		
Education level (%) [†]			255.723	<0.001
≤High School	17,597 (86.1)	2845 (13.9)		
College or above	18,955 (91.1)	1855 (8.9)		
BMI (Kg/m^2) [*†]			219.213	<0.001
≥30.0	102 (87.9)	14 (12.1)		
25.0–29.9	12,455 (90.5)	1304 (9.5)		
<25.0	11,298 (95.3)	557 (4.7)		
Moderate/severe physical activity (%) [†]			162.861	<0.001
Yes	14,859 (91.1)	1457 (8.9)		
No	21,719 (87.0)	3249 (13.0)		
Hypertension (%) [†]			537.915	<0.001
Yes	14,672 (84.7)	2648 (15.3)		
No	19,138 (92.2)	1611 (7.8)		
The doctor told you that you had diabetes (%)			18,424.978	<0.001
Yes	1711 (33.1)	3462 (66.9)		
Borderline	676 (76.2)	211 (23.8)		
No	34,207 (97.1)	1035 (2.9)		
Had at least 12 cups of alcoholic drink per year (%) [‡†]			157.612	<0.001
Yes	25,714 (89.8)	2932 (10.2)		
No	8981 (85.2)	1559 (14.8)		
Consumed over 100 cigarettes in lifetime (%) [†]			26.543	<0.001
Yes	16,589 (87.7)	2321 (12.3)		
No	19,979 (89.3)	2383 (10.7)		
Food security (%)			38.584	<0.001
Yes	26,893 (89.4)	3174 (10.6)		
No	5300 (86.7)	812 (13.3)		
PIR [*†]	2.2 (1.2–4.2)	1.8 (1.0–3.3)	6.236	<0.001
Energy (kcal)	1948.0 (1441.1–2612.0)	1725.0 (1257.0–2329.0)	7.599	<0.001
Protein (gm)	72.3 (51.8–100.7)	69.0 (49.3–94.0)	3.809	<0.001
Carbohydrate (gm)	236.6 (170.6–319.7)	204.5 (147.4–278.1)	8.295	<0.001
Total fat (gm)	71.3 (47.6–102.3)	64.6 (42.7–96.2)	4.666	<0.001
Dietary fiber (gm)	14.3 (9.3–21.2)	14.1 (9.3–20.8)	1.140	0.148
Thiamin (Vitamin B1) (mg)	1.4 (1.0–2.0)	1.4 (0.9–1.9)	2.685	<0.001
Riboflavin (Vitamin B2) (mg)	1.8 (1.3–2.6)	1.7 (1.2–2.3)	4.151	<0.001
Vitamin B6 (mg)	1.7 (1.1–2.5)	1.6 (1.1–2.3)	4.416	<0.001
Total folate (mcg)	341.0 (230.0–496.0)	320.0 (215.0–459.0)	3.558	<0.001
Vitamin B12 (mcg)	3.7 (2.1–6.2)	3.4 (1.9–5.6)	3.452	<0.001
Vitamin E (mg)	6.5 (4.2–10.0)	6.1 (3.8–9.3)	3.294	<0.001
Calcium (mg)	779.0 (496.0–1151.0)	713.0 (468.0–1040.8)	4.185	<0.001
Magnesium (mg)	265.0 (190.0–363.0)	249.0 (180.0–336.0)	4.041	<0.001
Iron (mg)	12.8 (8.9–18.4)	12.3 (8.5–17.5)	2.466	<0.001
Zinc (mg)	9.7 (6.6–14.1)	8.9 (6.1–13.0)	3.824	<0.001
Copper (mg)	1.1 (0.8–1.5)	1.0 (0.7–1.4)	4.124	<0.001
Insulin (uU/mL) [†]	9.5 (6.2–15.2)	14.7 (8.8–25.0)	10.705	<0.001
Glucose (mg/dL) [†]	91.0 (85.0–99.0)	149.0 (118.0–149.0)	45.353	<0.001
Hemoglobin (g/dL) [†]	14.2 (13.2–15.2)	13.9 (12.8–15.0)	5.840	<0.001

[#] The statistical description of the two groups was expressed in the form of a number (%)/median (25% percentile–75% percentile). [†] There were missing values in the two groups. [‡] One cup of alcoholic drink is equivalent to 12 ounces of beer, 4 ounces of wine, or an ounce of liquor. [*] BMI, body mass index; PIR, poverty income ratio; RGCS, recent glycemic control states.

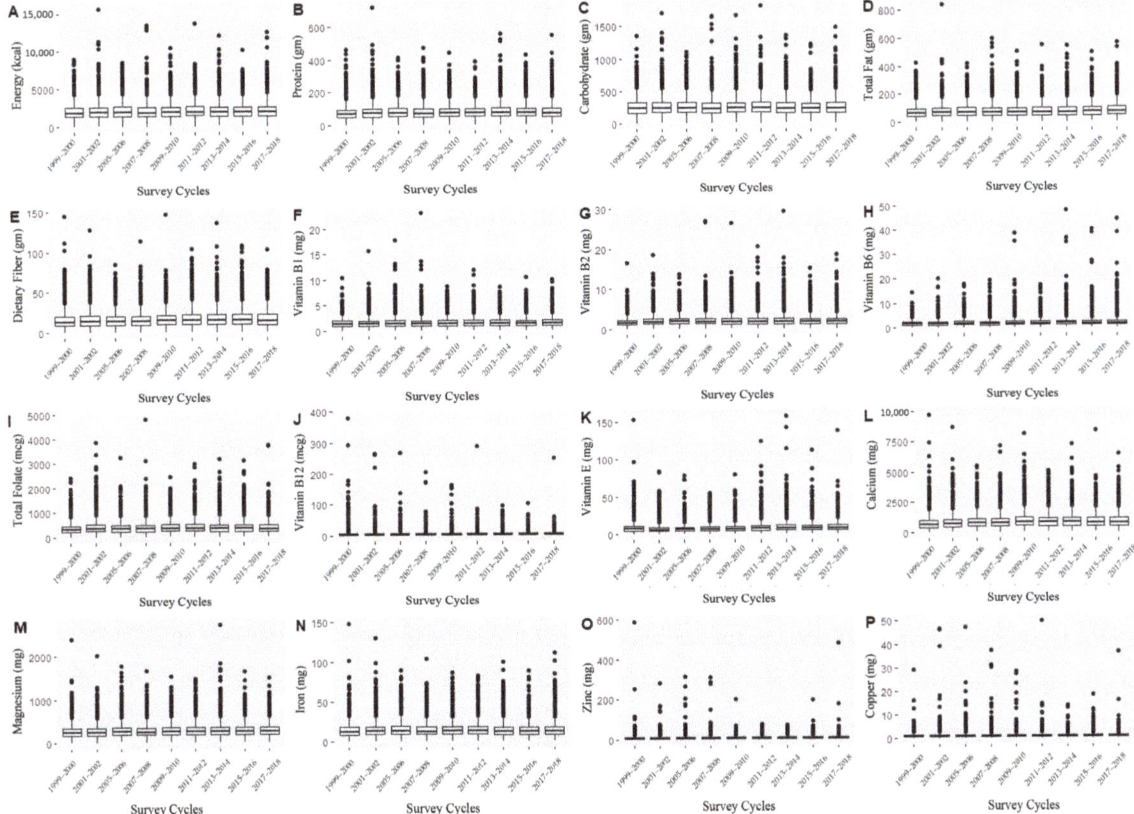

Figure 1. Distribution of daily total dietary energy and nutrient intakes in different investigation periods ((**A**) Energy (kcal); (**B**) Protein (gm); (**C**) Carbohydrate; (**D**) Total Fat (gm); (**E**) Dietary Fiber (gm); (**F**) Vitamin B1 (mg); (**G**) Vitamin B2 (mg); (**H**) Vitamin B6 (mg); (**I**) Total Folate (mg); (**J**) Vitamin B12 (mg); (**K**) Vitamin E (mg); (**L**) Calcium (mg); (**M**) Magnesium (mg); (**N**) Iron (mg); (**O**) Zinc (mg); (**P**) Copper (mg)).

3.2. Binary Logistic Regression Analysis

3.2.1. The Association between RGCS and Daily Total Dietary Energy, Macronutrients, Vitamins, and Minerals

For the crude model and adjusted model I, we found that energy, protein, total fat, dietary fiber, vitamin B1, vitamin B6, vitamin E, iron, and zinc intake were associated with RGCS, including good RGCS and poor RGCS (Figure 2A,B). However, after controlling of all covariates and time fixed effect (Figure 2C,D), opposite results were obtained from the former two models, for instance, three kinds of macronutrients, minerals, and dietary fiber actually had no statistical association with RGCS. Eventually, the statistical results in the robust check model (Figure 2D and Table 2), after controlling for the potential confounders and years fixed effect, suggested a significantly negative correlation between daily total dietary vitamin B6 intake and RGCS (adjusted OR = 0.848; 95% CI: 0.738, 0.973; *p*-value = 0.019).

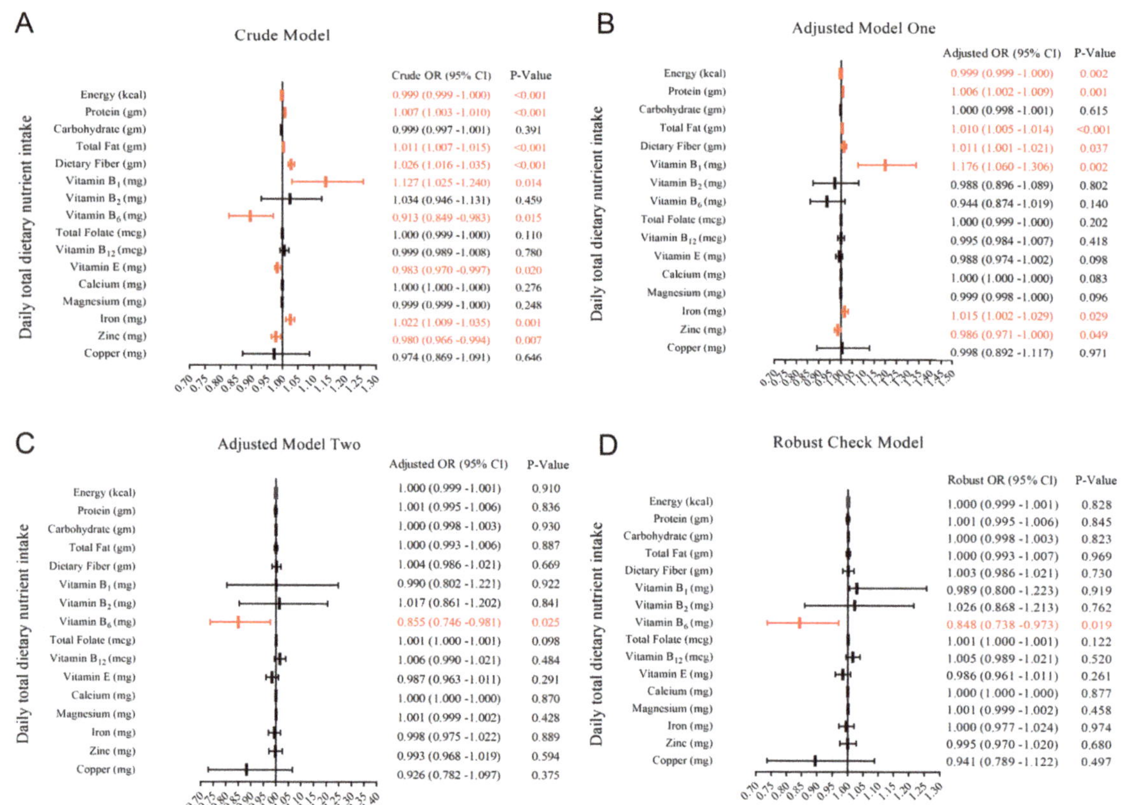

Figure 2. Forest plot for odds ratio (OR) and 95% confidence interval (CI) of daily total dietary nutrient and energy intake ((**A**) without covariates; (**B**) gender, age, and race were controlled; (**C**) all potential confounders in the study were controlled; (**D**) all potential confounders and the years fixed effect in the study were controlled).

Table 2. Binary logistic regression analysis between RGCS and dietary nutrient and energy intake among non-pregnant adults 20+ years old from NHANES 1999–2018 (except for 2003–2004).

Variables	Crude Model [a]	Model I [b]	Model II [c]	Robust Check Model [d]
	β (SE)	β (SE)	β (SE)	β (SE)
Energy (kcal)	−0.001 (0.0002) ***	−0.001 (0.0002) **	−0.00003 (0.0003)	−0.00006 (0.0003)
Protein (gm)	0.007 (0.002) ***	0.006 (0.002) **	0.001 (0.003)	0.001 (0.003)
Carbohydrate (gm)	−0.001 (0.001)	−0.0005 (0.001)	0.0001 (0.001)	0.0003 (0.001)
Total fat (gm)	0.011 (0.002) ***	0.010 (0.002) ***	−0.0005 (0.003)	−0.0001 (0.003)
Dietary fiber (gm)	0.025 (0.005) ***	0.011 (0.005) *	0.004 (0.009)	0.003 (0.009)
Thiamin (Vitamin B1) (mg)	0.120 (0.049) *	0.162 (0.053) **	−0.011 (0.107)	−0.011 (0.108)
Riboflavin (Vitamin B2) (mg)	0.034 (0.045)	−0.012 (0.050)	0.017 (0.085)	0.026 (0.085)
Vitamin B6 (mg)	−0.091 (0.037) *	−0.058 (0.039)	−0.157 (0.070) *	−0.165 (0.070) *
Total folate (mcg)	−0.0004 (0.0002)	−0.0003 (0.0002)	0.001 (0.0004)	0.001 (0.0004)
Vitamin B12 (mcg)	−0.001 (0.005)	−0.005 (0.006)	0.006 (0.008)	0.005 (0.008)
Vitamin E (mg)	−0.017 (0.007) *	−0.012 (0.007)	−0.013 (0.013)	−0.014 (0.013)
Calcium (mg)	−0.00008 (0.00008)	0.0001 (0.00008)	0.00002 (0.0001)	−0.00002 (0.0001)
Magnesium (mg)	−0.001 (0.0005)	−0.001 (0.0005)	0.001 (0.001)	0.001 (0.001)
Iron (mg)	0.022 (0.006) **	0.015 (0.007) *	−0.002 (0.012)	0.0004 (0.012)
Zinc (mg)	−0.020 (0.007) **	−0.015 (0.007) *	−0.007 (0.013)	−0.005 (0.013)
Copper (mg)	−0.027 (0.058)	−0.002 (0.057)	−0.077 (0.086) **	−0.061 (0.090)

Table 2. *Cont.*

Variables	Crude Model [a] β (SE)	Model I [b] β (SE)	Model II [c] β (SE)	Robust Check Model [d] β (SE)
Age (<40 years old)	-	Reference	Reference	Reference
Age (40−59 years old)	-	2.211 (0.103) ***	0.985 (0.190) ***	0.978 (0.191) ***
Age ($\geq$ 60 years old)	-	1.561 (0.104) ***	0.792 (0.189) ***	0.782 (0.189) ***
Gender (male)	-	0.230 (0.058) ***	0.322 (0.117) **	0.311 (0.118) **
Race (other races)	-	Reference	Reference	Reference
Race (Mexican American)	-	−0.551 (0.083) ***	−0.269 (0.150)	−0.229 (0.151)
Race (non-Hispanic Black)	-	0.298 (0.089) **	0.342 (0.163) *	0.396 (0.164) *
Race (non-Hispanic White)	-	0.209 (0.091) *	−0.024 (0.170)	0.043 (0.172)
Education level ($\leq$ high school)	-	-	0.179 (0.107)	0.187 (0.108)
BMI [†] (<25.0)	-	-	Reference	Reference
BMI (25.0–29.9)	-	-	0.726 (0.146) ***	0.714 (0.146) ***
BMI ($\geq$30.0)	-	-	0.081 (0.156)	0.076 (0.156)
Moderate/severe physical activity (no)	-	-	0.114 (0.103)	0.076 (0.104)
Hypertension (yes)	-	-	0.296 (0.100) **	0.323 (0.100)
The doctor told you that you had diabetes (no)	-	-	Reference	Reference
The doctor told you that you had diabetes (borderline)	-	-	2.501 (0.106) ***	2.491 (0.106) ***
The doctor told you that you had diabetes (yes)	-	-	1.167 (0.196) ***	1.141 (0.196) ***
Had at least 12 cups alcoholic drink per year (yes)	-	-	−0.057 (0.112)	−0.077 (0.113)
Consumed over 100 cigarettes in their lifetime (yes)	-	-	−0.085 (0.103)	−0.073 (0.104)
Food security (no)	-	-	0.076 (0.135)	0.047 (0.137)
PIR [†]	-	-	−0.049 (0.036)	−0.048 (0.036)
Insulin (uU/mL)	-	-	0.003 (0.002)	0.003 (0.002)
Glucose (mg/dL)	-	-	0.061 (0.002) ***	0.061 (0.002) ***
Hemoglobin (g/dL)	-	-	−0.095 (0.036) **	−0.086 (0.036) *
Years fixed effect	-	-	-	Included

[a] A total of 15 dietary variables were entered in the crude model: protein, carbohydrate, total fat, dietary fiber, vitamin b1, vitamin b2, vitamin b6, total folate, vitamin b12, vitamin e, calcium, magnesium, iron, zinc, copper. [b] Three variables were adjusted in model I: gender, age, race. [c] A total of 17 variables were adjusted in model II: gender, age, race, education level, BMI, moderate or severe physical activity, hypertension, the doctor informing them that they had diabetes, having at least 12 cups of alcoholic drink per year, consuming over 100 cigarettes in their lifetime, food security, PIR, energy, insulin, glucose, hemoglobin. [d] Robust check model: Based on model II, years fixed effect was adjusted. * *p*-value < 0.05; ** *p*-value < 0.01; *** *p*-value < 0.001. [†] BMI, body mass index; PIR, poverty income ratio; RGCS, recent glycemic control states; SE, standard error.

3.2.2. The Association between Adjusted Covariates and RGCS

The statistical results of the robust check model, all covariates, and time fixed effect being adjusted demonstrated that age (taking "<40 years old" as a reference, $OR_{[40–59 \text{ years old}]}$ = 2.659, *p*-value < 0.001; $OR_{[\geq 60 \text{ years old}]}$ = 2.186, *p*-value < 0.001), gender (taking "female" as a reference, $OR_{[Male]}$ = 1.365, *p*-value = 0.008), race (taking "other races" as a reference, $OR_{[Mexican American]}$ = 0.796, *p*-value = 0.131; $OR_{[Non-Hispanic Black]}$ = 1.486, *p*-value = 0.016; $OR_{[Non-Hispanic White]}$ = 1.044, *p*-value = 0.804), education level (taking ">high school" as a reference, $OR_{[\leq High School]}$ = 1.205, *p*-value = 0.083), BMI (taking "<25.0" as a reference, $OR_{[25.0–29.9]}$ = 2.042, *p*-value < 0.001; $OR_{[\geq 30.0]}$ = 1.079, *p*-value = 0.626), hypertension (taking "no" as a reference, $OR_{[Yes]}$ = 1.381, *p*-value = 0.001), the doctor informing them that they had diabetes (taking "no" as a reference, $OR_{[Borderline]}$ = 12.072, *p*-value < 0.001; $OR_{[Yes]}$ = 3.130, *p*-value < 0.001), insulin (OR = 1.003, *p*-value = 0.132), glucose (OR = 1.063, *p*-value < 0.001), and hemoglobin (OR = 0.918, *p*-value = 0.017) were significantly associated with RGCS in Table 2.

3.3. Model Fitting, Linear Discriminant Analysis, and ROC Analysis

3.3.1. Model Fitting and Linear Discriminant Analysis of Daily Total Dietary Vitamin B6 Intake, Glycohemoglobin, and RGCS

After smooth curve fitting of daily total dietary vitamin B6 intake and glycohemoglobin being conducted in Figure 3, the robust check model, a linear discriminant analysis of daily total dietary vitamin B6 intake and RGCS, was also fitted in Figure 4. The statistical analysis graphs showed that the established robust check model could not only distinguish American adults with different RGCS well, but pointed out that the negative correlation between daily total dietary vitamin B6 intake and RGCS did exist. It was indicated that daily total dietary vitamin B6 intake might have a potential predictive value for RGCS of American adults.

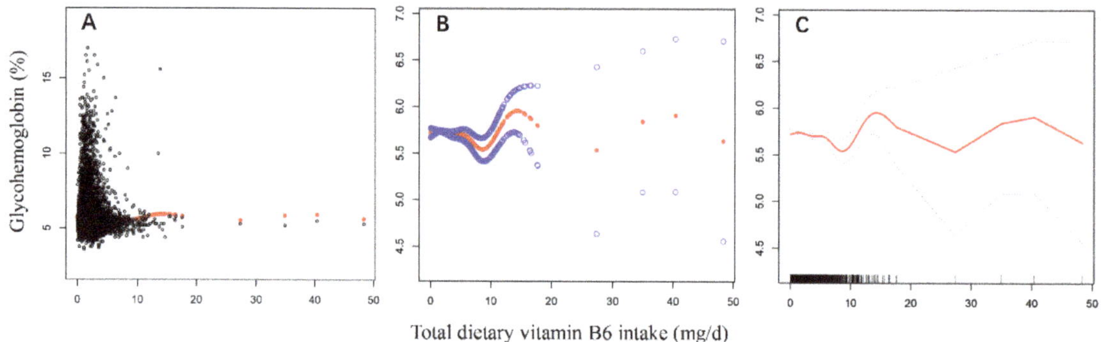

Figure 3. The model fitting processes of non-linear regression curve ((**A**,**B**), scatter plots; (**C**), the optimal smooth curve).

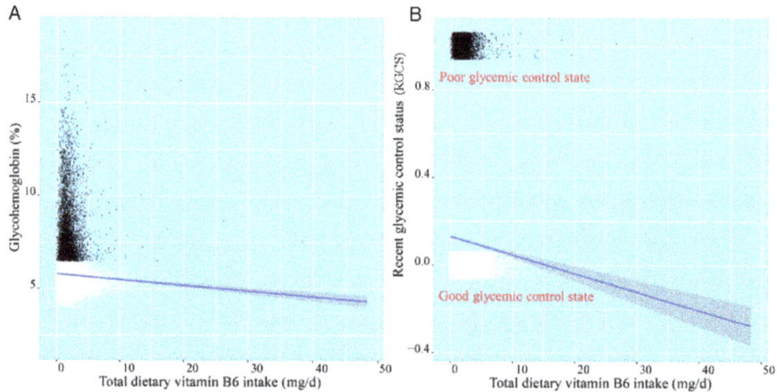

Figure 4. The linear discriminant analysis of daily total dietary vitamin B6 intake, glycohemoglobin (**A**), and RGCS (**B**).

3.3.2. ROC Analysis of Daily Total Dietary Vitamin B6 Intake

ROC analysis of daily total dietary vitamin B6 intake was performed to calculate the area under the curve (AUC), which was used to evaluate the discrimination accuracy among people with good and poor RGCS. As shown in Figure 5, after controlling for all potential confounders and the years fixed effect, the predictive potential or accuracy of the multivariate logistic regression robust check model (AUC = 0.977; 95% CI: 0.974, 0.980; p-value < 0.001) was higher than those of the crude model (AUC = 0.535; 95% CI: 0.519, 0.550; p-value < 0.001), adjusted model I (AUC = 0.710; 95% CI: 0.697, 0.723; p-value < 0.001), and adjusted model II (AUC = 0.975; 95% CI: 0.974, 0.979; p-value < 0.001). The test results of DeLong between robust check model and crude model, and adjusted model I and adjusted model II showed that there were two statistically significant results (robust check model vs. crude model, $Z = 53.54$, *p*-value < 0.001; robust check model vs. adjusted model I, $Z = 39.542$, *p*-value < 0.001; robust check model vs. adjusted model II, $Z = 0.751$, *p*-value $= 0.452$).

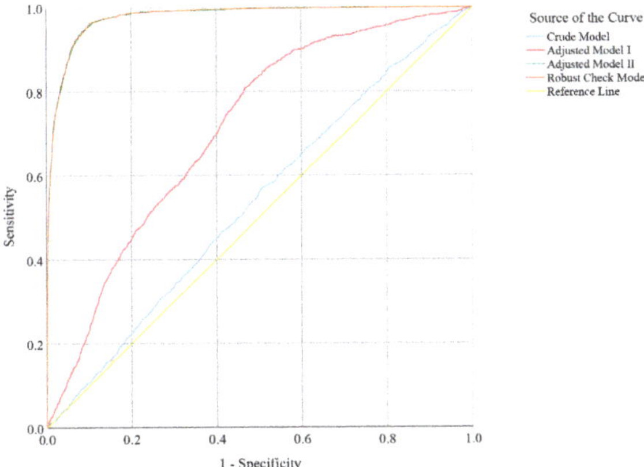

Figure 5. Receiver operator characteristic (ROC) curve indicator of poor RGCS (crude model: without covariates; adjusted model I: gender, age, and race were controlled; adjusted model II: all potential confounders in the study were controlled; robust check model: all potential confounders in the study were controlled, and the years fixed effect in the study was included).

4. Discussion

Although the reliable data of our study were from the national representative sample published by the Centers for Disease Control and Prevention of the United States, there were still some missing values in our collected data, which might have a subtle influence on our results of the statistical analysis. However, given the sufficient sample size of this study, the deviation caused by missing values could be reduced. Therefore, the reliability and authenticity of our findings were within acceptable limits. In addition, we did not ignore the interactions among nutrients when fitting the saturation model, but these interactions that might have biological significance (such as the interaction between vitamin B6 and vitamin B12) were not statistically significant when they were included in the robust check model.

The statistical model constructed in our research combined the specific macronutrients, minerals, vitamins, dietary fiber, and energy of the daily total diet, demographic, and medical indicators of American adults, because some statistical models mentioned in other studies might only be relevant for a small group of people with diabetes and not be suitable for American adults in terms of predicting their RGCS. Thus, our robust check model was closer to the real-world results than the models established by those research institutes [27,29].

Eventually, we found only daily total dietary vitamin B6 intake negatively correlated with RGCS, that is, the higher the daily total intake of dietary vitamin B6 was accompanied with better RGCS. Similarly, Mascolo et al. also concluded that the vitamin B6 level was significantly negatively associated with diabetes mellitus in diabetic people and suggested that vitamin B6 had a significantly protective effect on diabetic complications [30]. In addition, although covariates adjusted in our robust check model could not answer our research issues, they could still provide the theoretical foundation and scientific guidance for our health education related to glycemic control for American adults, which had a valuable public health significance.

The establishment of the robust check model of nutrients and RGCS was only the preliminary step of this study, which was mainly used to qualitatively find the associated factors affecting the RGCS. After screening the statistically significant daily total dietary vitamin B6 intake with this model, we further performed linear discriminant model and ROC analysis between RGCS and daily total dietary vitamin B6 intake as well as HbA1c, respectively (Figures 4 and 5), which could provide a quantitative reference and prediction accuracy of daily total dietary vitamin B6 intake for American adults who need to control blood glucose.

Vitamin B6 was an intriguing molecule that was involved in a wide range of metabolic, physiological, and developmental processes. Its active form, 5'-pyridoxal phosphate (PLP), was a co-factor for approximately 150 metabolic responses to glucose, lipid, amino acids, DNA, and neurotransmitters [30–34]. These studies showed that vitamin B6 had a potential to regulate body metabolism (including blood glucose). Although the United States, South Korea, and Japan published the recommended total dietary intake of vitamin B6 (fluctuating around 1.1~1.6 mg/d) for specific populations [35–37], it might not be suitable for American adults who need to control blood glucose. Therefore, it was necessary for the relevant health management agencies in the United States to formulate the recommended value of the total daily dietary vitamin B6 intake of RGC for American adults, so as to provide an effective way for them to obtain better RGCS. However, the formulation of total daily dietary vitamin B6 recommended intake remains to be further explored.

5. Conclusions

In summary, our results indicated that only daily total dietary vitamin B6 intake was significant negatively associated with RGCS among all dietary nutrients we studied. Although this study provided a ROC prediction result of daily total dietary vitamin B6 intake for RGCS, we might require further validation of whether it would have a positive and effective preventive effect and biological implications on RGCS of American adults.

Supplementary Materials: The following are available online at https://www.mdpi.com/article/10.3390/nu13114168/s1, Figure S1: Participant flow chart.

Author Contributions: The authors' responsibilities were as follows—Y.B., L.P.: contributed to data collection, analysis, and manuscript writing; H.Z., J.Y.: participated in the research design; L.P.: devoted to research design and manuscript writing. All authors have read and agreed to the published version of the manuscript.

Funding: The research received no sources of support such as commercial or non-commercial funding. The findings and conclusions expressed in this article were the authors' and do not necessarily represent the official position of the CDC or the U.S. Department of Health and Human Services. There was no private sponsor who played any role in the decision to design the study, collect data, analyze or interpret data, write reports, or submit manuscripts.

Institutional Review Board Statement: Ethical review and approval were waived for this study, since all the data from National Health and Nutrition Examination Survey is publicly accessible.

Informed Consent Statement: Informed consent from all subjects was obtained by National Health and Nutrition Examination Survey.

Data Availability Statement: Data described in the manuscript, codebook, and analytic code will not be made available because the data used in this study were from the NHANES database, which is a free and open database for all researchers around the world.

Conflicts of Interest: The authors stated that no conflict of interest would be deemed to prejudice the impartiality of the reported study.

Abbreviations

AUC: area under the curve; BMI, body mass index; CI, confidence interval; HbA1c, glycosylated hemoglobin; NCHS, National Center for Health Statistics; NHANES, National Health and Nutrition Examination Survey; OR, odds ratio; PIR, poverty income ratio; RGCS, recent glycemic control status; ROC, receiver operator characteristic; SE, standard error; USDA, United States Department of Agriculture; VIF, variance inflation factor.

References

1. Venn, B.J. Macronutrients and Human Health for the 21st Century. *Nutrients* **2020**, *12*, 2363. [CrossRef]
2. Franz, M.J. Diabetes Nutrition Therapy: Effectiveness, Macronutrients, Eating Patterns and Weight Management. *Am. J. Med Sci.* **2016**, *351*, 374–379. [CrossRef] [PubMed]
3. Scott, S.; Kempf, P.; Bally, L.; Stettler, C. Carbohydrate Intake in the Context of Exercise in People with Type 1 Diabetes. *Nutrients* **2019**, *11*, 3017. [CrossRef] [PubMed]
4. Fuller, S.; Beck, E.; Salman, H.; Tapsell, L. New Horizons for the Study of Dietary Fiber and Health: A Review. *Plant Foods Hum. Nutr.* **2016**, *71*, 1–12. [CrossRef] [PubMed]
5. Meyer, K.A.; Kushi, L.H.; Jacobs, D.R., Jr.; Slavin, J.; Sellers, T.A.; Folsom, A.R. Carbohydrates, dietary fiber, and incident type 2 diabetes in older women. *Am. J. Clin. Nutr.* **2000**, *71*, 921–930. [CrossRef]
6. Yu, K.; Ke, M.Y.; Li, W.H.; Zhang, S.Q.; Fang, X.C. The impact of soluble dietary fibre on gastric emptying, postprandial blood glucose and insulin in patients with type 2 diabetes. *Asia Pac. J. Clin. Nutr.* **2014**, *23*, 210–218. [CrossRef]
7. Lin, C.C.; Huang, Y.L. Chromium, zinc and magnesium status in type 1 diabetes. *Curr. Opin. Clin. Nutr. Metab. Care* **2015**, *18*, 588–592. [CrossRef]
8. Skalnaya, M.G.; Skalny, A.V.; Grabeklis, A.R.; Serebryansky, E.P.; Demidov, V.A.; Tinkov, A.A. Hair Trace Elements in Overweight and Obese Adults in Association with Metabolic Parameters. *Biol. Trace Elem. Res.* **2018**, *186*, 12–20. [CrossRef]
9. Soliman, A.T.; De Sanctis, V.; Yassin, M.; Soliman, N. Iron deficiency anemia and glucose metabolism. *Acta Bio-Med. Atenei Parm.* **2017**, *88*, 112–118. [CrossRef]
10. Deshmukh, S.V.; Prabhakar, B.; Kulkarni, Y.A. Water Soluble Vitamins and their Role in Diabetes and its Complications. *Curr. Diabetes Rev.* **2020**, *16*, 649–656. [CrossRef] [PubMed]
11. Kaur, B.; Henry, J. Micronutrient status in type 2 diabetes: A review. *Adv. Food Nutr. Res.* **2014**, *71*, 55–100. [CrossRef]
12. Li, X.; Liu, Y.; Zheng, Y.; Wang, P.; Zhang, Y. The Effect of Vitamin D Supplementation on Glycemic Control in Type 2 Diabetes Patients: A Systematic Review and Meta-Analysis. *Nutrients* **2018**, *10*, 375. [CrossRef] [PubMed]
13. Lips, P.; Eekhoff, M.; van Schoor, N.; Oosterwerff, M.; de Jongh, R.; Krul-Poel, Y.; Simsek, S. Vitamin D and type 2 diabetes. *J. Steroid Biochem. Mol. Biol.* **2017**, *173*, 280–285. [CrossRef]
14. Fazelian, S.; Rouhani, M.H.; Bank, S.S.; Amani, R. Chromium supplementation and polycystic ovary syndrome: A systematic review and meta-analysis. *J. Trace Elem. Med. Biol. Organ Soc. Miner. Trace Elem. (GMS)* **2017**, *42*, 92–96. [CrossRef] [PubMed]
15. Suksomboon, N.; Poolsup, N.; Yuwanakorn, A. Systematic review and meta-analysis of the efficacy and safety of chromium supplementation in diabetes. *J. Clin. Pharm. Ther.* **2014**, *39*, 292–306. [CrossRef]
16. Yin, R.V.; Phung, O.J. Effect of chromium supplementation on glycated hemoglobin and fasting plasma glucose in patients with diabetes mellitus. *Nutr. J.* **2015**, *14*, 14. [CrossRef]
17. Li, Z.; Xu, Y.; Huang, Z.; Wei, Y.; Hou, J.; Long, T.; Wang, F.; Hu, H.; Duan, Y.; Guo, H.; et al. Association between exposure to arsenic, nickel, cadmium, selenium, and zinc and fasting blood glucose levels. *Environ. Pollut.* **2019**, *255*, 113325. [CrossRef]
18. Wang, X.; Wu, W.; Zheng, W.; Fang, X.; Chen, L.; Rink, L.; Min, J.; Wang, F. Zinc supplementation improves glycemic control for diabetes prevention and management: A systematic review and meta-analysis of randomized controlled trials. *Am. J. Clin. Nutr.* **2019**, *110*, 76–90. [CrossRef] [PubMed]
19. Simental-Mendía, L.E.; Sahebkar, A.; Rodríguez-Morán, M.; Guerrero-Romero, F. A systematic review and meta-analysis of randomized controlled trials on the effects of magnesium supplementation on insulin sensitivity and glucose control. *Pharmacol. Res.* **2016**, *111*, 272–282. [CrossRef]
20. Volpe, S.L. Magnesium in disease prevention and overall health. *Adv. Nutr.* **2013**, *4*, 378s–383s. [CrossRef]
21. Yazdanpanah, S.; Rabiee, M.; Tahriri, M.; Abdolrahim, M.; Rajab, A.; Jazayeri, H.E.; Tayebi, L. Evaluation of glycated albumin (GA) and GA/HbA1c ratio for diagnosis of diabetes and glycemic control: A comprehensive review. *Crit. Rev. Clin. Lab. Sci.* **2017**, *54*, 219–232. [CrossRef] [PubMed]
22. Weykamp, C. HbA1c: A review of analytical and clinical aspects. *Ann. Lab. Med.* **2013**, *33*, 393–400. [CrossRef]
23. Konishi, K.; Wada, K.; Tamura, T.; Tsuji, M.; Kawachi, T.; Nagata, C. Dietary magnesium intake and the risk of diabetes in the Japanese community: Results from the Takayama study. *Eur. J. Nutr.* **2017**, *56*, 767–774. [CrossRef]
24. Bo, S.; Pisu, E. Role of dietary magnesium in cardiovascular disease prevention, insulin sensitivity and diabetes. *Curr. Opin. Lipidol.* **2008**, *19*, 50–56. [CrossRef]
25. Gannon, M.C.; Nuttall, F.Q. Effect of a high-protein, low-carbohydrate diet on blood glucose control in people with type 2 diabetes. *Diabetes* **2004**, *53*, 2375–2382. [CrossRef]
26. Intra, J.; Limonta, G.; Cappellini, F.; Bertona, M.; Brambilla, P. Glycosylated Hemoglobin in Subjects Affected by Iron-Deficiency Anemia. *Diabetes Metab. J.* **2019**, *43*, 539–544. [CrossRef] [PubMed]
27. Song, S.; Lee, J.E. Dietary Patterns Related to Triglyceride and High-Density Lipoprotein Cholesterol and the Incidence of Type 2 Diabetes in Korean Men and Women. *Nutrients* **2018**, *11*, 8. [CrossRef]
28. Ahluwalia, N.; Dwyer, J.; Terry, A.; Moshfegh, A.; Johnson, C. Update on NHANES Dietary Data: Focus on Collection, Release, Analytical Considerations, and Uses to Inform Public Policy. *Adv. Nutr.* **2016**, *7*, 121–134. [CrossRef] [PubMed]
29. Brandão-Lima, P.N.; Carvalho, G.B.; Santos, R.K.F.; Santos, B.D.C.; Dias-Vasconcelos, N.L.; Rocha, V.S.; Barbosa, K.B.F.; Pires, L.V. Intakes of Zinc, Potassium, Calcium, and Magnesium of Individuals with Type 2 Diabetes Mellitus and the Relationship with Glycemic Control. *Nutrients* **2018**, *10*, 1948. [CrossRef]

30. Mascolo, E.; Vernì, F. Vitamin B6 and Diabetes: Relationship and Molecular Mechanisms. *Int. J. Mol. Sci.* **2020**, *21*, 3669. [CrossRef] [PubMed]
31. Bender, D.A. Vitamin B6 requirements and recommendations. *Eur. J. Clin. Nutr.* **1989**, *43*, 289–309.
32. Ueland, P.M.; Ulvik, A.; Rios-Avila, L.; Midttun, Ø.; Gregory, J.F. Direct and Functional Biomarkers of Vitamin B6 Status. *Annu. Rev. Nutr.* **2015**, *35*, 33–70. [CrossRef] [PubMed]
33. Ueland, P.M.; McCann, A.; Midttun, Ø.; Ulvik, A. Inflammation, vitamin B6 and related pathways. *Mol. Asp. Med.* **2017**, *53*, 10–27. [CrossRef]
34. Hellmann, H.; Mooney, S. Vitamin B6: A molecule for human health? *Molecules* **2010**, *15*, 442–459. [CrossRef] [PubMed]
35. Horikawa, C.; Aida, R.; Kamada, C.; Fujihara, K.; Tanaka, S.; Tanaka, S.; Araki, A.; Yoshimura, Y.; Moriya, T.; Akanuma, Y.; et al. Vitamin B6 intake and incidence of diabetic retinopathy in Japanese patients with type 2 diabetes: Analysis of data from the Japan Diabetes Complications Study (JDCS). *Eur. J. Nutr.* **2020**, *59*, 1585–1594. [CrossRef]
36. Cho, Y.O.; Kim, B.Y. Vitamin B6 intake by Koreans should be based on sufficient amount and a variety of food sources. *Nutrition* **2005**, *21*, 1113–1119. [CrossRef] [PubMed]
37. Bolzetta, F.; Veronese, N.; De Rui, M.; Berton, L.; Toffanello, E.D.; Carraro, S.; Miotto, F.; Inelmen, E.M.; Donini, L.M.; Manzato, E.; et al. Are the Recommended Dietary Allowances for Vitamins Appropriate for Elderly People? *J. Acad. Nutr. Diet.* **2015**, *115*, 1789–1797. [CrossRef]

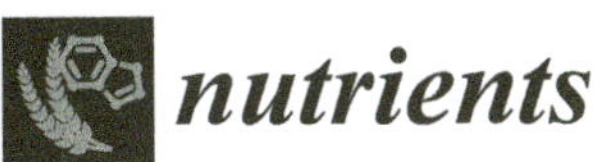

nutrients

Article

Dehulled Adlay Consumption Modulates Blood Pressure in Spontaneously Hypertensive Rats and Overweight and Obese Young Adults

Wan-Ju Yeh [1], Jung Ko [2], Wei-Yi Cheng [3] and Hsin-Yi Yang [4,*]

1 Graduate Program of Nutrition Science, National Taiwan Normal University, Taipei 106308, Taiwan; wandayeh@ntnu.edu.tw
2 Department of Applied Biological Chemistry, Graduate School of Agricultural and Life Sciences, The University of Tokyo, Tokyo 113-8657, Japan; 532732002@hotmail.com
3 Department of Nutrition, I-Shou University, Kaohsiung City 824005, Taiwan; wicheng@isu.edu.tw
4 Department of Nutritional Science, Fu Jen Catholic University, No.510, Zhongzheng Rd., Xinzhuang Dist., New Taipei City 242062, Taiwan
* Correspondence: b8506044@gmail.com; Tel.: +886-2-29053621; Fax: +886-2-29021215

Abstract: High blood pressure is a crucial risk factor for many cardiovascular diseases, and a diet rich in whole-grain foods may modulate blood pressure. This study investigated the effects of dehulled adlay consumption on blood pressure in vivo. We initially fed spontaneous hypertensive rats diets without (SHR group) or with 12 or 24% dehulled adlay (SHR + LA and SHR + HA groups), and discovered that it could limit blood pressure increases over a 12-week experimental period. Although we found no significant changes in plasma, heart, and kidney angiotensin-converting enzyme activities, both adlay-consuming groups had lower endothelin-1 and creatinine concentrations than the SHR group; the SHR + HA group also had lower aspartate aminotransferase and uric acid levels than the SHR group did. We later recruited 23 participants with overweight and obesity, and they consumed 60 g of dehulled adlay daily for a six-week experimental period. At the end of the study, we observed a significant decrease in the group's systolic blood pressure (SBP), and the change in SBP was even more evident in participants with high baseline SBP. In conclusion, our results suggested that daily intake of dehulled adlay had beneficial effects in blood-pressure management. Future studies may further clarify the possible underlying mechanisms for the consuming of dehulled adlay as a beneficial dietary approach for people at risk of hypertension.

Keywords: adlay; hypertension; blood pressure; ACE; ET-1

Citation: Yeh, W.-J.; Ko, J.; Cheng, W.-Y.; Yang, H.-Y. Dehulled Adlay Consumption Modulates Blood Pressure in Spontaneously Hypertensive Rats and Overweight and Obese Young Adults. *Nutrients* **2021**, *13*, 2305. https://doi.org/10.3390/nu13072305

Academic Editor: Lourdes Varela

Received: 11 June 2021
Accepted: 3 July 2021
Published: 4 July 2021

Publisher's Note: MDPI stays neutral with regard to jurisdictional claims in published maps and institutional affiliations.

1. Introduction

Hypertension is associated with mortality and morbidity related to various cardiovascular diseases [1]. Long-term high blood pressure may lead to cardiorenal remodeling and increased the risk of tissue injuries [2]. In a 2014 evidence-based guideline on the management of adult high blood pressure, adults with systolic blood pressure (SBP) and diastolic blood pressure (DBP) greater than 140 and 90 mmHg, respectively, were determined to have hypertension [3]. In addition, according to the American College of Cardiology/American Heart Association (ACC/AHA) 2017 Guideline for the Prevention, Detection, Evaluation, and Management of High Blood Pressure in Adults, adults with SBP and DBP above 130 and 80 mmHg, respectively, were defined as having hypertension, and individuals with SBP of 120–139 mmHg and DBP less than 80 mmHg were defined as having elevated blood pressure [4]. These guidelines served to increase awareness of hypertension; encourage proper antihypertensive medication usage, such as medications blocking the renin-angiotensin system; and lifestyle modification, such as adherence to the Dietary Approaches to Stop Hypertension (DASH) recommendations [5].

According to a 2019 meta-analysis survey, dietary consumption of whole grains rather than refined grains may aid in the prevention of non-communicable diseases [6]. The prospective study demonstrated that greater consumption of whole grains decreased the risk of hypertension in the Japanese population [7]. The blood-pressure-lowering DASH diet also recommends whole-grain foods because they contain fiber, minerals, vitamins, and other bioactive chemical components with health benefits [8,9]. Adlay (*Coix lachryma-jobi* L. var. *ma-yuen* Stapf) is a popular grain in Asian cuisine, and has been used as a traditional Chinese medicine for its antioxidative and anti-inflammatory potential [10]. Recent studies have also reported that adlay bran, which is rich in phenolic compounds, had beneficial effects on lipid metabolism and inflammatory responses in vivo [11,12]. Daily consumption of 60 g of adlay was also found to improve plasma lipid profiles in hyperlipidemic male patients [13]. However, evidence of adlay's effectiveness in blood-pressure modulation remains limited. Only one study reported that enzymatic hydrolyzed peptides derived from adlay seed exhibited the potential to inhibit angiotensin-converting enzyme (ACE) activity and to reduce blood pressure in rats [14]. Therefore, we aimed to investigate the effects of a diet rich in dehulled adlay instead of other refined cereals on blood-pressure regulation in both spontaneously hypertensive animals and in overweight and obese adults.

2. Materials and Methods

2.1. Animal Study

We purchased dehulled adlay powder (Taichung No. 3) from the Nantou County Tsao-Tun Production Association (Nantou County, Taiwan). Eight-week-old Wistar Kyoto (WKY) rats and spontaneously hypertensive rats (SHRs) were purchased from the National Laboratory Animal Breeding and Research Center. Rats were housed in the Experimental Animal Center as per guidelines reviewed by the Institutional Animal Care and Use Committee of I-Shou University (Approval ID: AUP-105-43-01). Rats were maintained in an environment with a constant temperature ($23 \pm 2\,^{\circ}$C) and humidity ($55 \pm 10\%$) and were exposed to a 12 h light–dark cycle in accordance with the Animal Protection Act and the regulations of the Animal Care and Use Committee of the Council of Agriculture, Executive Yuan. Rats were fed a standard rat chow diet for 1 week for acclimatization. Then, SHRs were randomly assigned to three groups: an SHR group fed a standard AIN-93M rodent diet ($n = 10$), an SHR + LA group fed AIN-93M with a low dose of 12% adlay powder (w/w), and an SHR + HA group fed AIN-93M with a high dose of 24% adlay powder (w/w), WKY rats were used as the normotensive control and also received a standard AIN-93M rodent diet ($n = 10$). We used adlay powder substituted for part of the components from the standard AIN-93M diet to ensure equal nutrient composition among the diets, as shown in Table 1. During the 12-week experimental period, food and water were provided ad libitum. Rats' food intake was recorded daily and their body weights recorded weekly. At the end of the study, we collected the previous 24 h of urine of rats using metabolic cages, and thereafter sacrificed the rats to obtain blood, heart, and kidney samples for analysis.

2.1.1. Measurement of Blood Pressure

SBP and DBP were measured using a noninvasive tail-cuff system (MK-2000ST, Muromachi Kikai, Tokyo, Japan) every 4 weeks. Rats were placed in restrainers, and we recorded at least five readings to calculate the mean of blood pressure over the course of the measurement.

Table 1. Dietary compositions (g/kg) of groups in the murine trial.

	WKY	SHR	SHR + LA	SHR + HA
Casein	140	140	118.2	96.3
Dextrin	155	155	155	155
Corn starch	465.7	465.7	389.4	313.1
Sucrose	100	100	100	100
Soy oil	40	40	38.4	36.9
Cellulose	50	50	29.7	9.4
L-cystine	1.8	1.8	1.8	1.8
AIN-93M mineral mix	35	35	35	35
AIN-93M vitamin mix	10	10	10	10
Choline bitartrate	2.5	2.5	2.5	2.5
Dehulled adlay	0	0	120	240

Corn starch, dextrin, casein, soy oil, cellulose (non-nutritive bulk), AIN-93M vitamin and mineral mixture were obtained from ICN Biochemicals (Aurora, OH, USA). Choline bitartrate and cystine were obtained from Sigma (St. Louis, MO, USA). Dehulled adlay (Taichung No. 3) powder was purchased from the Nantou County Tsao-Tun Production Association (Nantou County, Taiwan). SHR + LA, low-dose (12%, w/w) dehulled adlay powder in diet; SHR + HA, high-dose (24%, w/w) dehulled adlay powder in diet.

2.1.2. Blood Analysis

Blood samples were collected and centrifuged at $1500 \times g$ and 4 °C for 15 min for plasma separation. Plasma samples were collected to analyze the aspartate aminotransferase (AST), alanine aminotransferase (ALT), creatinine (Cr), uric acid, and phosphorus concentrations by using a Roche Modular P800 Autoanalyzer (Diagnostics Roche, Basel, Switzerland). ACE activity was analyzed according to the method previously described by Vermeirssen et al. [15]. C-reactive protein (CRP; Invitrogen, CA, USA), plasminogen activator inhibitor-1 (PAI-1; HYPHEN BioMed, Neuville-sur-Oise, France), and endothelin-1 (ET-1; Enzo Life Sciences, New York, USA) were analyzed using commercial kits as per the manufacturer's instructions.

2.1.3. Urine Analysis

The 24 h of urine samples were collected using metabolic cages. Urinary protein excretion, urine urea nitrogen (UUN), and Cr levels were analyzed using a Roche Modular P800 Autoanalyzer (Diagnostics Roche, Basel, Switzerland). All urine values were corrected in accordance with the Cr level.

2.1.4. Heart and Kidney Analysis

Heart and kidney samples were homogenized in a buffer solution (50 mM Tris-HCl, 150 mM NaCl, 0.1% SDS, 1% NP-40, pH 7.5), and suspensions were centrifuged at $1000 \times g$ at 4 °C for 10 min. ACE activity levels of the hearts and kidneys were determined using the method described by Yang et al. [16].

2.2. Human Study

Participants were recruited through announcement posters at the I-Shou University (Kaohsiung, Taiwan). People with diagnoses of diabetes, cardiovascular diseases, eating disorders, or liver, kidney, or other digestive diseases; medications and supplement users; pregnant or lactating individuals; and people with an adlay allergy were excluded. We recruited 25 volunteers, and among them, 23 participants with a body mass index (BMI, kg/m^2) within the range of 25 to 35 (inclusive) or waist circumference within an indicated sex-specific range (>90 cm for men and >80 cm for women) were included in the experiment as shown in Figure 1. We explained the purpose and design and of the study, as well as the risks involved to all participants, and obtained their written informed consent.

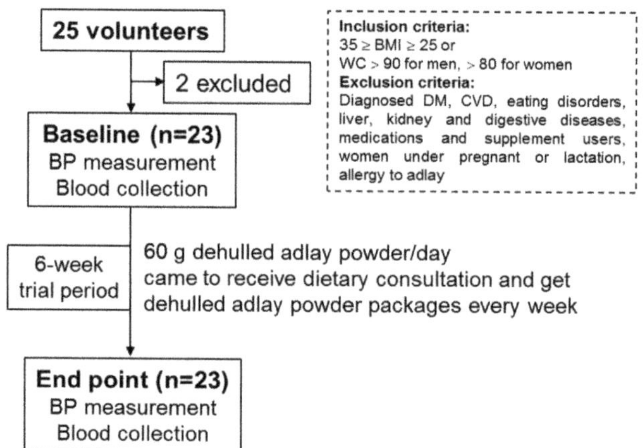

Figure 1. Flowchart illustrating the number of volunteers who were screened, included, and completed the study.

2.2.1. Experimental Design

We implemented this study following the protocol approved by the Institutional Review Board (IRB) of E-Da Hospital according to the guidelines in the Declaration of Helsinki (IRB No.: EMRP41104N). During the 6-week experimental period, 23 participants were asked to consume two packages (30 g/package) of dehulled adlay powder per day to replace three corresponding portions of cereal, according to the Food Exchange List of Taiwan and the dosage consumed daily in a previous study [13]. Those participants came to our center weekly to receive dietary consultation, bring back the used container, and obtain their adlay powder packages for the coming week. During the experimental period, the consumption of other supplements and foods not specified in the study was prohibited, and all participants were asked to maintain their normal dietary habits and physical activities.

2.2.2. Blood Pressure Measurement

Participants visited our research center at 07:30 a.m. at the baseline and the end of the study after a fasting period of at least 8 h. Blood pressure was measured using an automatic blood-pressure monitor on their right arm (Microlife, Taipei, Taiwan) after participants sat in a chair for at least 10 min. SBP and DBP were calculated as the average of three separate measurements.

2.2.3. Blood Analysis

At the baseline and end of the study, we collected plasma samples after blood-pressure measurement to measure ET-1 concentrations as described before.

2.3. Statistical Analysis

All data are presented as mean $\pm$ standard deviation (SD). Data from the animal study, and on changes in blood pressure among the three subgroups according to the guideline [4] (<120, 120–130, >130 mmHg) in the human study, were analyzed using one-way analysis of variance (ANOVA) with a post hoc Tukey test in SAS version 9.3. The differences in body weight and in blood pressure of animals at different time points and among groups were analyzed using repeated-measures ANOVA and Duncan's multiple-range test. The blood pressure and plasma ET-1 levels of participants at baseline and the end of the study were evaluated using a paired t-test. A p-value of <0.05 indicated a statistically significant difference.

3. Results

3.1. Effects of Dehulled Adlay Intake on Body Weight in SHRs

The results of the animal experiment demonstrated that using a diet containing dehulled adlay did not affect food and energy intake among groups. In addition, we also discovered no significant differences in body weight among the groups over the experiment period (Figure 2a).

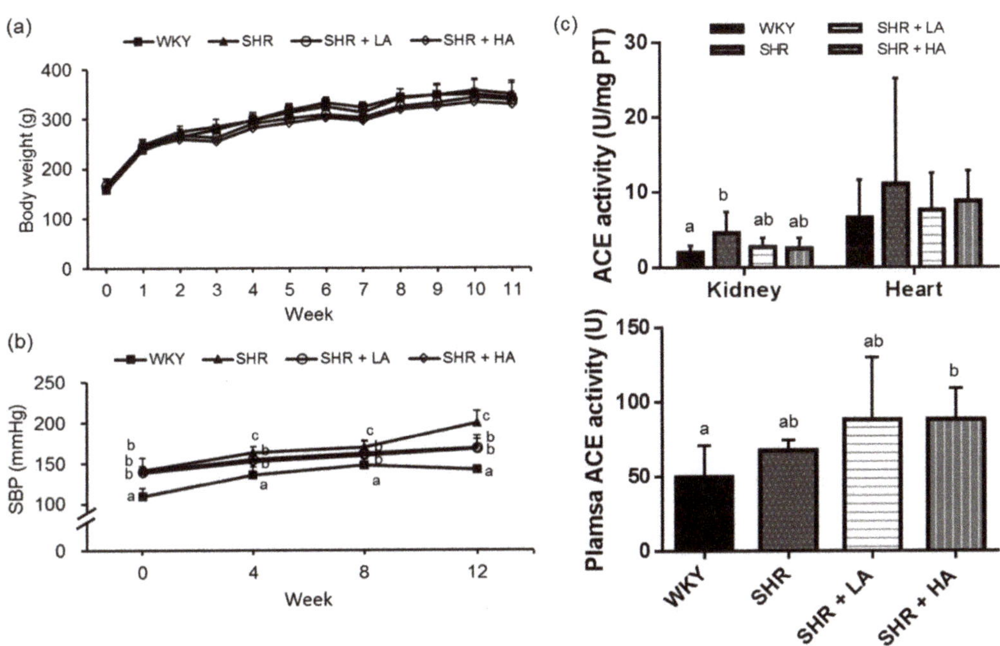

Figure 2. Food intake (**a**), SBP (**b**), and plasma and tissue ACE activities (**c**) of rats in different groups. Values are presented as mean ± SD ($n = 10$). [abc] Different superscript letters indicate a significant difference ($p < 0.05$). SBP, systolic blood pressure; ACE, angiotensin-converting enzyme. WKY, Wistar Kyoto) rats fed an AIN-93M diet; SHR, spontaneously hypertensive rats fed an AIN-93M diet; SHR + LA, SHRs fed an AIN-93M diet containing 12% dehulled adlay powder; SHR + HA, SHRs fed an AIN-93M diet containing 24% dehulled adlay powder.

3.2. Effects of Dehulled Adlay Intake on Blood Pressure and ACE Activity in SHRs

The SHR, SHR + LA, and SHR + HA groups all had higher SBP levels than the WKY group throughout the 12-week experimental period. Both the SHR + LA and SHR + HA groups had lower SBP than the SHR group after the fourth week, and this difference was maintained until the end of the study (Figure 2b). Although the SHR group had higher renal ACE activity than the WKY group (WKY vs. SHR, $p = 0.0004$), we found no significant difference in plasma, heart, and kidney ACE activity among the SHR, SHR + LA, and SHR + HA groups (Figure 2c). The results indicated that daily dehulled adlay intake in replacement of part of the diet composition could prevent blood-pressure increases among SHRs, but these effects may not be explained by the inhibition of ACE activity alone.

3.3. Effects of Dehulled Adlay Intake on AST, ALT, and Renal Functions in SHRs

At the end of the study, we found that the SHR group had higher plasma AST (WKY vs. SHR, $p < 0.0001$; SHR + LA vs. SHR, $p = 0.0011$; SHR + HA vs. SHR, $p = 0.0076$) and ALT (WKY vs. SHR, $p < 0.0001$) activities than the WKY group did, and that both the SHR + LA and SHR + HA groups had lower AST activities than the SHR group did (Figure 3a). In addition, plasma Cr concentrations (WKY vs. SHR, $p = 0.0289$) and the total protein-to-Cr ratios in the rat urine were significantly higher in the SHR groups than in WKY (WKY vs. SHR, $p = 0.0042$). Both dehulled adlay groups had lower plasma Cr concentrations than the SHR group did (SHR + LA vs. SHR, $p = 0.0020$; SHR + HA vs. SHR, $p < 0.0001$), but no significant differences were observed in total protein/Cr, UUN/Cr, and plasma phosphorus concentrations in urine among the three SHR groups. Additionally, plasma uric acid levels were significantly higher in the SHR group and lower in the HA group (WKY vs. SHR, $p = 0.0022$; SHR + HA vs. SHR, $p = 0.0002$) (Figure 3b,c). The results also indicated that elevation of blood pressure may increase the risk of renal tissue injuries, and that dehulled adlay consumption may ameliorate these risks.

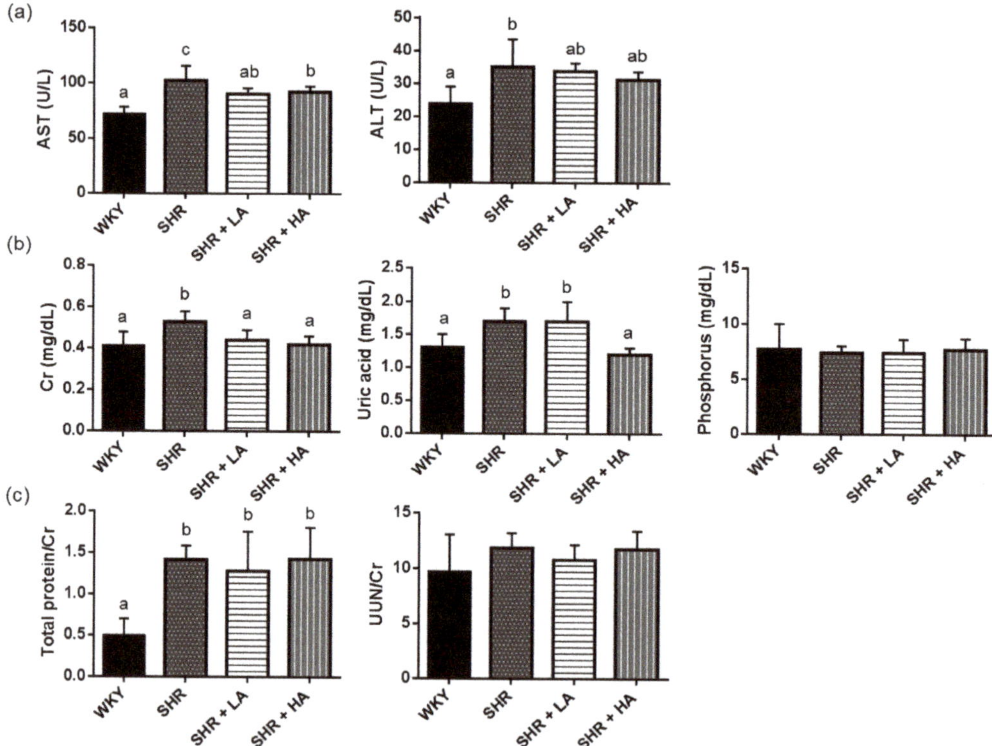

Figure 3. Plasma hepatic (**a**), renal function parameters (**b**), and urine analysis (**c**) of rats in different groups. Values are presented as mean ± SD ($n = 10$). [abc] Different superscript letters indicate a significant difference ($p < 0.05$). AST, aspartate aminotransferase; ALT, alanine aminotransferase; UUN, urine urea nitrogen. WKY Wistar Kyoto rats fed an AIN-93M diet; SHR, spontaneously hypertensive rats fed an AIN-93M diet; SHR + LA, SHRs fed an AIN-93M diet containing 12% dehulled adlay powder; SHR + HA, SHRs fed an AIN-93M diet containing 24% dehulled adlay powder.

3.4. Effects of Dehulled Adlay Intake on Indicators of Endothelial Function in SHRs

Over the course of the experiment, plasma CRP and PAI-1 levels tended to decrease in both the SHR + LA and SHR + HA groups when compared with the SHR group. Both dehulled-adlay-consuming groups also had lower plasma ET-1 levels than did the SHR group (SHR + LA vs. SHR, $p = 0.0164$; SHR + HA vs. SHE, $p = 0.0345$), and no significant difference in ET-1 level was observed compared with the WKY group (Figure 4). The results showed that adlay may retard the elevation of blood pressure through improving endothelial function.

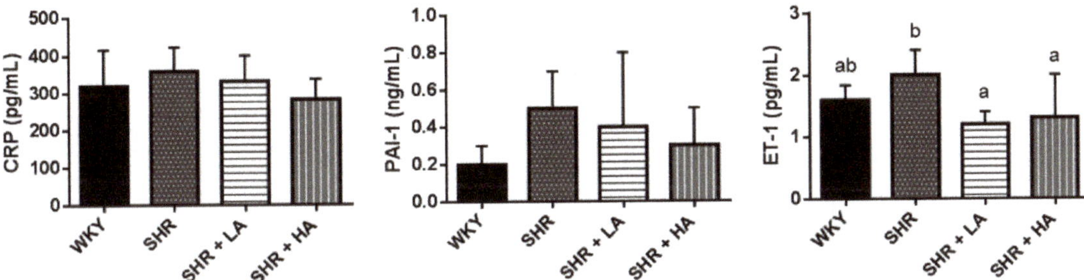

Figure 4. Plasma CRP, PAI-1, and ET-1 levels of rats in different groups. Values are presented as the mean $\pm$ SD ($n = 10$). [ab] Different superscript letters indicate a significant difference ($p < 0.05$). CRP, C-reactive protein; PAI-1, plasminogen activator inhibitor-1; ET-1, endothelin-1. WKYWistar Kyoto rats fed an AIN-93M diet; SHR, spontaneously hypertensive rats fed an AIN-93M diet; SHR + LA, SHRs fed an AIN-93M diet containing 12% dehulled adlay powder; SHR + HA, SHRs fed an AIN-93M diet containing 24% dehulled adlay powder.

3.5. Effects of Daily Dehulled Adlay Intake on Blood Pressure and Endothelial Function in Participants

Furthermore, we performed an interventional human study to observe the effects of a dehulled adlay-rich dietary pattern on blood-pressure regulation in participants. During the experimental period, participants were asked to maintain their normal dietary and physical activity, but to replace 60 g of refined grain products with dehulled adlay powder either in their beverage or meal under the guidance of a dietitian; subjects brought back the used and empty containers to our center every week, and no subjective adverse effects were reported. We learned that the SBP of our participants decreased over the 6-week experimental period (6-week vs. 0-week, $p = 0.006$) (Figure 5a). Additionally, we categorized participants into subgroups according to their baseline SBP (<120 mmHg, $n = 5$; 120–130 mmHg, $n = 11$; >130 mmHg, $n = 7$), and discovered that the effects of dehulled adlay consumption on blood-pressure change were more obvious in the participants with higher baseline SBP (ΔSBP: >130 vs. <120, $p = 0.0243$) (Figure 5b). We also noted a trend of decreasing plasma ET-1 levels in participants ($p = 0.07$) (Figure 5c). These results indicated a beneficial effect of dehulled adlay on blood-pressure modulation, and that these effects may be related to baseline SBP.

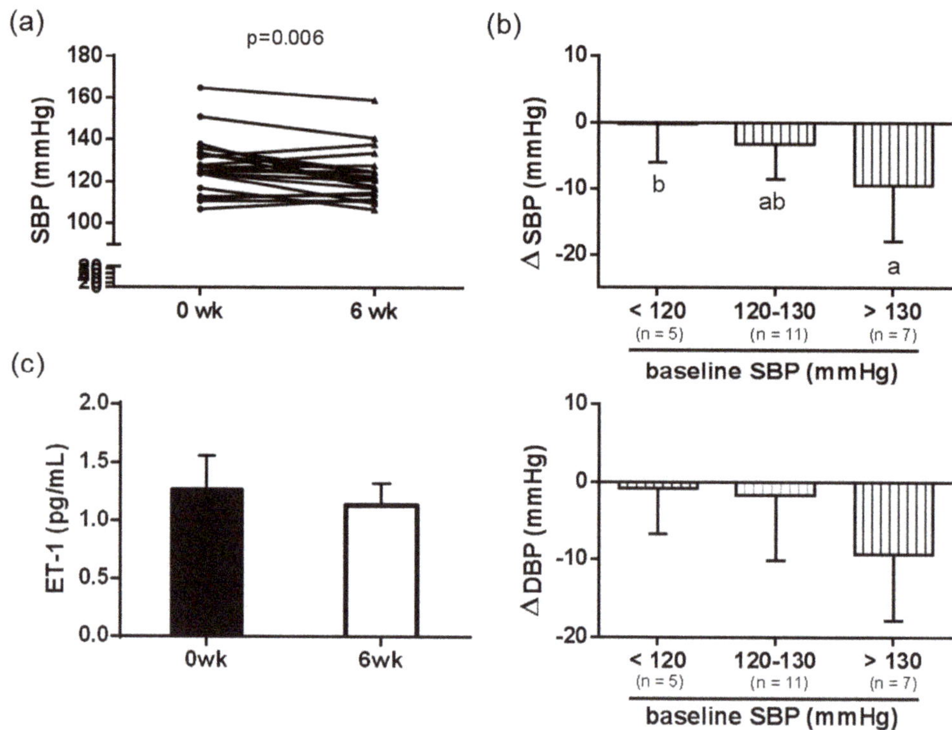

Figure 5. Baseline and end SBP (**a**) and ET-1 (**b**) levels, and changes in SBP and DBP (**c**) of participants subgrouping by baseline SBP after the 6-week dehulled adlay intervention. Values are presented as mean ± SD (*n* = 23). [a,b] Different superscript letters indicate a significant difference (*p* < 0.05). SBP, systolic blood pressure; DBP, diastolic blood pressure; ET-1, endothelin-1.

4. Discussion

In this study, we found that dehulled adlay consumption retarded the elevation of blood pressure in SHRs, and may be beneficial in blood pressure modulation in overweight and obese adults. Dietary intake of whole-grain foods may lower cardiovascular risks. A randomized controlled trial concluded that daily consumption of whole grains (50 g/1000 kcal) resulted in greater improvements in blood pressure than a refined grain diet did in adults with overweight and obesity [17]. Results from the Furukawa Nutrition and Health Study also indicated that higher intake of whole-grain foods may reduce hypertension risk [7]. Adlay is a common grain in Asian diets, and is used in traditional Chinese medicines to treat cardiovascular diseases. Studies have also reported that adlay has various beneficial effects. For example, adlay bran was discovered to have anti-inflammatory [18] and anti-tumor effects [19], and dehulled adlay also had a gastroprotective effect in vitro [20]. Although one previous study reported that adlay-derived peptides may have antihypertensive effects [14], studies focused on adlay's influence on blood-pressure management remains scarce. To our knowledge, this is the first study to explore the potential effects of daily consumption of dehulled adlay in reducing blood pressure in hypertensive rats and in overweight and obese participants.

Increased daily whole-grain consumption has positive effects on blood-pressure control. The 2020 International Society of Hypertension's Global Hypertension Practice Guidelines also include a suggestion to eat a healthy diet rich in whole grains to treat hypertension [21]. Dehulled adlay is one of the ingredients recommended to replace polished rice in some Asian diets. According to the Nutrient Composition Database of the Food and Drug Administration of the Ministry of Health and Welfare, every 100 g of adlay seed contains 199 mg of magnesium, which is approximately 10 times of the level in white rice. Magnesium has been shown to regulate blood pressure through directly stimulating prostacyclin and nitric oxide production [22]. These blood-pressure-reducing effects may be caused by endothelium-dependent and endothelium-independent vasodilation [23,24]. Furthermore, magnesium may also prevent vascular injury due to its antioxidant and anti-inflammatory effects [25]. In the present study, we discovered that in hypertensive rats, partial dietary replacement with dehulled adlay could limit the progression of hypertension without affecting food intake or body weight in hypertensive rats. We also found that daily intake of 60 g dehulled adlay could lower blood pressure in human participants with high baseline SBP. These results suggested that dehulled adlay has potential use for the treatment or prevention of hypertension.

Blood pressure is regulated by numerous mechanisms in vivo, and the renin-angiotensin system is one of such major regulatory mechanism. Increased ACE activity reveals the formation of angiotensin II, which leads to vessel constriction and elevated blood pressure. In 2017, Li et al. [14] observed potent anti-hypertensive peptides in Coix glutelin. However, we found no significant effect of dehulled adlay on plasma, kidney, and heart ACE activities in SHRs; these rats did, however, have significantly lower SBP at the end of the 12-week experimental period. Therefore, the lowered blood pressure associated with consuming dehulled adlay cannot be explained by its ACE inhibitory activity. Conversely, we found that both dehulled adlay intervention groups had significant lower plasma ET-1 and Cr concentrations than the non-treated SHR group did. Studies have indicated that ET-1 secretion raises blood pressure and accelerates the progression of nephropathy by stimulating vasoconstriction and the retention of water and sodium [26]. Therefore, our results indicated that dehulled adlay may not only retard the elevation of blood pressure in hypertensive rats, but also reduce the risk of kidney injury. In addition, we discovered, through human trials, that replacing part of daily staple food intake with dehulled adlay intake for up to six weeks produced positive effects of lower blood pressure. However, no significant change in ET-1 was found six 6 weeks. On the basis of these results, future studies should extend the experimental period or increase the sample size to further clarify the mechanisms underlying such outcomes.

Recent studies have found that uric acid is strongly linked to high blood pressure. A cross-sectional study reported that each 1 mg/dL increase in plasma uric acid increases the risk of hypertension by 20% [27]. Uric acid may directly cause endothelial dysfunction. When uric acid crystals are deposited in blood vessels, vascular inflammation and endothelial damage arise [28]. Moreover, uric acid could also affect vascular function through crystalline-independent pathways. Otani et al. [29] revealed that uric acid has the potential to reduce the phosphorylation of endothelial nitric oxide synthase and to damage endothelial function. Furthermore, hyperuricemia leads to increased ET-1 expression and renal injury [30]. In a hyperuricemic rat model, dehulled adlay extract effectively decreased serum uric acid levels by inhibiting xanthine oxidase [31]. In this study, we observed that rats fed high-dose dehulled adlay exhibited lower plasma uric acid levels than the SHR group, but the level was not significantly different from those of the WKY group. In addition, we ascertained that levels of the inflammatory-response indicators CRP and PAI-1 tended to decline as a result of consumption of an adlay-rich diet. These results indicated that the blood-pressure reduction associated with dehulled adlay may be related to moderating effects on uric acid and ET-1 levels.

This is the first study to apply dehulled adlay intake in the daily diet of participants with a high risk of hypertension, and we observed that replacing 60 g of staple food in daily diet with dehulled adlay helped moderate high blood pressure. In the animal study, we also discovered that dehulled adlay intake curbed blood-pressure elevation and lessened uric acid and ET-1 levels. However, some limitations were present in our study and may be rectified by further studies. First, we used a non-invasive tail-cuff method with a four-week interval to investigate the change of blood pressure in this study. A telemetry system may be more ideal, and could be used to record more hemodynamic information in future long-lasting experiments. Second, the number of human participants in this study was limited and lacked a control group. The single-arm study design followed by a pre-post evaluation can only offer preliminary information, and may not completely exclude the placebo effects of the intervention [32]. Although there currently are not enough previous references available about the effects of adlay on blood pressure, the results of this study can be used as a basis for further research. Future studies may increase the number of participants, extend the duration of the intervention period, use a control group consuming refined cereals, and measure dietary intake throughout the intervention to better observe more influential results and to clarify the related underlying mechanisms. Third, we used participants with high risks of cardiovascular diseases, such as overweight and obesity, in this study, and discovered that the effects of dehulled adlay intake on blood-pressure reduction was more evident in participants with high basal blood pressure. Therefore, future studies also could focus on patients diagnosed as having hypertension to further explore whether combining drug treatment with daily dehulled adlay consumption would have synergistic effects. The pathways related to uric acid and ET-1 also could be emphasized in future investigations.

5. Conclusions

In conclusion, our results suggested that daily intake of 60 g dehulled adlay had beneficial effects on blood-pressure management. Future studies could further clarify the possible underlying mechanisms for the consuming of dehulled adlay as a beneficial dietary approach for people at risk of hypertension.

Author Contributions: W.-J.Y. and H.-Y.Y. designed the study; W.-J.Y., J.K., W.-Y.C., and H.-Y.Y. conducted the experiments; and W.-J.Y., J.K., and H.-Y.Y. wrote the manuscript. All authors have read and agreed to the published version of the manuscript.

Funding: This research was funded by E-Da Hospital (Kaohsiung, Taiwan), grant number ISU 104-IUC-03. The APC received no external funding.

Institutional Review Board Statement: The study was conducted according to the guidelines of the Declaration of Helsinki, and approved by the Institutional Review Board of E-Da Hospital (EMRP41104N 2016/02/04).

Informed Consent Statement: Informed consent was obtained from all subjects involved in the study.

Conflicts of Interest: The authors declare no conflict of interest, and all authors adhered to the Committee on Publication Ethics' guidelines on research and publication ethics.

References

1. Lawes, C.M.; Vander Hoorn, S.; Rodgers, A. International Society of H. Global burden of blood-pressure-related disease. *Lancet* **2008**, *371*, 1513–1518. [CrossRef]
2. Touyz, R.M.; Alves-Lopes, R.; Rios, F.J.; Camargo, L.L.; Anagnostopoulou, A.; Arner, A.; Montezano, A.C. Vascular smooth muscle contraction in hypertension. *Cardiovasc. Res.* **2018**, *114*, 529–539. [CrossRef]
3. James, P.A.; Oparil, S.; Carter, B.L.; Cushman, W.C.; Dennison-Himmelfarb, C.; Handler, J.; Lackland, D.T.; LeFevre, M.L.; MacKenzie, T.D.; Ogedegbe, O.; et al. 2014 evidence-based guideline for the management of high blood pressure in adults: Report from the panel members appointed to the Eighth Joint National Committee (JNC 8). *JAMA* **2014**, *311*, 507–520. [CrossRef]
4. Whelton, P.K.; Carey, R.M.; Aronow, W.S.; Casey, D.E., Jr.; Collins, K.J.; Dennison Himmelfarb, C.; DePalma, S.M.; Gidding, S.; Jamerson, K.A.; Jones, D.W.; et al. 2017 ACC/AHA/AAPA/ABC/ACPM/AGS/APhA/ASH/ASPC/NMA/PCNA Guideline for the Prevention, Detection, Evaluation, and Management of High Blood Pressure in Adults: A Report of the American College of Cardiology/American Heart Association Task Force on Clinical Practice Guidelines. *J. Am. Coll. Cardiol.* **2018**, *71*, e127–e248.
5. Muntner, P.; Carey, R.M.; Gidding, S.; Jones, D.W.; Taler, S.J.; Wright, J.T., Jr.; Whelton, P.K. Potential US Population Impact of the 2017 ACC/AHA High Blood Pressure Guideline. *Circulation* **2018**, *137*, 109–118. [CrossRef]
6. Reynolds, A.; Mann, J.; Cummings, J.; Winter, N.; Mete, E.; Te Morenga, L. Carbohydrate quality and human health: A series of systematic reviews and meta-analyses. *Lancet* **2019**, *393*, 434–445. [CrossRef]
7. Kashino, I.; Eguchi, M.; Miki, T.; Kochi, T.; Nanri, A.; Kabe, I.; Mizoue, T. Prospective association between whole grain consumption and hypertension: The Furukawa nutrition and health study. *Nutrients* **2020**, *12*, 902. [CrossRef] [PubMed]

8. Cohen, J.F.W.; Lehnerd, M.E.; Houser, R.F.; Rimm, E.B. Dietary Approaches to Stop Hypertension Diet, Weight Status, and Blood Pressure among Children and Adolescents: National Health and Nutrition Examination Surveys 2003–2012. *J. Acad. Nutr. Diet.* **2017**, *117*, 1437–1444.e2. [CrossRef]

9. Borneo, R.; Leon, A.E. Whole grain cereals: Functional components and health benefits. *Food Funct.* **2012**, *3*, 110–119. [CrossRef] [PubMed]

10. Tsai, W.H.; Yang, C.C.; Li, P.C.; Chen, W.C.; Chien, C.T. Therapeutic potential of traditional chinese medicine on inflammatory diseases. *J. Tradit. Complement. Med.* **2013**, *3*, 142–151. [CrossRef] [PubMed]

11. Li, Y.; Tian, X.; Li, S.; Chang, L.; Sun, P.; Lu, Y.; Yu, X.; Chen, S.; Wu, Z.; Xu, Z.; et al. Total polysaccharides of adlay bran (Coix lachryma-jobi L.) improve TNF-alpha induced epithelial barrier dysfunction in Caco-2 cells via inhibition of the inflammatory response. *Food Funct.* **2019**, *10*, 2906–2913. [CrossRef]

12. Tseng, Y.H.; Chang, C.W.; Chiang, W.; Hsieh, S.C. Adlay bran oil suppresses hepatic gluconeogenesis and attenuates hyperlipidemia in type 2 diabetes rats. *J. Med. Food* **2019**, *22*, 22–28. [CrossRef] [PubMed]

13. Yu, Y.M.; Chang, W.C.; Liu, C.S.; Tsai, C.M. Effect of young barley leaf extract and adlay on plasma lipids and LDL oxidation in hyperlipidemic smokers. *Biol. Pharm. Bull.* **2004**, *27*, 802–805. [CrossRef] [PubMed]

14. Li, B.; Qiao, L.; Li, L.; Zhang, Y.; Li, K.; Wang, L.; Qiao, Y. A novel antihypertensive peptides derived from adlay (Coix larchryma-jobi L. var. ma-yuen Stapf) Glutelin. *Molecules* **2017**, *22*, 123. [CrossRef] [PubMed]

15. Vermeirssen, V.; Van Camp, J.; Verstraete, W. Optimisation and validation of an angiotensin-converting enzyme inhibition assay for the screening of bioactive peptides. *J. Biochem. Biophys. Methods* **2002**, *51*, 75–87. [CrossRef]

16. Yang, H.Y.; Wu, L.Y.; Yeh, W.J.; Chen, J.R. Beneficial effects of beta-conglycinin on renal function and nephrin expression in early streptozotocin-induced diabetic nephropathy rats. *Br. J. Nutr.* **2014**, *111*, 78–85. [CrossRef]

17. Kirwan, J.P.; Malin, S.K.; Scelsi, A.R.; Kullman, E.L.; Navaneethan, S.D.; Pagadala, M.R.; Haus, J.M.; Filion, J.; Godin, J.P.; Kochhar, S.; et al. A whole-grain diet reduces cardiovascular risk factors in overweight and obese adults: A randomized controlled trial. *J. Nutr.* **2016**, *146*, 2244–2251. [CrossRef]

18. Chen, H.J.; Chung, C.P.; Chiang, W.; Lin, Y.L. Anti-inflammatory effects and chemical study of a flavonoid-enriched fraction from adlay bran. *Food Chem.* **2011**, *126*, 1741–1748. [CrossRef]

19. Chung, C.P.; Hsu, H.Y.; Huang, D.W.; Hsu, H.H.; Lin, J.T.; Shih, C.K.; Chiang, W. Ethyl acetate fraction of adlay bran ethanolic extract inhibits oncogene expression and suppresses DMH-induced preneoplastic lesions of the colon in F344 rats through an anti-inflammatory pathway. *J. Agric. Food Chem.* **2010**, *58*, 7616–7623. [CrossRef]

20. Chung, C.P.; Hsia, S.M.; Lee, M.Y.; Chen, H.J.; Cheng, F.; Chan, L.C.; Kuo, Y.H.; Lin, Y.L.; Chiang, W. Gastroprotective activities of adlay (Coix lachryma-jobi L. var. ma-yuen Stapf) on the growth of the stomach cancer AGS cell line and indomethacin-induced gastric ulcers. *J. Agric. Food Chem.* **2011**, *59*, 6025–6033. [CrossRef] [PubMed]

21. Unger, T.; Borghi, C.; Charchar, F.; Khan, N.A.; Poulter, N.R.; Prabhakaran, D.; Ramirez, A.; Schlaich, M.; Stergiou, G.S.; Tomaszewski, M.; et al. 2020 International Society of Hypertension Global Hypertension Practice Guidelines. *Hypertension* **2020**, *75*, 1334–1357. [CrossRef] [PubMed]

22. Satake, K.; Lee, J.D.; Shimizu, H.; Uzui, H.; Mitsuke, Y.; Yue, H.; Ueda, T. Effects of magnesium on prostacyclin synthesis and intracellular free calcium concentration in vascular cells. *Magnes. Res.* **2004**, *17*, 20–27.

23. Landau, R.; Scott, J.A.; Smiley, R.M. Magnesium-induced vasodilation in the dorsal hand vein. *BJOG Int. J. Obstet. Gynaecol.* **2004**, *111*, 446–451. [CrossRef]

24. Soltani, N.; Keshavarz, M.; Sohanaki, H.; Zahedi, A.S.; Dehpour, A.R. Relaxatory effect of magnesium on mesenteric vascular beds differs from normal and streptozotocin induced diabetic rats. *Eur. J. Pharmacol.* **2005**, *508*, 177–181. [CrossRef] [PubMed]

25. Blache, D.; Devaux, S.; Joubert, O.; Loreau, N.; Schneider, M.; Durand, P.; Prost, M.; Gaume, V.; Adrian, M.; Laurant, P.; et al. Long-term moderate magnesium-deficient diet shows relationships between blood pressure, inflammation and oxidant stress defense in aging rats. *Free Radic. Biol. Med.* **2006**, *41*, 277–284. [CrossRef] [PubMed]

26. Deng, L.Y.; Day, R.; Schiffrin, E.L. Localization of sites of enhanced expression of endothelin-1 in the kidney of DOCA-salt hypertensive rats. *J. Am. Soc. Nephrol.* **1996**, *7*, 1158–1164. [CrossRef]

27. Kuwabara, M.; Niwa, K.; Nishi, Y.; Mizuno, A.; Asano, T.; Masuda, K.; Komatsu, I.; Yamazoe, M.; Takahashi, O.; Hisatome, I. Relationship between serum uric acid levels and hypertension among Japanese individuals not treated for hyperuricemia and hypertension. *Hypertens. Res.* **2014**, *37*, 785–789. [CrossRef] [PubMed]

28. Kuwabara, M.; Kanbay, M.; Hisatome, I. Uric acid and hypertension because of arterial stiffness. *Hypertension* **2018**, *72*, 582–584. [CrossRef] [PubMed]

29. Otani, N.; Toyoda, S.; Sakuma, M.; Hayashi, K.; Ouchi, M.; Fujita, T.; Anzai, N.; Tanaka, A.; Node, K.; Uemura, N.; et al. Effects of uric acid on vascular endothelial function from bedside to bench. *Hypertens. Res.* **2018**, *41*, 923–931. [CrossRef]

30. Romi, M.M.; Arfian, N.; Tranggono, U.; Setyaningsih, W.A.W.; Sari, D.C.R. Uric acid causes kidney injury through inducing fibroblast expansion, endothelin-1 expression, and inflammation. *BMC Nephrol.* **2017**, *18*, 326. [CrossRef]

31. Zhao, M.; Zhu, D.; Sun-Waterhouse, D.; Su, G.; Lin, L.; Wang, X.; Dong, Y. In vitro and in vivo studies on adlay-derived seed extracts: Phenolic profiles, antioxidant activities, serum uric acid suppression, and xanthine oxidase inhibitory effects. *J. Agric. Food Chem.* **2014**, *62*, 7771–7778. [CrossRef] [PubMed]

32. Evans, S.R. Clinical trial structures. *J. Exp. Stroke Transl. Med.* **2010**, *3*, 8.

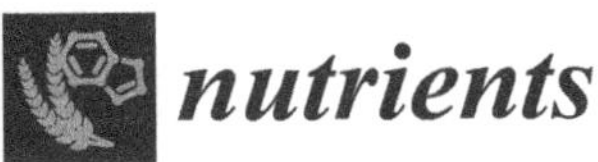

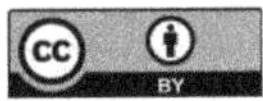

Article

Self-Reported Lifetime History of Eating Disorders and Mortality in the General Population: A Canadian Population Survey with Record Linkage

Pardis Pedram [1,2,3,*], Scott B. Patten [2,3,4,5,6], Andrew G. M. Bulloch [2,3,4,5], Jeanne V. A. Williams [4] and Gina Dimitropoulos [1,2,3,5,7]

[1] Department of Psychiatry, University of Calgary, 2500 University Drive NW, Calgary, AB T2N 1N4, Canada; gdimit@ucalgary.ca

[2] Mathison Centre for Mental Health Research & Education, Foothills Medical Centre, 3280 Hospital Drive NW, Calgary, AB T2N 4Z6, Canada; patten@ucalgary.ca (S.B.P.); bulloch@ucalgary.ca (A.G.M.B.)

[3] Hotchkiss Brain Institute, University of Calgary Foothills, 3330 Hospital Drive NW, Calgary, AB T2N 4N1, Canada

[4] Department of Community Health Sciences, University of Calgary, 2500 University Drive NW, Calgary, AB T2N 1N4, Canada; jvawilli@ucalgary.ca

[5] O'Brien Institute for Public Health, University of Calgary Foothills, 3280 Hospital Drive NW, Calgary, AB T2N 4Z6, Canada

[6] Cuthbertson & Fischer Chair in Pediatric Mental Health, 2500 University Drive NW, Calgary, AB T2N 1N4, Canada

[7] Faculty of Social Work, University of Calgary, 2500 University Drive NW, Calgary, AB T2N 1N4, Canada

* Correspondence: pardis.pedram@ucalgary.ca

Citation: Pedram, P.; Patten, S.B.; Bulloch, A.G.M.; Williams, J.V.A.; Dimitropoulos, G. Self-Reported Lifetime History of Eating Disorders and Mortality in the General Population: A Canadian Population Survey with Record Linkage. *Nutrients* **2021**, *13*, 3333. https://doi.org/10.3390/nu13103333

Academic Editor: Lourdes Varela

Received: 31 July 2021
Accepted: 19 September 2021
Published: 23 September 2021

Publisher's Note: MDPI stays neutral with regard to jurisdictional claims in published maps and institutional affiliations.

Abstract: Eating disorders (EDs) are often reported to have the highest mortality of any mental health disorder. However, this assertion is based on clinical samples, which may provide an inaccurate view of the actual risks in the population. Hence, in the current retrospective cohort study, mortality of self-reported lifetime history of EDs in the general population was explored. The data source was the Canadian Community Health Survey: Mental Health and Well-Being (CCHS 1.2), linked to a national mortality database. The survey sample was representative of the Canadian household population (mean age = 43.95 years, 50.9% female). The survey inquired about the history of professionally diagnosed chronic conditions, including EDs. Subsequently, the survey dataset was linked to the national mortality dataset (for the date of death) up to 2017. Cox proportional hazards models were used to explore the effect of EDs on mortality. The unadjusted-hazard ratio (HR) for the lifetime history of an ED was 1.35 (95% CI 0.70–2.58). However, the age/sex-adjusted HR increased to 4.5 (95% CI 2.33–8.84), which was over two times higher than age/sex-adjusted HRs for other mental disorders (schizophrenia/psychosis, mood-disorders, and post-traumatic stress disorder). In conclusion, all-cause mortality of self-reported lifetime history of EDs in the household population was markedly elevated and considerably higher than that of other self-reported disorders. This finding replicates prior findings in a population-representative sample and provides a definitive quantification of increased risk of mortality in EDs, which was previously lacking. Furthermore, it highlights the seriousness of EDs and an urgent need for strategies that may help to improve long-term outcomes.

Keywords: eating disorder; all-cause mortality; epidemiology; hazard ratio; general population; Canada

1. Introduction

Eating disorders (EDs) are serious and persistent psychiatric disorders characterized by severe disturbance in body weight and eating behavior [1]. Based on the Diagnostic and Statistical Manual of Mental Disorders-Fifth Edition (DSM-5) classification, EDs include anorexia nervosa, bulimia nervosa, binge eating disorder, other specified feeding or eating disorders, and avoidant/restrictive food intake disorder [2]. Based on the systematic review of 33 studies, the lifetime prevalence of EDs (total) is 8.4% for women and 2.2% for men [1], that of anorexia nervosa is 1.4% for women and 0.2% for men, that of bulimia nervosa is 1.9% for women and 0.6% for men, and finally, that of binge eating disorder is 2.8% for women and 1.0% for men [1]. EDs are associated with significantly impaired health-related quality of life compared with the healthy population and even with those with other psychiatric conditions [3]. These disorders encompass a range of problematic behaviors, including starvation, binge eating, and purging, leading to an increased risk of premature death [4]. Many factors in these patients have also been identified as predictors of mortality, such as type of ED diagnosis, low body mass index (BMI), suicide behaviors, alcohol abuse, and comorbidities [5–7]. In addition, the age of onset and age of treatment are also two important death-predictive factors in patients with EDs, as evidence has shown that older individuals (25–44 age group) have an elevated risk of mortality for all types of EDs compared to youth (15–24 age group) [8]. Mortality data on EDs are important and considered an indicator of illness severity [9]. Most mortality studies in EDs have focused on anorexia nervosa; however, a few studies of bulimia nervosa and other specified feeding or eating disorders, and even fewer for binge eating disorder, have been published [4]. The standard measures for mortality are the crude mortality rate (CMR) (CMR is the proportion of death within the study population over a specific period) [10], the standardized mortality rate (SMR) (SMR is calculated using the number of observed deaths in a targeted population at a certain point of time divided by the number of expected deaths in the general population while taking into account certain demographic variables) [11], and hazard ratios (HR) (the HR in survivorship curves is the temporal progression of death within a group and defined as the hazard in the groups with EDs divided by the hazard in the control groups) [12,13].

The ED mortality studies are largely based on cohorts from inpatient settings or case registers covering a circumscribed geographical area, such as the catchment area of a hospital, while relatively less is known about the general population [9,14,15]. For example, a retrospective Canadian cohort study, using administrative healthcare data of 19,041 individuals with ED from 1990–2013, showed that individuals with EDs identified in hospital settings had roughly a five-fold higher mortality rate relative to the general population [16]. The age, sex, and place of residence-adjusted HR for all-cause mortality of EDs in a longitudinal study in Finland among 2450 adults referred to a tertiary care-level ED unit was 3.54 (95%CI 2.52–4.96) [14]. The mortality associated with different types of mental disorders, including EDs, schizophrenia, mood disorders, personality disorders, and behavioral disorders, was also investigated in a recent population-based cohort study in Denmark on 7,369,926 people (23,196 persons with ED) younger than 95 years of age from 1995–2015. Similar to the previous studies, diagnosed individuals in this study also only included those with mental disorders registered in psychiatric inpatient, outpatient, and emergency settings. Therefore, one of the limitations of this cohort was a vulnerability to selection bias arising from a lack of representation of patients who are only treated by a general practitioner or who do not seek specialized help for their mental health. The CMR per 1000 person-year for EDs in this study was 3.0; however, those for schizophrenia and mood disorders were higher (28.1 and 31.2, respectively) [17]. Nevertheless, these aforementioned findings on mortality of EDs may not be representative of a general population and may not be generalizable to a greater range of cases of EDs. They may represent a very small and distinct proportion of the wider EDs population [18–20]. Since it has been revealed that despite the elevated contact with health care services among people with EDs, somewhere between 67% and 83% of cases fail to engage with treatment after referral [21,22]. A wide range of factors lead to this unmet need for treatment, such as difficulty accessing specialist services, the financial cost of treatment, perceived shame, and stigma attached to EDs [19,21]. Therefore, an important question to be answered is whether EDs are associated with higher mortality in the general population.

For epidemiological surveys of EDs in the general population, a self-reported current and lifetime screening tool using single-item questions, such as "Have you ever had anorexia", has been shown to have a reliable specificity and sensitivity [23]. Moreover, the validity of self-reported health in population-based studies has repeatedly been confirmed and even found to be a stronger predictor of associated mortality than instruments explicitly designed for this purpose [24]. However, to our knowledge, there is no empirical research available to assess the mortality of EDs based on the self-reported current and lifetime history of EDs in the general population. Nevertheless, these findings will assist health care providers and policymakers in public health messages about the serious consequences of eating disorders. While this study was conducted in Canada, the results are likely to apply to the general populations of other developed countries. However, to the extent that cultural, health system, or other between-country differences may affect the association of EDs with mortality, the results are most directly supportive of a need to address the issue of mortality in people with EDs in Canada. Hence, the main objective of the current study was to investigate the mortality of self-reported lifetime history of EDs among participants in the population-representative Canadian Community Health Survey linked to national mortality data, which covers all of the general Canadian population.

2. Materials and Methods

2.1. Data Source

The data source was the Canadian Community Health Survey (CCHS) 1.2, also known as the CCHS mental health and well-being survey conducted by Statistics Canada [25]. The CCHS is a cross-sectional survey that collects information related to mental health status, mental health care utilization, and mental health determinants for the Canadian population. This survey was conducted in 2002 (between May and December), and the sample size was 36,984 with a 77% response rate (Figure 1) [26]. The sampling method was a multi-stage stratified cluster design. The inclusion criteria in this national survey consisted of noninstitutionalized people aged 15 years or older living in private dwellings in the 10 Canadian provinces [26,27]. The exclusion criteria contained individuals residing in the three territories, on reserves and other Aboriginal settlements in the provinces, the clientele of institutions, children aged 15–17 that are living in foster care, the full-time members of the Canadian Forces, and residents of some remote areas, groups that, in total, exclude less than 3% of the general population [26,28]. A "share file" that included the participants who provided consent for their data to be linked to other data sources was subsequently linked, by Statistics Canada, to the Canadian Vital Statistics Database (CVSD), allowing confirmation of vital status and, where relevant, and date of death, see Figure 1. A detailed description of data linkage procedures and their quality assessment has been reported elsewhere [29,30]. The linked data are available to researchers through the Canadian Research Data Centres Network. The current analysis took place in the Prairie Regional Data Centre on the University of Calgary Campus [29,31].

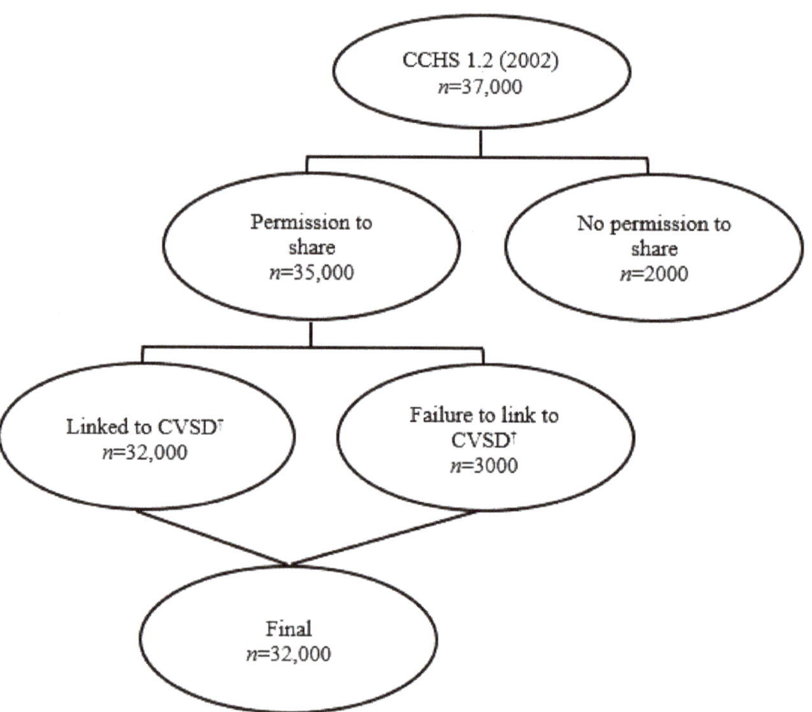

Figure 1. Flow diagrams for data linkage (estimates are rounded in keeping with Statistics Canada data release guidelines). † CVSD, Canadian Vital Statistics Database.

2.2. Measures

The demographic information of the entire population, including age, sex, employment status (currently working versus not employed), the highest educational level, and marital status in three groups: "Married/Common-law" (in Canada, common-law and legally married spouses have very similar legal standing [29]), "Single", i.e., never married, and "Widow/Separated/Divorced" were collected using field-tested items. Diagnosis of the EDs, schizophrenia, and mood disorders such as depression, bipolar disorder, mania or dysthymia, and post-traumatic stress disorder (PTSD), were assessed in each survey's "chronic conditions" module. The wording of the item was similar in each survey: "Remember, we're interested in conditions diagnosed by a health professional". For example: "Do you have an eating disorder such as anorexia or bulimia?". The interview questions for these disorders were those of a Canadian adaptation of the World Mental Health version of the Composite International Diagnostic Interview (WMH-CIDI) [26]. The WMH-CIDI is a lay-administered psychiatric interview that generates a lifetime profile of a person with a disorder defined partly according to both the 10th version of the International Statistical Classification of Diseases and Related Health Problems (ICD-10) and the Diagnostic and Statistical Manual of Mental Disorders, 4th Edition (DSM-IV) [26].

BMI was calculated by dividing the self-reported participants' weight in kilograms by the square of their self-reported height in meters (kg/m^2). The low BMI for participants younger than 18 years old was defined as less than the tenth percentile for age and sex [32], and for older participants below 18.5 kg/m^2, as recommended by the World Health Organization (WHO) criteria [33,34]. Binge drinking was assessed with a question in the CCHS survey "How often in the past 12 months have you had five or more drinks on one occasion?". Binge drinking was defined if the response was "more than once a month". Smoking to cope with stress was determined based on the question "When dealing with stress, how often do you try to feel better by smoking more cigarettes than usual?" if the response was "sometimes" or more.

All of the variables mentioned above were assessed using field-tested survey modules developed by Statistics Canada, which were made available in multiple languages. Detailed information on each of the surveys, questionnaires, and user guides are available from the 2002 mental health survey documentation [25,29,35].

2.3. Data Analysis

The interview date for each participant is recorded in the survey, which is considered the baseline time point. The participants were classified as exposed or not exposed to EDs according to their answers in the survey. Time to death was calculated as the difference between the date of death and the interview date. In the linked data, both the date and underlying cause of death for those who subsequently died were recorded. Time to the event (death) was calculated by subtracting the date of the baseline interview from the date of death [29]. Those surviving up to the linkage date (31 December 2017) were censored at that date. Covariates were derived from the survey dataset and were, therefore, all recorded at baseline. No information on time-varying covariates was available.

The stratified multi-stage sampling procedure used in CCHS leads to unequal selection probabilities. Therefore, the estimates should be analyzed using a set of 500 replicate bootstrap-sampling weights to ensure population representativeness. A procedure for bootstrap-weighting recommended by Statistics Canada was used in this analysis [28].

As in most studies of mortality, a time-to-event method of analysis was considered most appropriate due to its ability to address differing person time contributions by study participants. Therefore, after confirming the proportional hazard assumption, a Cox proportional hazards model was used to estimate hazard ratios from the time to event data [36] using Stata version 16. An unadjusted HR (crude HR) was estimated using a model that contained EDs but not covariates. While the CCHS dataset contains a rich set of covariates, the number of participants with EDs who died was too small to produce models with multiple covariate adjustments; therefore, covariates in this study included age (treated as a continuous variable) and sex. Confounding was observed only by age; however, to be consistent with other EDs mortality studies, the impact of sex and both age and sex were also assessed by adding each variable (along with an interaction term) one at a time to the model. For all analyses, the alpha level was set at 0.05.

3. Results

This study sample was restricted to respondents age 15 years and older at the time of the survey (consisting of approximately 31,130 respondents and mean age = 43.95 years). As shown in Table 1, 0.5% reported a positive lifetime history of EDs. About 14.4% of these individuals died, 89% were female, 52.5% were single, most had a post-secondary graduate degree (64.4%), and 11.5% reported a low BMI.

A Cox proportional hazard model showed that the unadjusted HR (crude HR) for the lifetime history of an ED was 1.35 (95% CI 0.70–2.58). When the model was adjusted for age and then both age and sex, the HR increased to 4.4 (95% CI 2.2–8.0) (data not shown) and 4.54 (95% CI 2.33–8.84, Table 2), respectively.

Table 1. Characteristics of the population [†].

		Entire Population (95% CI)	History of Eating Disorder (95% CI)
History of an Eating Disorder (%)		0.47 (0.47–0.47)	-
Mean Age (Year)		43.95	32.96
All-Cause Death (%)		12.9 (12.9–13)	14.4 (14.2–14.6)
Sex (%)	Male	49.15 (49.13–49.17)	11.86 (11.68–12.05)
	Female	50.85 (50.83–50.87)	88.98 (88.80–89.16)
Marital Status (%)	Married/Common-law	62.04 (62.02–62.06)	29.66 (29.40–29.92)
	Single	25.11 (25.09–25.12)	52.54 (52.26–52.83)
	Widow/Separated/Divorced	12.85 (12.84–12.87)	17.8 (17.58–18.02)
Employment Status in the Past Week (%)	Working	63.84 (63.82–63.86)	44.44 (44.16–44.73)
	Absent	4.73 (4.72–4.74)	6.83 (6.69–6.98)
	No job/Permanently Unable to Work	31.44 (31.42–31.46)	47.86 (47.58–48.15)
Education (%)	<Secondary Graduate	11.54 (11.53–11.56)	15.25 (15.05–15.46)
	Secondary Graduate	13.15 (13.13–13.16)	11.02 (10.83–11.20)
	Some Post-Secondary	7.08 (7.07–7.09)	10.17 (10.00–10.34)
	Post-Secondary Graduate	68.23 (68.21–68.25)	64.41 (64.13–64.68)
Low BMI (%)		1.98 (1.98–1.99)	11.54 (11.32–11.76)

[†] CI—Confidence Interval, BMI—Body Mass Index (definition of low BMI: for ages <18, below the 10th percentile for age and sex, and for ages >18, below 18.5 kg/m^2).

Table 2. Crude and age/sex-adjusted effect of the self-reported major mental health problems on mortality [†].

	Crude HR (95% CI)	Age/Sex-Adjusted HR (95% CI)
Eating Disorder	1.35 (0.70–2.58)	4.54 * (2.33–8.84)
Schizophrenia/Psychosis	1.44 * (1.04–1.99)	2.02 * (1.24–3.31)
Mood disorder	0.60 (0.26–1.39)	1.07 (0.49–2.35)
PTSD	1.11 (0.80–1.55)	1.45 * (1.03–2.03)
Binge Drinking	0.55 (0.49–0.63)	1.39 * (1.20–1.62)
Smoking to Cope with Stress	0.91 (0.83–0.99)	1.82 * (1.65–2.00)
Low BMI	1.92 * (1.27–2.90)	2.97 * (1.93–4.59)

[†] CI—Confidence Interval, HR—Hazard Ratio, PTSD—Post-Traumatic Stress Disorder, BMI—Body Mass Index (definition of low BMI: for ages < 18, below the 10th percentile for age and sex, and for ages >18, below 18.5 kg/m^2). * Indicates statistical significance at the $p < 0.05$ level.

For purposes of comparison, we generated unadjusted and age/sex-adjusted HR for other self-reported history of mental health disorders and low BMI in the same population. As shown in Table 2, the unadjusted HR for schizophrenia/psychosis (1.44, 95% CI 1.04–1.99) was higher than the crude HR for ED, however, the age/sex-adjusted HR (2.02, 95% CI 1.24–3.31) was smaller than the age/sex-adjusted HR for EDs. Similarly, the age/sex-adjusted HR for the self-reported history of mood disorder and PTSD was lower than that of eating disorders. For comparison, age/sex-adjusted HRs for other potential determinants of mortality are also presented in Table 2: binge drinking, smoking to cope with stress (which is here considered a proxy for smoking), and low BMI.

4. Discussion

To our knowledge, this is the first study that evaluated all-cause mortality of self-reported lifetime history of all EDs in a general population. This study confirms the high mortality in individuals with a lifetime history of ED that is not due to the selection of severely ill respondents as in prior studies of clinical individuals. However, as the prevalence of EDs was low, it is likely that these general population estimates also reflect a subset of the entire population with EDs. Previous studies reported mortality in a broad category of EDs [8,16,17] or with DSM or ICD diagnosis of anorexia nervosa [37,38], bulimia nervosa [37,38], other specified feeding or eating disorders [37], or binge eating disorder [14] based on a selective population, such as health-administrative data, inpatients-settings, or outpatients care. Therefore, the generalization of these results to all patients with EDs was limited only to those in treatment settings [14]. The current study helps to confirm that mortality is substantially elevated in members of the general population who report that they have been diagnosed with an ED, including those with subclinical eating disorders or those who failed to engage with treatment once referred. There is widespread stigma toward people affected by EDs by the general public, medical professionals, and service users due to the attribution of personal responsibility for illness behaviors [39]. Therefore, the seriousness of EDs may be underreported as a result of individuals who trivialize and minimize associated psychological and medical challenges [40]. There is also a self-stigma in people with EDs that leads them to deny, minimize, or assign positive meaning to their behaviors [39,41]. The effect of public/self-stigma may lead people to be reluctant to seek treatment, leave treatment prematurely, or experience a loss in the necessary components of recovery [42]. The current findings could be integrated into psychoeducation material for adolescents/adults with ED and their caregivers to help challenge the view that these illnesses are not serious, necessitating treatment. Public health campaigns could further highlight the high mortality rate of EDs [43].

Evidence has shown that mortality in EDs is influenced by age, sex, and case severity [6,9,16,44]. Generally, older individuals have an elevated risk of mortality for all types of EDs compared to the mortality of younger individuals [8], probably reflecting the strong effect of age and chronicity of illness on mortality. Consistent with this, age-adjusted estimates show a strong association with mortality. In a dataset of English national Hospital Episode Statistics, the SMR for the 15–24 age group diagnosed with anorexia nervosa or bulimia nervosa was found to be 11.5 and 4.1, respectively [8]. The SMR for the 25–44 age group diagnosed with anorexia nervosa or bulimia nervosa was found to be 14.0 and 7.7, respectively [8]. A number of studies have also reported sex differences in ED mortality [44–46]. Although the lifetime prevalence of EDs among males is lower than females, the CMR and SMR observed in males are almost two-fold higher than in females [16,17]. These provide evidence for the potential impact of age and sex as covariates in the all-cause EDs mortality assessment. Therefore, in the current study, the HR for eating disorders was reported as adjusted for age, sex, and both age and sex.

A naïve interpretation of crude HRs suggests only a weak effect of EDs (1.35, 95% CI 0.70–2.58, since the low end of the interval is below one); however, the age/sex-adjusted HR for EDs is much higher than that of other major mental health problems. This indicates that the unadjusted estimates were strongly confounded by age and sex, information that will be useful in planning the analysis of future studies. The direction of the confounding is predictable, since EDs were reported more often by younger people and by women (see Table 1), both of whom have lower rates of mortality.

In this study, only for the purpose of comparison, the mortality associated with some self-reported lifetime major mental health problems, and low BMI calculated based on self-reported height and weight were also evaluated. Evidence shows that low BMI associated with EDs may affect mortality [4,7,47]. About 12% of the individuals with a self-reported lifetime history of ED and 2% of the entire population reported a low BMI. However, the causes of this low BMI are not distinguishable between those who were initially underweight and those who became underweight due to malnutrition, over-exercising, or other comorbidities [48]. The present study aimed to evaluate all-cause mortality of self-reported history of EDs; however, numerous previous studies have reported a different degree of malnutrition in patients with EDs [49–51]. Several lines of evidence on the effect of low BMI caused by malnutrition on mortality meets the key Bradford Hill's criteria to establish this causal relationship [52–55].

In the current study, the age/sex-adjusted HR for lifetime history of EDs was over two-fold higher than the age/sex-adjusted HR for self-reported lifetime schizophrenia/psychosis. In this study, the self-reported lifetime schizophrenia/psychosis was based on the question asking whether they have schizophrenia or any other psychosis as diagnosed by a health professional (response options, yes or no). A previous study on the CCHS1.2 survey has shown that the prevalence estimates of these two self-report survey items provide what appears to be a plausible epidemiologic pattern [56]. Accordingly, the mortality associated with these two items might also follow the same pattern. A nationally representative cohort study in the UK using primary care electronic health records on over 11 million people reported a very similar adjusted HR (accounting for age, gender, calendar year, area-level deprivation, ethnicity, and the average number of visits to the physician per year of follow-up) for schizophrenia (2.08, 95% CI 1.98–2.19) to our study [57]. In the current study, the results in the general population are in line with the previous studies on the clinical samples that observed lower crude HR and higher sex/age-adjusted HR in EDs than schizophrenia [8,17,58,59].

Although the sex ratio of the participants in this study was 1:1, males reported a history of lifetime ED nearly eight times less than females (11.86% vs. 88.98%). This difference is much larger than the existing literature on the lifetime prevalence of EDs among different sexes measured with a standardized tool (2.2% vs. 8.4%) [1]. This discrepancy may be associated with the difference between females and males in diagnosis, self-identifying, and self-reporting lifetime EDs due to the immense stigmatization toward males with EDs, stereotypes linked to EDs, and a misdiagnosis by a specialist treatment center [60–62]. These current findings may indicate the importance of gendered issues in diagnosing and treating patients with EDs and the necessity of tailored services to the patient's need, such as the same-sex therapeutic groups [61].

In the current study, mood disorders were not associated with mortality, which is surprising since CCHS respondents (linking data from four surveys: CCHS 1.1 (2000/2001), CCHS 1.2 (2002), CCHS 2.1 (2003/2004), and CCHS 3.1 (2005/2006)) with symptoms of major depressive episodes (according to versions of Composite International Diagnostic Interview, a structured interview that does not depend on help-seeking) do have elevated all-cause mortality [29]. As the variable included in this analysis was self-reported diagnoses of mood disorders, it is possible that help-seeking and potentially treated individuals with major depression do not have elevated mortality, in contrast to what was reported here for EDs.

Limitations

In this study, not all the potential confounding effects in the analysis were considered. Relevant variables include the age of onset and duration of EDs, specific type of ED, information on treatment, dietary intake, suicidal ideation/attempts, and potential comorbidities. Prior studies on ED patients suggested that these factors predicted the time to death [4,63]. According to Statistics Canada regulations, the number of these variables in the current study was insufficient to release the data (such as suicidal ideation/attempts) or were not measured in the data source. However, the current study was not designed to make a causal statement of the effects of EDs, independent of other variables, on mortality, but rather to describe the pattern of mortality in this population.

Another limitation is the lack of information regarding if the EDs cases also include binge eating disorder and other specified feeding or eating disorders, since in this study, the screening of current and lifetime EDs was based on a dichotomous question "Do you have an eating disorder such as anorexia or bulimia?". While the self-reported current and lifetime-screening questions have a reliable specificity and sensitivity, bulimia nervosa compared to other ED types has poorer reliability in identifying true cases [23], which might be one of the reasons that the prevalence of EDs in our population is lower than other reports based on psychometric questionnaires. However, another possible reason for this prevalence discrepancy might be because they represent more severe groups, i.e., those who have sought professional help [23].

CCHS in Canada represents over 97% of the Canadian population aged $\geq$15, which covers the ten provinces and the three territories, while excluding those persons who meet the exclusion criteria [25,26]. Therefore, these findings cannot be generalized to these groups. Furthermore, in Canada, health care is based on a universal healthcare system, meaning that it is largely based on need rather than the ability to pay, permitting Canadians to have access to most healthcare services [64]. A universal healthcare system reduces, though does not eliminate, the potential inequalities in accessing care for the initial diagnosis of EDs by a healthcare provider among people with different socioeconomic backgrounds [64,65].

5. Conclusions

To our knowledge, the current study, for the first time, has reported the all-cause mortality of self-reported lifetime history of EDs in a population-based study. This finding highlights the seriousness of these disorders and supports the idea that there is an urgent need for strategies that may help to improve long-term outcomes, such as a need for public education for early diagnosis and a long-term plan for adequate early intervention. Different types of research would be needed to understand the underlying causal mechanism and, consequently, formulate a preventive strategy.

Author Contributions: P.P. is the first author: analyzing the data and interpreting the results and leading in the preparation of the manuscript; S.B.P.: conceiving the original idea, contributing to the design and implementation of the research, supervising the project, interpreting the results, and providing critical feedback; A.G.M.B.: contributing to interpreting the results and providing critical feedback to the final manuscript; J.V.A.W.: analyzing the data, contributing to interpreting the results, and providing critical feedback; G.D. is the senior author and an expert in eating disorders: contributing to the design and implementation of the research, interpreting the results, and revising the manuscript. All authors have read and agreed to the published version of the manuscript.

Funding: This work was supported by the Cuthbertson and Fischer Chair in Pediatric Mental Health, held by Scott Patten at the University of Calgary.

Institutional Review Board Statement: Ethical review and approval were waived for this study, due to the Canadian Interagency Advisory Panel on Research Ethics, Tri-Council Policy Statement 2 (2018), chapter 5, Article 5.5A. Information is available at: https://ethics.gc.ca/eng/tcps2-eptc2_2018_chapter5-chapitre5.html#5a (access on 21 September 2021).

Informed Consent Statement: Informed consent was obtained from all subjects involved in the study.

Data Availability Statement: The data used in this analysis are available through the Research Data Centers Program. Information is available at: http://www.statcan.gc.ca/eng/rdc/index (accessed on 21 September 2021).

Acknowledgments: This study was supported by a pilot grant from the Mathison Centre for Mental Health Research & Education. The analysis was conducted at the Prairie Regional Data Centre, which is part of the Canadian Research Data Centre Network (CRDCN). The services and activities provided by the CRDCN are made possible by the financial or in-kind support of the SSHRC, the CIHR, the CFI, Statistics Canada, and participating universities, whose support is gratefully acknowledged. The views expressed in this paper do not necessarily represent the CRDCN's or those of its partners.

Conflicts of Interest: The authors have no conflict of interest to declare.

References

1. Galmiche, M.; Déchelotte, P.; Lambert, G.; Tavolacci, M.P. Prevalence of eating disorders over the 2000–2018 period: A systematic literature review. *Am. J. Clin. Nutr.* **2019**, *109*, 1402–1413. [CrossRef]
2. American Psychiatric Association. *Diagnostic and Statistical Manual of Mental Disorders*, 5th ed.; American Psychiatric Association: Washington, DC, USA, 2013; Volume 21.
3. Ágh, T.; Kovács, G.; Supina, D.; Pawaskar, M.; Herman, B.K.; Vokó, Z.; Sheehan, D.V. A systematic review of the health-related quality of life and economic burdens of anorexia nervosa, bulimia nervosa, and binge eating disorder. *Eat. Weight Disord. Stud. Anorex. Bulim. Obes.* **2016**, *21*, 353–364. [CrossRef]
4. Fichter, M.M.; Quadflieg, N. Mortality in eating disorders—Results of a large prospective clinical longitudinal study. *Int. J. Eat. Disord.* **2016**, *49*, 391–401. [CrossRef]
5. Keel, P.K.; Dorer, D.J.; Eddy, K.T.; Franko, D.; Charatan, D.L.; Herzog, D.B. Predictors of mortality in eating disorders. *Arch. Gen. Psychiatry* **2003**, *60*, 179–183. [CrossRef]
6. Guinhut, M.; Godart, N.; Benadjaoud, M.; Melchior, J.; Hanachi, M. Five-year mortality of severely malnourished patients with chronic anorexia nervosa admitted to a medical unit. *Acta Psychiatr. Scand.* **2021**, *143*, 130–140. [CrossRef]
7. Button, E.J.; Chadalavada, B.; Palmer, R.L. Mortality and predictors of death in a cohort of patients presenting to an eating disorders service. *Int. J. Eat. Disord.* **2009**, *43*, 387–392. [CrossRef] [PubMed]
8. Crow, S.J.; Peterson, C.B.; Swanson, S.A.; Raymond, N.C.; Specker, S.; Eckert, E.D.; Mitchell, J.E. Increased mortality in bulimia nervosa and other eating disorders. *Am. J. Psychiatry* **2009**, *166*, 1342–1346. [CrossRef]
9. Smink, F.R.E.; van Hoeken, D.; Hoek, H.W. Epidemiology of eating disorders: Incidence, prevalence and mortality rates. *Curr. Psychiatry Rep.* **2012**, *14*, 406–414. [CrossRef]
10. Hoek, H.W. Incidence, prevalence and mortality of anorexia nervosa and other eating disorders. *Curr. Opin. Psychiatry* **2006**, *19*, 389–394. [CrossRef]
11. Franko, D.L.; Keel, P.K. Suicidality in eating disorders: Occurrence, correlates, and clinical implications. *Clin. Psychol. Rev.* **2006**, *26*, 769–782. [CrossRef]
12. George, A.; Stead, T.S.; Ganti, L. What's the risk: Differentiating risk ratios, odds ratios, and hazard ratios? *Cureus* **2020**, *12*, e10047. [CrossRef]
13. Hernán, M.A. The hazards of hazard ratios. *Epidemiology* **2010**, *21*, 13–15. [CrossRef] [PubMed]
14. Suokas, J.T.; Suvisaari, J.; Gissler, M.; Löfman, R.; Linna, M.S.; Raevuori, A.; Haukka, J. Mortality in eating disorders: A follow-up study of adult eating disorder patients treated in tertiary care, 1995–2010. *Psychiatry Res.* **2013**, *210*, 1101–1106. [CrossRef] [PubMed]
15. van Hoeken, D.; Hoek, H.W. Review of the burden of eating disorders: Mortality, disability, costs, quality of life, and family burden. *Curr. Opin. Psychiatry* **2020**, *33*, 521. [CrossRef] [PubMed]
16. Iwajomo, T.; Bondy, S.J.; de Oliveira, C.; Colton, P.; Trottier, K.; Kurdyak, P. Excess mortality associated with eating disorders: Population-based cohort study. *Br. J. Psychiatry* **2020**, *219*, 487–493. [CrossRef]
17. Plana-Ripoll, O.; Pedersen, C.B.; Agerbo, E.; Holtz, Y.; Erlangsen, A.; Canudas-Romo, V.; Andersen, P.K.; Charlson, F.; Christensen, M.K.; Erskine, H.E.; et al. A comprehensive analysis of mortality-related health metrics associated with mental disorders: A nationwide, register-based cohort study. *Lancet* **2019**, *394*, 1827–1835. [CrossRef]
18. Mayes, S.D.; Fernandez-Mendoza, J.; Baweja, R.; Calhoun, S.; Mahr, F.; Aggarwal, R.; Arnold, M. Correlates of suicide ideation and attempts in children and adolescents with eating disorders. *Eat. Disord.* **2014**, *22*, 352–366. [CrossRef]
19. Cachelin, F.M.; Striegel-Moore, R.H.; Regan, P.C. Factors associated with treatment seeking in a community sample of European American and Mexican American women with eating disorders. *Eur. Eat. Disord. Rev.* **2006**, *14*, 422–429. [CrossRef]
20. Mitchison, D.; Hay, P.; Mond, J.; Slewa-Younan, S. Self-reported history of anorexia nervosa and current quality of life: Findings from a community-based study. *Qual. Life Res.* **2012**, *22*, 273–281. [CrossRef]
21. Hart, L.M.; Granillo, M.T.; Jorm, A.F.; Paxton, S.J. Unmet need for treatment in the eating disorders: A systematic review of eating disorder specific treatment seeking among community cases. *Clin. Psychol. Rev.* **2011**, *31*, 727–735. [CrossRef]
22. Bell, L. What predicts failure to engage in or drop out from treatment for bulimia nervosa and what implications does this have for treatment? *Clin. Psychol. Psychother. Int. J. Theory Pract.* **2001**, *8*, 424–435. [CrossRef]
23. Keski-Rahkonen, A.; Sihvola, E.; Raevuori, A.; Kaukoranta, J.; Bulik, C.M.; Hoek, H.; Rissanen, A.; Kaprio, J. Reliability of self-reported eating disorders: Optimizing population screening. *Int. J. Eat. Disord.* **2006**, *39*, 754–762. [CrossRef]
24. Lorem, G.; Cook, S.; Leon, D.A.; Emaus, N.; Schirmer, H. Self-reported health as a predictor of mortality: A cohort study of its relation to other health measurements and observation time. *Sci. Rep.* **2020**, *10*, 4886. [CrossRef]

25. Statistics-Canada, Canadian Community Health Survey Cycle 1.2 Mental Health and Well-Being Public Use Microdata File Documentation. Available online: https://www23.statcan.gc.ca/imdb-bmdi/document/3226_DLI_D1_T22_V2-eng.pdf (accessed on 30 July 2021).
26. Gravel, R.; Béland, Y. The Canadian Community Health Survey: Mental health and well-being. *Can. J. Psychiatry* **2005**, *50*, 573–579. [CrossRef]
27. Satyanarayana, S.; Enns, M.W.; Cox, B.J.; Sareen, J. Prevalence and correlates of chronic depression in the Canadian Community Health Survey: Mental health and well-being. *Can. J. Psychiatry* **2009**, *54*, 389–398. [CrossRef]
28. Statistics-Canada, Canadian Community Health Survey—Annual Component (CCHS). Available online: https://www23.statcan.gc.ca/imdb/p2SV.pl?Function=getSurvey&SDDS=3226 (accessed on 30 July 2021).
29. Patten, S.B.; Williams, J.V.; Bulloch, A.G. Major depressive episodes and mortality in the Canadian household population. *J. Affect. Disord.* **2018**, *242*, 165–171. [CrossRef]
30. Sanmartin, C.; Decady, Y.; Trudeau, R.; Dasylva, A.; Tjepkema, M.; Finès, P.; Burnett, R.; Ross, N.; Manuel, D.G. Linking the Canadian Community Health Survey and the Canadian Mortality Database: An enhanced data source for the study of mortality. *Health Rep.* **2016**, *27*, 10–18.
31. Canadian-Research-Data-Centre-Network, Prairie Regional RDC. Available online: https://crdcn.org/prairie-regional-rdc-history (accessed on 30 July 2021).
32. Hebebrand, J.; Wehmeier, P.M.; Remschmidt, H. Weight criteria for diagnosis of anorexia nervosa. *Am. J. Psychiatry* **2000**, *157*, 1024. [CrossRef]
33. StatisticsCanada, Body Mass Index (BMI) Nomogram. Available online: https://www.canada.ca/en/health-canada/services/food-nutrition/healthy-eating/healthy-weights/canadian-guidelines-body-weight-classification-adults/body-mass-index-nomogram.html (accessed on 30 July 2021).
34. World Health Organization. Body Mass Index—BMI. Available online: https://www.euro.who.int/en/health-topics/disease-prevention/nutrition/a-healthy-lifestyle/body-mass-index-bmi (accessed on 21 September 2021).
35. Canadian Community Health Survey-Annual Component (CCHS), Variable(s). 2019. Available online: https://www23.statcan.gc.ca/imdb/p2SV.pl?Function=getSurvVariableList&Id=1208978 (accessed on 8 September 2021).
36. Hoang, U.; Goldacre, M.; James, A. Mortality following hospital discharge with a diagnosis of eating disorder: National record linkage study, England, 2001–2009. *Int. J. Eat. Disord.* **2014**, *47*, 507–515. [CrossRef]
37. Franko, D.L.; Keshaviah, A.; Eddy, K.T.; Krishna, M.; Davis, M.C.; Keel, P.K.; Herzog, D.B. A longitudinal investigation of mortality in anorexia nervosa and bulimia nervosa. *Am. J. Psychiatry* **2013**, *170*, 917–925. [CrossRef]
38. Griffiths, S.; Mond, J.M.; Murray, S.B.; Thornton, C.; Touyz, S. Stigma resistance in eating disorders. *Soc. Psychiatry Psychiatr. Epidemiol.* **2015**, *50*, 279–287. [CrossRef]
39. Dimitropoulos, G.; McCallum, L.; Colasanto, M.; Freeman, V.E.; Gadalla, T. The effects of stigma on recovery attitudes in people with anorexia nervosa in intensive treatment. *J. Nerv. Ment. Dis.* **2016**, *204*, 370–380. [CrossRef]
40. Griffiths, S.; Mond, J.; Murray, S.B.; Touyz, S. The prevalence and adverse associations of stigmatization in people with eating disorders. *Int. J. Eat. Disord.* **2014**, *48*, 767–774. [CrossRef]
41. Hackler, A.H.; Vogel, D.L.; Wade, N.G. Attitudes toward seeking professional help for an eating disorder: The role of stigma and anticipated outcomes. *J. Couns. Dev.* **2010**, *88*, 424–431. [CrossRef]
42. Becker, C.B.; Plasencia, M.; Kilpela, L.S.; Briggs, M.; Stewart, T. Changing the course of comorbid eating disorders and depression: What is the role of public health interventions in targeting shared risk factors? *J. Eat. Disord.* **2014**, *2*, 15. [CrossRef]
43. Gueguen, J.; Godart, N.; Chambry, J.; Brun-Eberentz, A.; Foulon, C.; Divac, S.M.; Guelfi, J.-D.; Rouillon, F.; Falissard, B.; Huas, C.; et al. Severe anorexia nervosa in men: Comparison with severe AN in women and analysis of mortality. *Int. J. Eat. Disord.* **2012**, *45*, 537–545. [CrossRef]
44. Møller-Madsen, S.; Nystrup, J.; Nielsen, S. Mortality in anorexia nervosa in Denmark during the period 1970–1987. *Acta Psychiatr. Scand.* **1996**, *94*, 454–459. [CrossRef]
45. Lorem, G.F.; Schirmer, H.; Emaus, N. What is the impact of underweight on self-reported health trajectories and mortality rates: A cohort study. *Health Qual. Life Outcomes* **2017**, *15*, 191. [CrossRef]
46. Keshaviah, A.; Edkins, K.; Hastings, E.R.; Krishna, M.; Franko, D.L.; Herzog, D.B.; Thomas, J.J.; Murray, H.B.; Eddy, K.T. Re-examining premature mortality in anorexia nervosa: A meta-analysis redux. *Compr. Psychiatry* **2014**, *55*, 1773–1784. [CrossRef]
47. Rosling, A.M.; Sparén, P.; Norring, C.; Von Knorring, A.-L. Mortality of eating disorders: A follow-up study of treatment in a specialist unit 1974–2000. *Int. J. Eat. Disord.* **2011**, *44*, 304–310. [CrossRef]
48. Himmerich, H.; Kan, C.; Au, K.; Treasure, J. Pharmacological treatment of eating disorders, comorbid mental health problems, malnutrition and physical health consequences. *Pharmacol. Ther.* **2020**, *217*, 107667. [CrossRef] [PubMed]
49. Mattar, L.; Huas, C.; Duclos, J.; Apfel, A.; Godart, N. Relationship between malnutrition and depression or anxiety in Anorexia Nervosa: A critical review of the literature. *J. Affect. Disord.* **2011**, *132*, 311–318. [CrossRef]
50. DiVasta, A.D.; Walls, C.E.; Feldman, H.A.; Quach, A.E.; Woods, E.R.; Gordon, C.M.; Alexander, M.E. Malnutrition and hemodynamic status in adolescents hospitalized for anorexia nervosa. *Arch. Pediatr. Adolesc. Med.* **2010**, *164*, 706–713. [CrossRef]
51. Schwinger, C.; Golden, M.H.; Grellety, E.; Roberfroid, D.; Guesdon, B. Severe acute malnutrition and mortality in children in the community: Comparison of indicators in a multi-country pooled analysis. *PLoS ONE* **2019**, *14*, e0219745. [CrossRef]

52. Bell, C.L.; Tamura, B.K.; Masaki, K.H.; Amella, E.J. Prevalence and measures of nutritional compromise among nursing home patients: Weight loss, low body mass index, malnutrition, and feeding dependency, a systematic review of the literature. *J. Am. Med. Dir. Assoc.* **2013**, *14*, 94–100. [CrossRef] [PubMed]

53. Maeda, K.; Ishida, Y.; Nonogaki, T.; Mori, N. Reference body mass index values and the prevalence of malnutrition according to the Global Leadership Initiative on Malnutrition criteria. *Clin. Nutr.* **2019**, *39*, 180–184. [CrossRef]

54. Tamura, B.K.; Bell, C.; Masaki, K.H.; Amella, E. Factors associated with weight loss, low BMI, and malnutrition among nursing home patients: A systematic review of the literature. *J. Am. Med. Dir. Assoc.* **2013**, *14*, 649–655. [CrossRef]

55. Supina, A.L.; Patten, S.B. Self-reported diagnoses of schizophrenia and psychotic disorders may be valuable for monitoring and surveillance. *Can. J. Psychiatry* **2006**, *51*, 256–259. [CrossRef]

56. Hayes, J.F.; Marston, L.; Walters, K.; King, M.B.; Osborn, D.P.J. Mortality gap for people with bipolar disorder and schizophrenia: UK-based cohort study 2000–2014. *Br. J. Psychiatry* **2017**, *211*, 175–181. [CrossRef]

57. Arcelus, J.; Mitchell, A.J.; Wales, J.; Nielsen, S. Mortality rates in patients with anorexia nervosa and other eating disorders: A meta-analysis of 36 studies. *Arch. Gen. Psychiatry* **2011**, *68*, 724–731. [CrossRef]

58. Chesney, E.; Goodwin, G.M.; Fazel, S. Risks of all-cause and suicide mortality in mental disorders: A meta-review. *World Psychiatry* **2014**, *13*, 153–160. [CrossRef] [PubMed]

59. Murray, S.B.; Nagata, J.; Griffiths, S.; Calzo, J.; Brown, T.A.; Mitchison, D.; Blashill, A.; Mond, J. The enigma of male eating disorders: A critical review and synthesis. *Clin. Psychol. Rev.* **2017**, *57*, 1–11. [CrossRef] [PubMed]

60. Grillot, C.L.; Keel, P.K. Barriers to seeking treatment for eating disorders: The role of self-recognition in understanding gender disparities in who seeks help. *Int. J. Eat. Disord.* **2018**, *51*, 1285–1289. [CrossRef] [PubMed]

61. Strother, E.; Lemberg, R.; Stanford, S.C.; Turberville, D. Eating disorders in men: Underdiagnosed, undertreated, and misunderstood. *Eat. Disord.* **2012**, *20*, 346–355. [CrossRef] [PubMed]

62. Martin, D.; Miller, A.P.; Quesnel-Vallée, A.; Caron, N.R.; Vissandjée, B.; Marchildon, G.P. Canada's universal health-care system: Achieving its potential. *Obstet. Gynecol. Surv.* **2018**, *73*, 509–511. [CrossRef]

63. Pisetsky, E.M.; Thornton, L.M.; Lichtenstein, P.; Pedersen, N.L.; Bulik, C.M. Suicide attempts in women with eating disorders. *J. Abnorm. Psychol.* **2013**, *122*, 1042–1056. [CrossRef]

64. Plana-Ripoll, O.; Musliner, K.L.; Dalsgaard, S.; Momen, N.C.; Weye, N.; Christensen, M.K.; Agerbo, E.; Iburg, K.M.; Laursen, T.M.; Mortensen, P.B.; et al. Nature and prevalence of combinations of mental disorders and their association with excess mortality in a population-based cohort study. *World Psychiatry* **2020**, *19*, 339–349. [CrossRef]

65. Veugelers, P.J.; Yip, A.M. Socioeconomic disparities in health care use: Does universal coverage reduce inequalities in health? *J. Epidemiol. Community Health* **2003**, *57*, 424–428. [CrossRef]

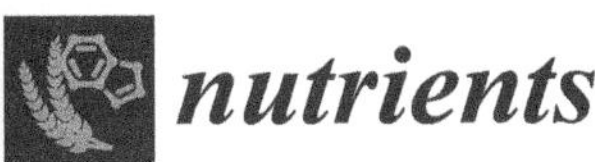

Article

The Structure of Relationships between the Human Exposome and Cardiometabolic Health: The Million Veteran Program

Kerry L. Ivey [1,2,3,*], Xuan-Mai T. Nguyen [1,4,5], Daniel Posner [1], Geraint B. Rogers [2], Deirdre K. Tobias [3,6], Rebecca Song [1,7], Yuk-Lam Ho [1], Ruifeng Li [3], Peter W. F. Wilson [8,9], Kelly Cho [1,4,5], John Michael Gaziano [1,4,5,10], Frank B. Hu [3,11,12], Walter C. Willett [3,11,12] and Luc Djoussé [1,4,5,†]

[1] Massachusetts Veterans Epidemiology and Research Information Center (MAVERIC), Boston Veterans Affairs Healthcare System, Boston, MA 02130, USA; xuan-mai.nguyen@va.gov (X.-M.T.N.); dcposner@bu.edu (D.P.); Rebecca.Song@va.gov (R.S.); Yuk-Lam.Ho@va.gov (Y.-L.H.); Kelly.Cho@va.gov (K.C.); michael.gaziano@va.gov (J.M.G.); ldjousse@rics.bwh.harvard.edu (L.D.)
[2] South Australian Health and Medical Research Institute, Infection and Immunity Theme, Adelaide 5000, Australia; Geraint.Rogers@sahmri.com
[3] Department of Nutrition, Harvard T.H. Chan School of Public Health, Boston, MA 02115, USA; dtobias@bwh.harvard.edu (D.K.T.); rli@hsph.harvard.edu (R.L.); fhu@hsph.harvard.edu (F.B.H.); wwillett@hsph.harvard.edu (W.C.W.)
[4] Division of Aging, Department of Medicine, Brigham and Women's Hospital, Boston, MA 02115, USA
[5] Department of Medicine, Harvard Medical School, Boston, MA 02115, USA
[6] Division of Preventive Medicine, Department of Medicine, Brigham and Women's Hospital, Boston, MA 02115, USA
[7] Department of Epidemiology, Boston University School of Public Health, Boston, MA 02118, USA
[8] Atlanta Veterans Affairs Medical Center, Decatur, GA 30033, USA; pwwilso@emory.edu
[9] Department of Medicine, Division of Cardiovascular Disease, Emory University Schools of Medicine and Public Health, Atlanta, GA 30322, USA
[10] Division of General Internal Medicine, Department of Medicine, Brigham and Women's Hospital, Boston, MA 02115, USA
[11] Department of Epidemiology, Harvard T.H. Chan School of Public Health, Boston, MA 02115, USA
[12] Channing Division of Network Medicine, Department of Medicine, Brigham and Women's Hospital, Harvard Medical School, Boston, MA 02115, USA
[*] Correspondence: kivey@hsph.harvard.edu
[†] On behalf of the VA Million Veteran Program.

Citation: Ivey, K.L.; Nguyen, X.-M.T.; Posner, D.; Rogers, G.B.; Tobias, D.K.; Song, R.; Ho, Y.-L.; Li, R.; Wilson, P.W.F.; Cho, K.; et al. The Structure of Relationships between the Human Exposome and Cardiometabolic Health: The Million Veteran Program. *Nutrients* **2021**, *13*, 1364. https://doi.org/10.3390/nu13041364

Academic Editor: Rosa Casas

Received: 10 March 2021
Accepted: 14 April 2021
Published: 19 April 2021

Publisher's Note: MDPI stays neutral with regard to jurisdictional claims in published maps and institutional affiliations.

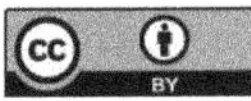

Abstract: The *exposome* represents the array of dietary, lifestyle, and demographic factors to which an individual is exposed. Individual components of the exposome, or groups of components, are recognized as influencing many aspects of human physiology, including cardiometabolic health. However, the influence of the whole exposome on health outcomes is poorly understood and may differ substantially from the sum of its individual components. As such, studies of the complete exposome are more biologically representative than fragmented models based on subsets of factors. This study aimed to model the system of relationships underlying the way in which the diet, lifestyle, and demographic components of the overall exposome shapes the cardiometabolic risk profile. The current study included 36,496 US Veterans enrolled in the VA Million Veteran Program (MVP) who had complete assessments of their diet, lifestyle, demography, and markers of cardiometabolic health, including serum lipids, blood pressure, and glycemic control. The cohort was randomly divided into training and validation datasets. In the training dataset, we conducted two separate exploratory factor analyses (EFA) to identify common factors among exposures (diet, demographics, and physical activity) and laboratory measures (lipids, blood pressure, and glycemic control), respectively. In the validation dataset, we used multiple normal regression to examine the combined effects of exposure factors on the clinical factors representing cardiometabolic health. The mean ± SD age of participants was 62.4 ± 13.4 years for both the training and validation datasets. The EFA revealed 19 Exposure Common Factors and 5 Physiology Common Factors that explained the observed (measured) data. Multivariate regression in the validation dataset revealed the structure of associations between the Exposure Common Factors and the Physiology Common Factors. For example, we found that the factor for fruit consumption was inversely associated with the factor summarizing total cholesterol and low-density lipoprotein cholesterol (LDLC, $p = 0.008$), and the latent construct describing light levels of physical activity was inversely associated with the blood pressure latent construct ($p < 0.0001$). We also found that a factor summarizing that participants who frequently consume whole milk are less likely to frequently consume skim milk, was positively associated with the latent constructs representing total cholesterol and LDLC as well as systolic and diastolic blood pressure ($p = 0.0006$ and <0.0001, respectively). Multiple multivariable-adjusted regression analyses of exposome factors allowed us to model the influence of the exposome as a whole. In this metadata-rich, prospective cohort of US Veterans, there was evidence of structural relationships between diet, lifestyle, and demographic exposures and subsequent markers of cardiometabolic health. This methodology could be applied to answer a variety of research questions about human health exposures that utilize electronic health record data and can accommodate continuous, ordinal, and binary data derived from questionnaires. Further work to explore the potential utility of including genetic risk scores and time-varying covariates is warranted.

Keywords: exposome; diet; lifestyle; demographics; cardiovascular disease; cholesterol; triglycerides; blood pressure; glycemic control

1. Background

Cardiovascular disease (CVD) is the leading cause of adult mortality globally [1] Strategies aimed at reducing CVD rates involve modulation of markers of CVD risk. In particular, elevated circulating cholesterol and triglyceride levels are associated with higher CVD risk and mortality and are principal targets for risk reduction [2,3]. Further, elevated blood pressure is one of the leading non-communicable disease risk factors [4], and elevated glycated hemoglobin is also a predictor of cardiovascular disease [5–8]. As such, strategies aimed at improving lipid profile, blood pressure, and glycemic control are urgently needed.

The array of external factors an individual is exposed to, referred to as the exposome, represents a complex network of interrelationships within and between different components comprising diet, lifestyle, and demographics. Despite the well-documented ability of individual exposome components, or groups of exposome components, to influence many aspects of human physiology [9–11], surprisingly little is known about how the complex array of exposures as a whole shape the cardiometabolic risk profile. Reductionist approaches, such as single-exposure models, are unable to account for the complex interactions between the many potential exposome components and their effect on physiology [12]. The absence of models that integrate the many different components undermines the capacity of current studies of exposome components to draw robust generalizations. This project therefore aims to model the system of relationships underlying the way in which the exposome, as a whole, shapes the cardiometabolic risk profile. To achieve this aim, we utilized a truly unique dataset generated from an exposome assessment, as well as longitudinally assessed markers of cardiometabolic health in the Million Veteran Program.

2. Methods

2.1. Study Population

Between January 2011 and November 2019, approximately 800,000 Veterans enrolled in the Million Veteran Program (MVP) [13]. The current prospective study draws from the approximately 350,000 Veterans that had enrolled in the MVP between January 2011 and 2016. Of the 297,937 participants that had exposure data, 182,363 participants were excluded if they were using antilipemic, antihypertensive, and/or hypoglycemic medications during either the exposure-assessment or outcome-assessment periods (Supplementary Table S1). A further 79,078 participants were excluded as they had incomplete exposure and/or physiology data. Consequently, the final analysis included 36,496 MVP participants. Consent was obtained in accordance with all VA policies and under the authority of the VA Central IRB [13].

2.2. Exposome Assessment

Variables representing the exposome were observed (measured) using various questionnaires. At enrollment, participants completed a baseline questionnaire in which they reported their date of birth, height, smoking status, gender, ethnicity, and race. Participants also completed a lifestyle questionnaire in which they reported body weight, frequency of light, moderate, and vigorous physical activities both during and outside of work hours, smoking status, and number of hours per week spent in sedentary activities (watching television, DVDs, or videos, using a computer, or playing video games). Body mass index (BMI) was calculated as weight (kg)/height (m) [2].

A food frequency questionnaire (FFQ) was used to assess habitual dietary intake over the year preceding lifestyle questionnaire administration. Participants were asked to describe the average consumption frequency of 67 different foods. "For each food listed, please mark the column indicating how often, on average, you have used the amount specified during the past year". Pre-specified answers were as follows: "Never or less than once a month; 1 to 3 per month; once a week; 2 to 4 per week; 5 to 6 per week; once (1) a day; 2 to 3 per day; 4 to 5 per day; or 6+ per day".

For this study, we included 83 measured (observed) variables to represent the exposome. This is a large number of individual variables, many of which are not independent from one another due to patterns of behaviors amongst participants. In order to make sense of the numerous individual measured (observed) exposome variables, it was imperative that we reduce the dimensionality of the exposome variables to a smaller set of common factors representing groups of covarying measured (observed) variables. The methods to achieve this dimension reduction are detailed in the statistical analysis section.

2.3. Assessment of Physiological Markers of Cardiometabolic Health

A panel of clinicians reviewed lab measurements across all VA locations and adjudicated discrepancies to ensure lab measure consistency. Electronic medical records, adjudicated by two clinicians, were used to ascertain the markers of cardiometabolic health, which included systolic and diastolic blood pressures, as well as the concentration of total cholesterol, low-density lipoprotein cholesterol (LDLC), high density lipoprotein cholesterol (HDLC), triglycerides, HbA1c, and glucose.

This study included the physiological variables that were assessed during the 1–4 years post lifestyle questionnaire administration. For each individual marker of cardiometabolic health, analyses utilized the mean measurement of all of the assessments taken during this period, as well as the maximum recorded measurement during this time period. For each physiology parameter, measurements were excluded if they were taken within 4 days of a previous measurement [14], if they had negative values, or if they had values that were three interquartile ranges from the 25th and 75th percentiles. Data from casually obtained specimens were used in the analysis without regard to fasting status.

2.4. Assessment of Medication Usage

Electronic medical records were used to ascertain antilipemic agent usage during the 1 year preceding exposure assessment and during the outcome assessment period. Two clinicians adjudicated the list of antilipemic agents and included specific medications and doses from the following Generic Adjudication Classes: alirocumab; atorvastatin; atromid; bezafibrate; bezalip retard; cholestyramine; choloxin; clofibrate; colesevelam; colestipol; dextrothyroxine; evolocumab; ezetimibe; ezetimibe/simvastatin; fenofibrate; fenofibric acid; fish oil; gemfibrozil; icosapent ethyl; lomitapide; mevacor; mipomersen; niacinamide; omega-3; omega-3 acid; probucol; rosuvastatin; and statin. The same method of adjudication was used to ascertain usage of antihypertensive medications and combinations, as well as use of hypoglycemic agents.

2.5. Statistical Analysis

Before analysis, participants were randomly divided into one of two groups: a training dataset containing 66.6% of participants ($n = 24,411$) or a validation dataset containing the remaining 33.3% of participants ($n = 12,085$). See Supplementary Figure S1 for details.

The advent of multidimensional cohorts that both assess the exposome and are linked to electronic health records has resulted in large and complex datasets that comprise normally and non-normally distributed data that can be continuous, ordinal, categorical, and binary. There are many techniques available for reducing data dimensionality, which can be broadly categorized into supervised analyses (such as decision trees) and unsupervised analyses. Of the unsupervised analytic approaches, methods such as cluster analysis were not implemented as they would have reduced the number of observations (participants) by grouping them into a smaller set of clusters. Instead, we were aiming to achieve a reduction in the number of variables by grouping them into a smaller set of factors. We achieved this aim through implementation of common exploratory factor analysis. In fact, the use of common exploratory factor analysis in biomedical research is well-tested and effective [15,16], representing an established method whereby "hidden" relationships between the assumed latent variables and the initial observed (measured) variables can be uncovered [17]. To make sense of these data, this study aimed to (i) holistically examine the complex networks of interrelationships that define the exposome and clinical cardiometabolic risk profile; (ii) represent theoretical constructs that are unmeasurable or unmeasured; (iii) include parameter-specific measurement error; and (iv) integrate a number of techniques into one framework, accounting for the range of distributions, units, and relations within and between exposures and cardiometabolic health. Through applying tetrachoric and polychoric, common exploratory factor analysis followed by multivariable-adjusted regression analysis, our methods allowed us to observe the structure of relationships within and between the human exposome and subsequent markers of cardiometabolic health in this large, metadata-rich, prospective cohort of adult US Veterans.

The first stage of the analysis identified the latent constructs (common factors) that best described the shared covariance of the observed (measured) exposures and the physiological variables in the training dataset. These unobservable latent constructs are essentially hypothetical constructs that are used to represent groups of interconnected measured variables [18]. Exploratory factor analyses were used to evaluate the latent constructs and underlying structure because there were multiple hypotheses and extremely limited *a priori* knowledge of how observed (measured) variables might cluster, and because we aimed to develop a measurement model of latent variables, and not to merely identify a linear combination of variables, as is the case in principal component analysis.

For exposure variables, the exploratory factor analysis used tetrachoric and polychoric correlation coefficients between measures of exposure and oblique promax rotation and the varimax prerotation method to make exposure factors more parsimonious [19]. For physiology variables, Spearman's correlation coefficients were estimated and utilized a common exploratory factor analysis using the orthogonal parsimax rotation [20]. Factors were estimated with maximum likelihood methods [20,21]. As a sensitivity analysis, we implemented an alternative method for extracting factors: iterated principal factor analysis. We determined the number of factors to extract through parallel analysis, where each of the eigenvalues of the input correlation matrix was compared against an empirical distribution of eigenvalues. The empirical distribution of eigenvalues was obtained from 10,000 simulations of generated random correlation matrices. We retained all factors with corresponding eigenvalues that exceeded the one-sided critical value ($\alpha = 0.01$) of the empirical eigenvalue distribution [20,22].

The eigenvalues and vectors were then used to compute the standardized (mean = 0, standard deviation = 1) latent constructs in the validation dataset, upon which multivariable-adjusted regression analysis that simultaneously adjusted for all of the exposure latent constructs could be applied to identify the structure of relationships between exposure latent constructs and latent constructs representing cardiometabolic health. These interrelationships were visualized using Cytoscape Version 3.7.2, with the following criteria dictating which associations were displayed: rotated factor pattern (standardized regression coefficients ≥ 0.5); uniqueness (display = all); inter-factor correlations (correlation coefficient ≥ 0.4); and multivariable-adjusted regression coefficients (significance under the Bonferroni criterion).

All analyses were conducted using SAS version 9.4, maintenance release #6.

3. Results

3.1. Participant Characteristics

All of the exposome variables that were included in the models are detailed in Table 1 and Supplementary Table S2. Of the 36,496 MVP participants analyzed, 86% were men, 85% were Caucasians and 11% were African-Americans (Table 1). The mean $\pm$ SD body mass index was 28 ± 5 kg/m^2 (Supplementary Table S2). Markers of cardiometabolic health are presented in Table 2.

Table 1. Key baseline characteristics of all Million Veteran Program participants included in this study.

	Value
DEMOGRAPHICS	
Age (years)	62.40 ± 13.41
Gender (% males)	86
Caucasian (%)	85
Current smoking (number of cigarettes smoked/day)	0.26 ± 0.77
SUPPLEMENT USE	
Omega-3 supplement use (%)	23
Vitamin D supplement use (%)	36
Multivitamin supplement use (%)	54
DIETARY INTAKE	
Dairy	
Whole milk (serves/day)	0.17 ± 0.55
Skim milk (serves/day)	0.51 ± 0.87
Meat	
Red meat in main dish (serves/day)	0.20 ± 0.28
Red meat in mixed dish (serves/day)	0.19 ± 0.26
Hamburgers (serves/day)	0.16 ± 0.24
Processed meat (serves/day)	0.16 ± 0.28
Hot dogs (serves/day)	0.08 ± 0.19
Bacon (serves/day)	0.15 ± 0.29
Sweets and other foods	
French fries (serves/day)	0.12 ± 0.23
Potato chips (serves/day)	0.18 ± 0.32
Cake (serves/day)	0.06 ± 0.15
Home-made pie (serves/day)	0.05 ± 0.13
Ready-made pie (serves/day)	0.05 ± 0.14
Alcoholic beverages	
Liquor (serves/day)	0.15 ± 0.52
Beer (serves/day)	0.31 ± 0.84
Wine (serves/day)	0.17 ± 0.49
Fruit	
Peaches (serves/day)	0.13 ± 0.32
Oranges (serves/day)	0.19 ± 0.37
Apples (serves/day)	0.27 ± 0.43
Vegetables	
Peas (serves/day)	0.14 ± 0.25
Spinach (serves/day)	0.15 ± 0.32
Yams (serves/day)	0.09 ± 0.23
Squash (serves/day)	0.07 ± 0.21
Cooked carrot (serves/day)	0.13 ± 0.25

Table 1. *Cont.*

	Value
Corn (serves/day)	0.15 ± 0.25
String beans (serves/day)	0.17 ± 0.26
Beans (serves/day)	0.18 ± 0.32
Cabbage (serves/day)	0.14 ± 0.28
Broccoli (serves/day)	0.19 ± 0.31
PHYSICAL ACTIVITY	
Vigorous physical activity during leisure time (hours/day)	0.85 ± 1.68
Moderate physical activity during leisure time (hours/day)	1.20 ± 1.92
Vigorous physical activity at home (hours/day)	0.85 ± 1.51
Moderate physical activity at home (hours/day)	1.14 ± 1.75
Vigorous physical activity at work (hours/day)	0.9 ± 1.87
Moderate physical activity at work (hours/day)	1.77 ± 2.53
Light physical activity during leisure time (hours/day)	2.37 ± 2.65
Light physical activity at home (hours/day)	2.93 ± 2.71
Light physical activity at work (hours/day)	2.96 ± 3.19

Number of participants: 36,496. Results are mean ± standard deviation or %, where appropriate.

Table 2. Physiological markers of cardiometabolic health in all included Million Veteran Program participants.

	Mean ± SD
Total cholesterol	
Mean of measurements (mg/dL)	177.40 ± 33.96
Maximum measurement (mg/dL)	187.28 ± 36.98
Low-density lipoprotein cholesterol	
Mean of measurements (mg/dL)	104.57 ± 29.36
Maximum measurement (mg/dL)	113.15 ± 31.90
Triglycerides	
Mean of measurements (mg/dL)	123.48 ± 63.96
Maximum measurement (mg/dL)	145.81 ± 80.31
High-density lipoprotein cholesterol	
Mean of measurements (mg/dL)	49.79 ± 13.94
Maximum measurement (mg/dL)	53.02 ± 15.10
Systolic blood pressure	
Mean of measurements (mmHg)	130.27 ± 12.43
Maximum measurement (mmHg)	145.71 ± 17.93
Diastolic blood pressure	
Mean of measurements (mmHg)	76.72 ± 7.67
Maximum measurement (mmHg)	85.74 ± 10.24
HbA1c	
Mean of measurements (DCCT %)	5.64 ± 0.58
Maximum measurement (DCCT %)	5.74 ± 0.66
Glucose	
Mean of measurements (mg/dL)	101.92 ± 17.70
Maximum measurement (mg/dL)	113.45 ± 26.93

Number of participants: 36,496. Mean of measurements reflects mean value for all measurements, whereas maximum measurement reflects the maximum value for all measurements.

Two-thirds of participants (n = 24,411) were randomly assigned to the training dataset and the remaining one-third (n = 12,085) were randomly assigned to the validation dataset. The mean ± SD age of the participants in the training and validation datasets was identical (62.4 ± 13.4 years).

3.2. Latent Constructs Describing the Exposure Variables in the Training Dataset

Tetrachoric and polychoric, common exploratory factor analysis in the training dataset revealed 19 common factors that explained shared exposure observed (measured) variable covariance. The common factors could be broadly categorized according to the measured (observed) variables they represented (Figure 1 and Supplementary Figure S2). For example, the Common Exposure Factor E1 represented shared covariance in the intakes of many commonly consumed vegetables. Furthermore, Common Exposure Factor E17 had strong positive weighting for intake of whole milk but a strong negative weighting for intake of skim milk, representing the fact that, in this cohort, participants who frequently consumed whole milk were less likely to frequently consume skim milk.

Different types of physical activity were grouped together in three separate Common Exposure Factors. In particular, Common Exposure Factor E6 represented moderate and vigorous physical activity at home and during leisure time, Common Exposure Factor E7 represented moderate and vigorous physical activity at work, and Common Exposure Factor E10 represented light levels of physical activity at home, during leisure and at work.

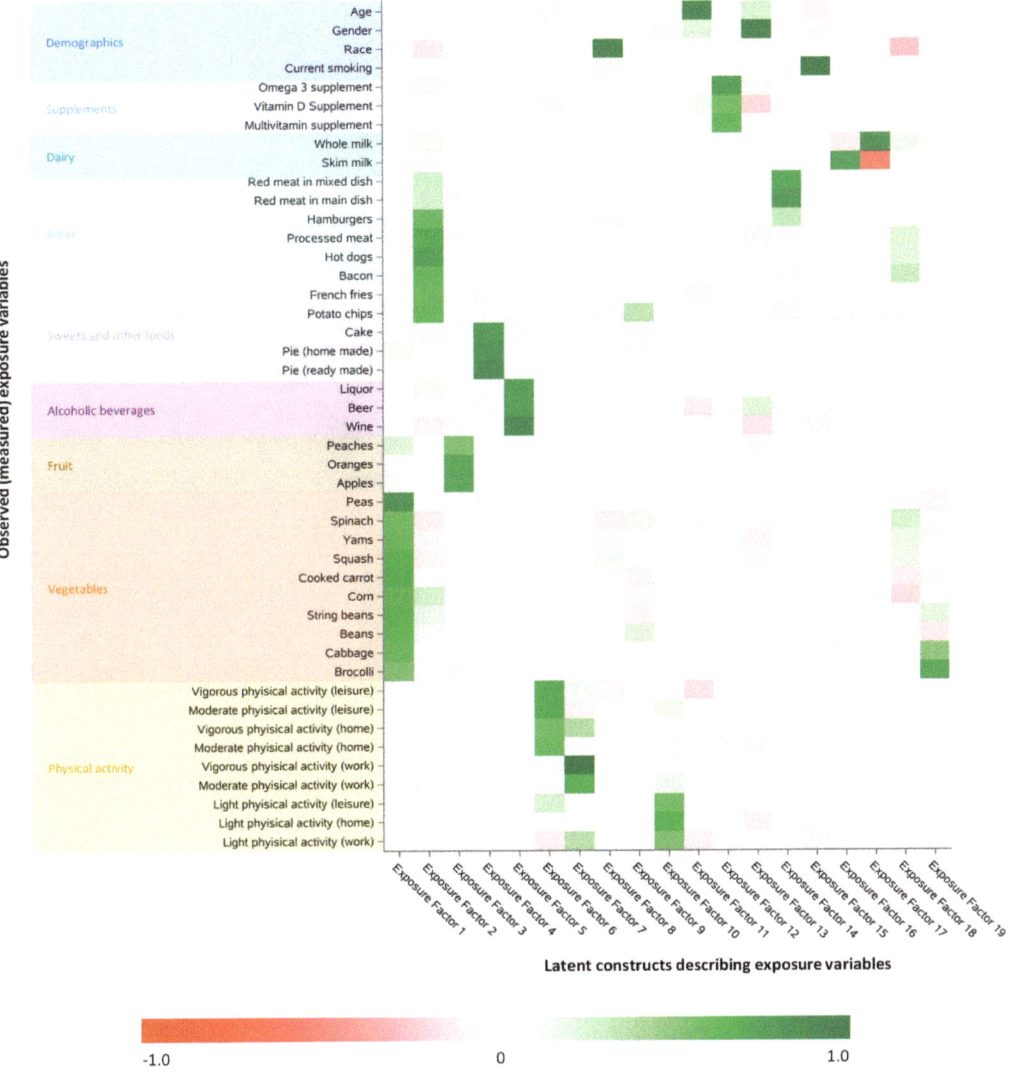

Figure 1. Rotated factor pattern based on tetrachoric and polychoric, common exploratory factor analysis of measured exposure variables in the training dataset; limited to observed (measured) variables that had a standardized regression coefficient ≥ 0.5 for at least one latent construct. These latent constructs (common factors) are those that best described the shared covariance of the observed (measured) exposures in the training, dataset. Number of participants: 24,411. Standardized regression coefficient.

3.3. Latent Constructs Describing the Physiological Variables in the Training Dataset

Common exploratory factor analysis in the training dataset revealed 5 common factors that explained shared physiology variable covariance. These broadly represented (i) total cholesterol and LDLC; (ii) glycemic control; (iii) blood pressure; (iv) HDLC; and (v) triglycerides (Figure 2). Common Physiology Factor P1 had positive loadings for all measures of total cholesterol and LDLC, and Common Physiology Factor P3 had high loadings for all of the measures of blood pressure. In fact, the final model applied similar loadings to mean and maximum values of the observed (measured) variables. As sensitivity analysis, we implemented an iterated principal factor analysis as the extraction method and observed similar factor loadings with the exception of mean and maximum glucose, which went from having a factor loading < 0.5 for Common Physiology Factor P2 in the primary analysis to having a factor loading > 0.5 (0.64 and 0.60, respectively) for Common Physiology Factor P2 in the sensitivity analysis.

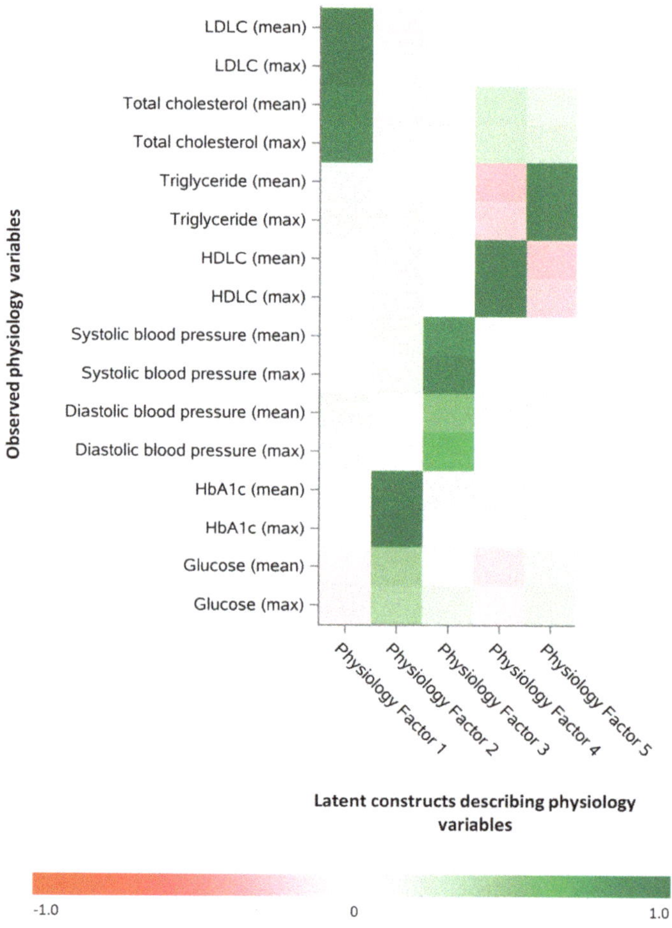

Figure 2. Rotated factor pattern based on common exploratory factor analysis of measured physiology variables in the training dataset. These latent constructs (common factors) are those that best described the shared covariance of the observed (measured) physiology variables in the training dataset.Number of participants: 24,411, "Mean" represents the mean measurement of all assessments. "Max" represents the maximum value of all the assessments. Abbreviations: LDLC: low-density lipoprotein cholesterol; HDLC: high-density lipoprotein cholesterol; HbA1c: glycated hemoglobin. Key:Standardized regression coefficient.

3.4. Relationships between Human Exposures and Physiology in the Validation Dataset

Identification of the 19 Common Exposure Factors was done without knowledge of the physiological variables. Likewise, the creation of the 5 Common Physiology Factors was independent of the exposure variables. In Figure 3a–e, we present the complex patterns underlying the structure of relationships between Common Exposure Factors and Common Physiology Factors that remain after taking into account the non-independence of the assessed exposome. Some Common Exposure Factors had no association with the Common Physiology Factors, whereas others showed a strong association, both inversely and positively. Specifically, even though the Common Exposure Factor describing intake of processed meat and fried potato (E2) was associated with the Common Physiology Factors describing total cholesterol and LDLC (P1), triglycerides (P5), blood pressure (P3), and glycemic control (P2), the Common Exposure Factor representing red meat intake from main and mixed dishes (E14) was not associated with any of the physiological common factors. Similarly, although the Common Exposure Factor describing intake of moderate and vigorous physical activity at home and during leisure (E6) was associated with the Common Physiology Factors describing total cholesterol and LDLC (P1), triglycerides (P5), and HDLC (P4), the Common Exposure Factor representing moderate and vigorous physical activity at work (E7) was not associated with any of the physiological common factors.

When considering individual physiology factors, the fruit latent construct (Common Exposure Factor E3), but not the vegetable latent constructs (Common Exposure Factors E1 and E19) was inversely associated (estimate: -0.03, P: 0.0077) with the latent construct summarizing total cholesterol and LDLC (Common Physiology Factor P1) (Figure 3a). Conversely, the latent construct with a positive weighting for intake of whole milk but a strong negative weighting for intake of skim milk (Common Exposure Factor E17) had a positive association with Common Physiology Factor P1, as well as with Common Physiology Factor P3, the latent construct summarizing measures of blood pressure (Figure 3d). The latent construct describing light levels of physical activity (Common Exposure Factor E10) was inversely associated with the blood pressure latent construct.

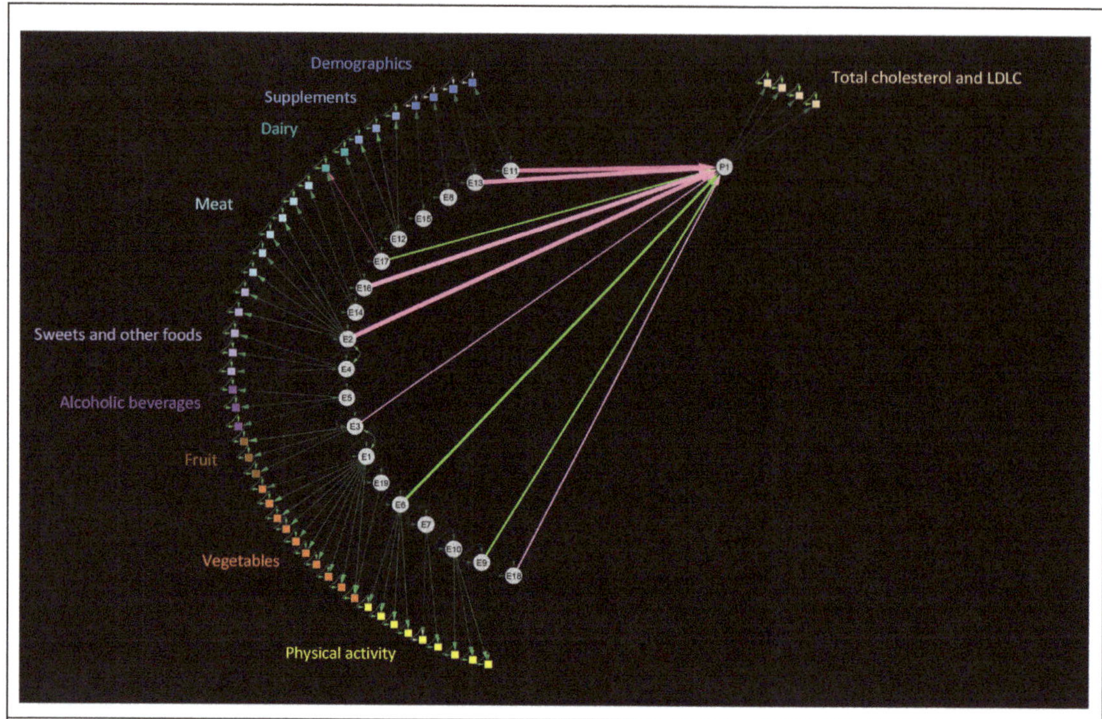

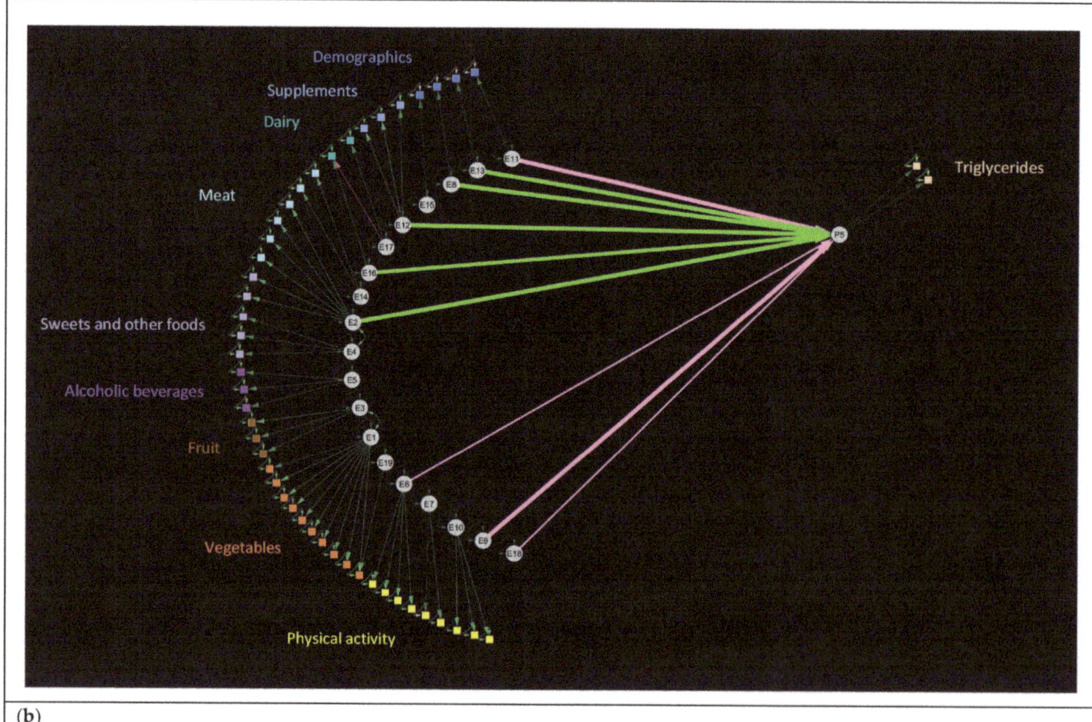

Figure 3. *Cont.*

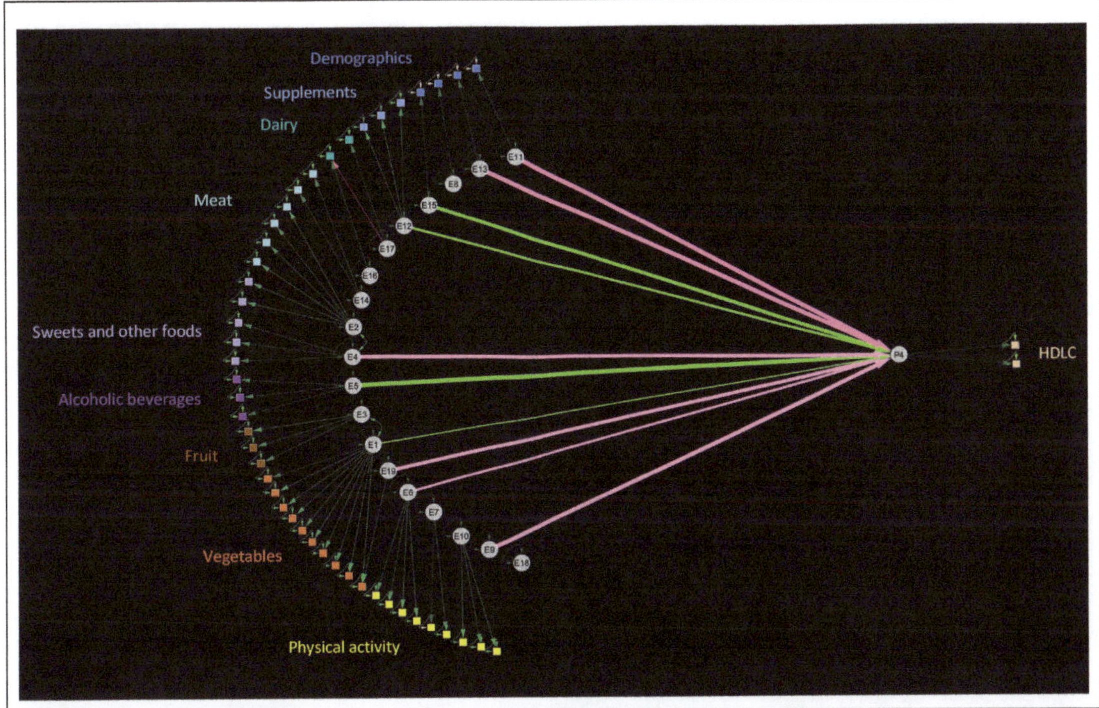

(c)

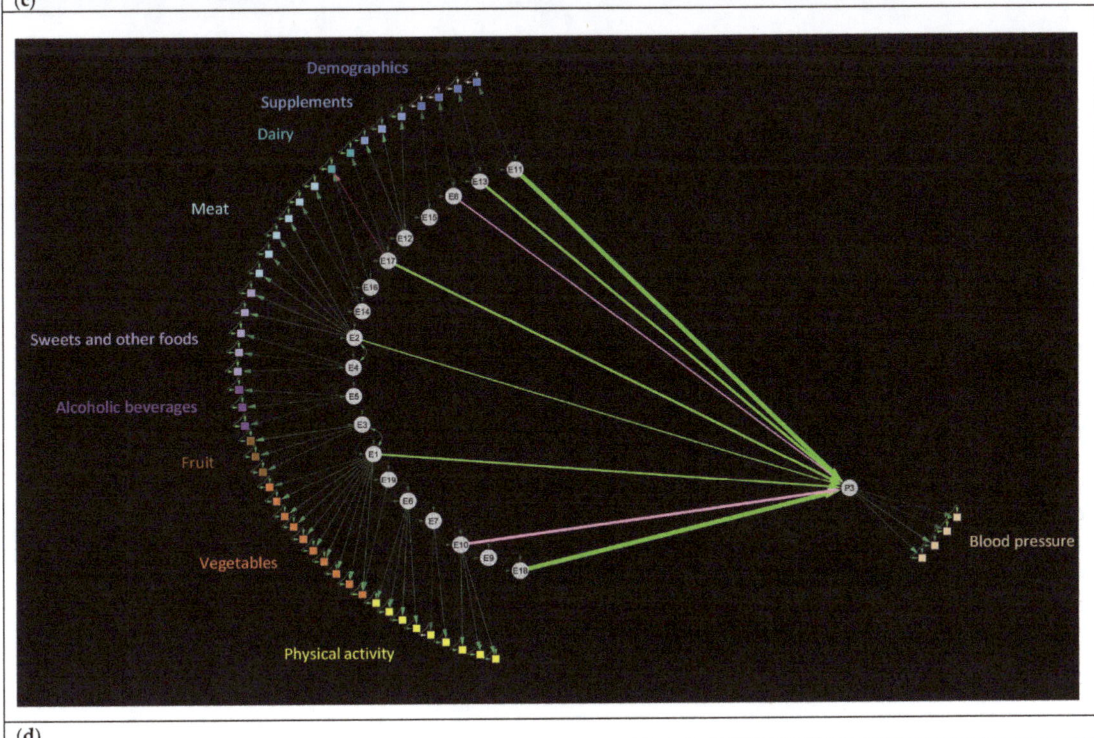

(d)

Figure 3. *Cont.*

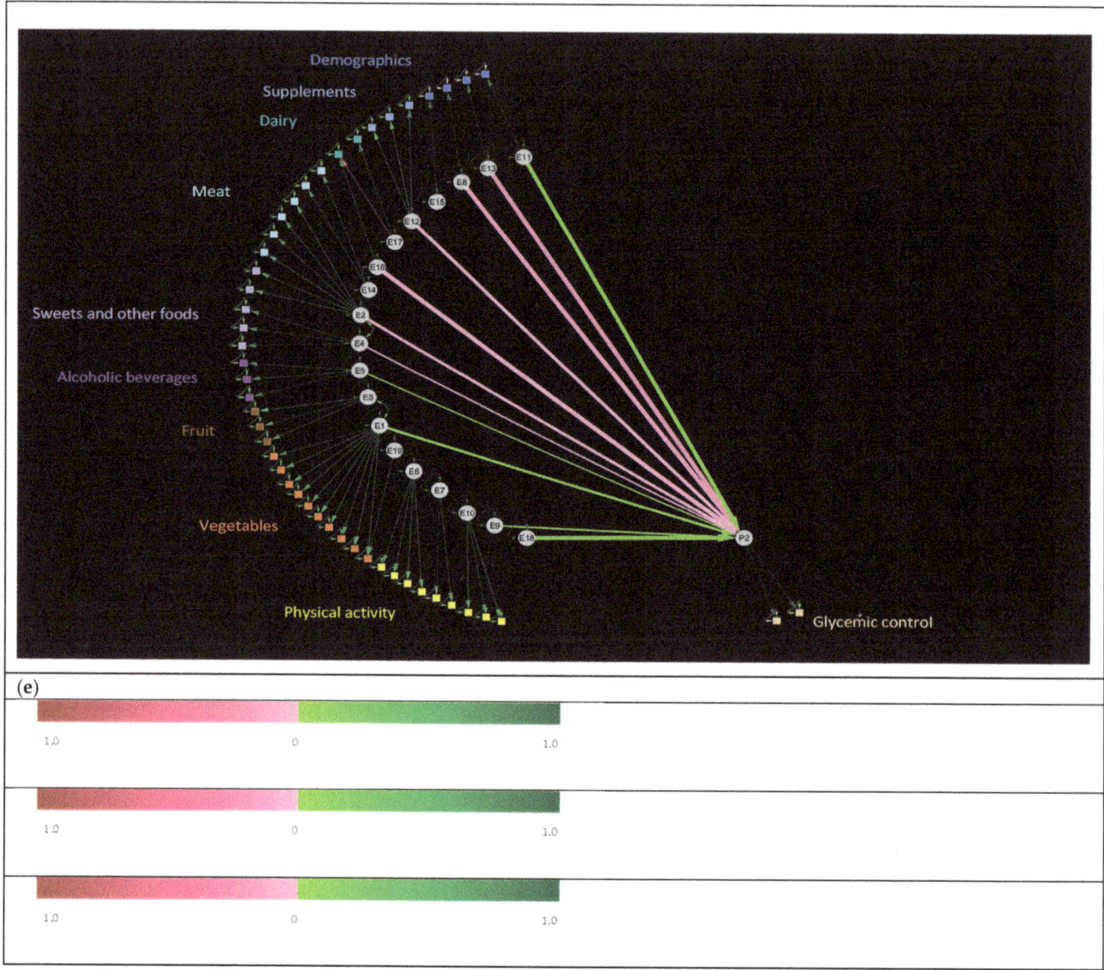

Figure 3. Common exploratory factor analysis (training dataset) and multiple regression analysis (validation dataset) outlining the interrelationships between human exposures and markers of cardiometabolic health. (**a**) Association of latent constructs representing exposure to various dietary and lifestyle common factors with the latent construct that explains the shared covariance in total cholesterol and low-density lipoprotein cholesterol (LDLC) concentrations. (**b**) Association of latent constructs representing exposure to various dietary and lifestyle common factors with the latent construct representing triglyceride concentrations. (**c**) Association of latent constructs representing exposure to various dietary and lifestyle common factors with the latent construct representing high-density lipoprotein cholesterol (HDLC) concentrations. (**d**) Association of latent constructs representing exposure to various dietary and lifestyle common factors with the latent construct representing blood pressure. (**e**) Association of latent constructs representing exposure to various dietary and lifestyle common factors with the latent construct representing glycemic control. Number of participants for the common exploratory factor analysis that was conducted in the training dataset: n = 24,411. Number of participants for the multivariable-adjusted regression analysis that was conducted in the validation dataset: n = 12,085. Observed (measured) exposure and physiology variables are presented in the order in which they appear in Figures 1 and 2, respectively. Criteria for displaying measured (observed) variables: rotated factor pattern: Standardized regression coefficient ≥ 0.5. Criteria for displaying association lines: uniqueness (display all); inter-factor correlations (correlation coefficient ≥ 0.4); and multivariable, adjusted regression coefficients (*p* value significant using the Bonferroni threshold). For multivariable-adjusted regression coefficients, the line thickness represents the value of the -log10(*p* value), range: 2.11, 9.05.

4. Discussion

In this prospective cohort study of U.S. male and female Veterans, we reported an association between the exposome and markers of cardiometabolic health. Specifically, using factors identified in a training dataset, multiple multivariable-adjusted regression analyses revealed significant positive and inverse associations between exposure latent constructs and latent constructs describing observed (measured) physiology variables when applied to a separate validation dataset containing different participants. This provided us with critical insights and observations that represent steps forward in enhancing our understanding of how the exposome, as a holistic entity, shapes human physiology.

We employed common exploratory factor analysis to reveal the structure of interrelationships between individual exposures and physiology variables in a way that substantially advances our understanding of how observed (measured) exposome variables relate to the cardiometabolic risk profile. For example, a Common Exposure Factor was created to reflect the close relationship in study participants between high levels of moderate and vigorous physical activity at home and high levels of moderate and vigorous physical activity during leisure time. This relationship was not strongly correlated with levels of moderate and vigorous physical activity at work, which was represented by a different Common Exposure Factor. This suggests that the amount of moderate to vigorous physical activity participants perform at work did not covary with the amount of moderate to vigorous physical activity performed during leisure and at home [23]. By unveiling "hidden" relationships between the latent constructs and the observed (measured) variables they represent that matched our understanding of biology and variable representation, the utility of common exploratory factor analysis for both questionnaire-derived assessments of exposome and electronic medical record-derived assessments of cardiometabolic health was highlighted. However, it is unclear what the causal implications for these relationships are.

Very few studies have attempted to determine the influence of the exposome as a whole on cardiometabolic risk (as determined through electronic medical records). Modelling the system of relationships underlying the way in which the exposome, as a whole, shaped the cardiometabolic risk profile was therefore an important aim of our investigation. In addition to revealing the structure of the exposome and the structure of physiology variables, this study also revealed the structure of relationships between the exposome and cardiometabolic risk profile through multiple regression of latent constructs. An example of this was the creation of a latent construct in the training dataset that represented the reciprocal relationship between consumption of whole and skim milk. In other words, any associations of whole milk with cardiometabolic disease risk could not be separated from the effects of skim milk and should not be interpreted in isolation. When applied to separate validation datasets, this milk-based latent construct was positively associated with the latent constructs representing total cholesterol and LDLC as well as systolic and diastolic blood pressure. This observation is supported by randomized controlled trials directly comparing non-fermented whole milk to non-fermented skim milk that suggest adverse effects of whole milk, compared to skim milk, on total cholesterol and LDLC [24,25]. Further, skim but not whole milk has been shown to exhibit antihypertensive properties [26,27]. It is not yet clear whether dairy fat intake increases cardiovascular disease risk [28]. Despite this, results of our exposome analysis support the 2006 American Heart Association to Diet and Lifestyle Recommendations and the 2015–2020 Dietary Guidelines for Americans, which both encourage adults to select milk products that are either fat-free or low in fat rather than whole milk products [29,30]. The finding that individual components of the exposome are both numerically and biologically intertwined highlights the urgent need to implement analytic techniques that holistically examine the complex networks of interrelationships within and between observed (measured) variables. This was achieved through the representation of unmeasurable or unmeasured theoretical constructs as well as parameter-specific measurement error in order to draw robust generalizations regarding the complex interactions between the many exposome components and human physiology.

The use of latent factors to describe interrelationships between individual exposome and physiology components was able to shed light on hypothesized relationships. For example, the factor describing fruit consumption was inversely associated with the factor describing concentrations of total cholesterol and LDLC. This is supported by (i) our previous findings from the National Heart, Lung, and Blood Institute Family Heart Study, which found that consumption of fruit and vegetables was inversely related to LDLC in both men and women [31] and (ii) results from other cohort studies and randomized controlled trials [32,33]. Although the benefits of fruit consumption on cholesterol concentrations are not conclusive, with some studies showing no benefit of fruit consumption [34], the high fiber content of fruit has been attributed to its cholesterol-lowering capacity [35,36]. In this study, peaches, oranges, and apples contributed to the fruit factor. Apples have been shown to increase the clearance of plasma cholesterol by enhancing the fecal excretion of bile acids and cholesterol [37], and the peel of peaches has been shown to lower total cholesterol and LDLC in rats fed a high-sucrose diet. Further, the polyphenols in apples have been shown to have beneficial effects on cholesterol metabolism [38–41], as too have the pectins of apples and oranges [42]. A randomized controlled trial testing the effect of the combination of peaches, oranges, and apples on serum lipid profile is needed in order to ascertain causality of this observed association. It is important to note that there were cases where hypothesized relationships were not observed. For example, despite vegetables being a rich source of dietary fiber and higher consumption of vegetables being associated with lower risk of all-cause mortality and cardiovascular mortality [43], the vegetable consumption factors in this study were not significantly associated with the factor describing total cholesterol and LDLC. The absence of confirmatory findings regarding vegetables in this study may be explained by the absence of data on intake of nutrients, such as fiber, which can summarize contributions from many different foods that are biologically important. Another reason may be that the measurement error may be lower in fruits as opposed to vegetables. However, another interpretation may be that, after controlling for other exposome components, vegetables are not associated with total cholesterol and LDLC concentrations in this cohort. Further studies using longitudinal data are needed to confirm these findings.

Although the methods implemented were well-tested and effective, it is important to note that diet was self-reported, health outcomes were captured through electronic medical records, there was a lack of data on medication adherence, and there were a limited number of women and non-whites in this U.S. Veteran cohort. Additionally, causality of observed relationships could not be established due to the observational nature of the study. Nevertheless, it is important to note that the exposome was measured at least one year prior to any of the physiologic variables being assessed, which, although not ruling it out, does reduce the likelihood and impact of reverse causation. An additional factor to consider when interpreting the results is the possibility of false-positive findings, which was reduced through implementation of the conservative Bonferroni correction [44]. Furthermore, although residual or unmeasured confounders cannot be ruled out, the common exploratory methods implemented in this study do aim to represent unmeasured and/or immeasurable variables through the creation of latent constructs. This analytic approach also enabled us to model the measurement error inherent when using self-reported exposome assessments as well as collations from electronic medical records, even when there are some exposome variables, such as environmental variables, that are not measured directly. By conducting the analysis in both a training and a validation dataset, we were able to demonstrate the utility of our analytic strategy for use in the increasingly prevalent type of cohort that has extensive questionnaire-based assessments of the exposome as well as markers of human physiology derived from electronic medical records. However, further replication in separate datasets is warranted.

It is becoming increasingly recognized that studies of the complete exposome are more biologically representative than fragmented models based on subsets of factors. There is no more clear example of this than the position of the Academy of Nutrition and Dietetics, which plainly states that the "total diet or overall pattern of food eaten is the most important focus of healthy eating" [45]. In recognition of this, as opposed to focusing on individual nutrient recommendations, the Dietary Guidelines for Americans highlight key elements of healthy eating patterns [30]. Some patterns, such as the Mediterranean Dietary Pattern, are based on a priori knowledge of how individual dietary components influence human health, and are often represented by a pattern score that reflects relative adherence to the dietary pattern, as is the case for the Healthy Eating Index [46,47]. Although hypothesis-driven, there is no general consensus in the scientific or clinical community as to what is the ideal dietary pattern for optimal health [48]. Importantly, these dietary patterns typically reflect only a select group of dietary components, and not necessarily the diet as a whole [46,47]. Given that the aim of the present paper was to identify the importance of the entire exposome in influencing cardiometabolic health, we chose to adopt a data-driven approach which allowed us to identify existing patterns in the population, and how individual foods, lifestyle factors, and demographic features related to each other at a population level. In this study, the measured exposome variables were represented by 19 common factors that were created independently from the physiological variables. We observed heterogeneous patterns of association of exposome constructs with each of the physiological constructs, which represented measured biomarkers that are important indicators of cardiometabolic health. As such, even though the exposome overall contributed to cardiometabolic health, each facet of the exposome had differential implications for different aspects of cardiometabolic health. It is evident that the overall complex exposome that individuals are exposed to needs to be studied more in order to more fully understand what is contributing to cardiometabolic risk profiles in communities of free-living individuals. To be more comprehensive, a logical extension to this current work would be to incorporate more environmental exposome variables, such as air pollution and access to green space, into the current models.

In conclusion, we observed a complex pattern of associations between the exposome and markers of cardiometabolic health. Given that we are increasingly recognizing the potential of the exposome as a whole to have far-reaching health implications beyond the effects associated with the sum of its parts, it is more important than ever that we make available analytic tools and approaches that are capable of dealing with this directly. It should be noted that the analytic strategy implemented in this paper could be applied to address a range of research questions that utilize data from questionnaire and electronic health record data, thus bringing us one step closer to understanding how the exposome, as a whole, impacts human health.

Supplementary Materials: The following are available online at https://www.mdpi.com/article/10.3390/nu13041364/s1, Table S1: Number of participants excluded based on use of antilipemic, antihypertensive and/or hypoglycemic medications during either the exposure-assessment or outcome-assessment periods, Table S2: Additional baseline characteristics of all Million Veterans Program participants included in this study, Figure S1: Schematic overview of the training and validation datasets, Figure S2: Rotated factor pattern based on tetrachoric and polychoric, common exploratory factor analysis of measured exposure variables in the training dataset; limited to observed (measured) variables that did not have a standardized regression coefficient ≥ 0.5 for at least one latent construct.

Author Contributions: K.L.I. conducted analyses and wrote the manuscript. X.-M.T.N., K.C., J.M.G. and L.D. collected data. All authors critically reviewed the manuscript for content and clarity. K.L.I., X.-M.T.N., D.P., G.B.R., D.K.T., R.S., Y.-L.H., R.L., P.W.F.W., K.C., J.M.G., F.B.H., W.C.W. and L.D. All authors have read and agreed to the published version of the manuscript.

Funding: This research is based on data from the Million Veteran Program supported by the MVP001 and MVP#000 awards from the Department of Veterans Affairs. This research was also supported by the VA Merit Award I01 BX003340-01. Support for VA/CMS data was provided by the Department of Veterans Affairs, VA Health Services Research and Development Service, VA Information Resource Center (Project Numbers SDR 02-237 and 98-004). This research is based on data from the VA Million Veteran Program supported by award MVP#000 from the Department of Veterans

Affairs. This publication does not represent the views of the Department of Veterans Affairs or the U.S. government.

Institutional Review Board Statement: The study was conducted according to the guidelines of the Declaration of Helsinki and approved by the VA Central IRB [13] (protocol code MVP001 approved in 2010).

Informed Consent Statement: Written informed consent has been obtained from the participants in accordance with all VA policies and under the authority of the VA Central IRB [13].

Data Availability Statement: Data described in the article, code book, and analytic code will not be made available to other researchers for purposes of reproducing the results or replicating the procedure, in order to comply with current VA privacy regulations pursuant to the US Department of Veterans Administration policies on compliance with the confidentiality of US veterans' data.

Acknowledgments: The authors thank the members of the Million Veteran Program Core, those who have contributed to the Million Veteran Program, and especially the Veteran participants for their generous contributions. This work was supported using resources and facilities of the Department of Veterans Affairs (VA) Informatics and Computing Infrastructure (VINCI), VA HSR RES 13-457. More information could be found in Appendix A.

Conflicts of Interest: No authors have any relevant conflict of interest.

Appendix A

MVP Executive Committee

- Co-Chair: J. Michael Gaziano, M.D., M.P.H.
  - VA Boston Healthcare System, 150 S. Huntington Avenue, Boston, MA 02130, USA
- Co-Chair: Sumitra Muralidhar, Ph.D.
  - US Department of Veterans Affairs, 810 Vermont Avenue NW, Washington, DC 20420, USA
- Rachel Ramoni, D.M.D., Sc.D., Chief VA Research and Development Officer
  - US Department of Veterans Affairs, 810 Vermont Avenue NW, Washington, DC 20420, USA
- Jean Beckham, Ph.D.
  - Durham VA Medical Center, 508 Fulton Street, Durham, NC 27705, USA
- Kyong-Mi Chang, M.D.
  - Philadelphia VA Medical Center, 3900 Woodland Avenue, Philadelphia, PA 19104, USA
- Christopher J. O'Donnell, M.D., M.P.H.
  - VA Boston Healthcare System, 150 S. Huntington Avenue, Boston, MA 02130, USA
- Philip S. Tsao, Ph.D.
  - VA Palo Alto Health Care System, 3801 Miranda Avenue, Palo Alto, CA 94304, USA
- James Breeling, M.D., Ex-Officio
  - US Department of Veterans Affairs, 810 Vermont Avenue NW, Washington, DC 20420, USA
- Grant Huang, Ph.D., Ex-Officio
  - US Department of Veterans Affairs, 810 Vermont Avenue NW, Washington, DC 20420, USA
- Juan P. Casas, M.D., Ph.D., Ex-Officio
  - VA Boston Healthcare System, 150 S. Huntington Avenue, Boston, MA 02130, USA

MVP Program Office

- Sumitra Muralidhar, Ph.D.
  - o US Department of Veterans Affairs, 810 Vermont Avenue NW, Washington, DC 20420, USA
- Jennifer Moser, Ph.D.
  - o US Department of Veterans Affairs, 810 Vermont Avenue NW, Washington, DC 20420, USA

MVP Recruitment/Enrollment

- Recruitment/Enrollment Director/Deputy Director, Boston—Stacey B. Whitbourne, Ph.D.; Jessica V. Brewer, M.P.H.
  - VA Boston Healthcare System, 150 S. Huntington Avenue, Boston, MA 02130, USA
- MVP Coordinating Centers
  - Clinical Epidemiology Research Center (CERC), West Haven—Mihaela Aslan, Ph.D.
  - West Haven VA Medical Center, 950 Campbell Avenue, West Haven, CT 06516, USA
  - Cooperative Studies Program Clinical Research Pharmacy Coordinating Center, Albuquerque—Todd Connor, Pharm.D.; Dean P. Argyres, B.S., M.S.
  - New Mexico VA Health Care System, 1501 San Pedro Drive SE, Albuquerque, NM 87108, USA
  - Genomics Coordinating Center, Palo Alto—Philip S. Tsao, Ph.D.
  - VA Palo Alto Health Care System, 3801 Miranda Avenue, Palo Alto, CA 94304, USA
  - MVP Boston Coordinating Center, Boston—J. Michael Gaziano, M.D., M.P.H.
  - VA Boston Healthcare System, 150 S. Huntington Avenue, Boston, MA 02130, USA
  - MVP Information Center, Canandaigua—Brady Stephens, M.S.
  - Canandaigua VA Medical Center, 400 Fort Hill Avenue, Canandaigua, NY 14424, USA
- VA Central Biorepository, Boston—Mary T. Brophy M.D., M.P.H.; Donald E. Humphries, Ph.D.; Luis E. Selva, Ph.D.
  - VA Boston Healthcare System, 150 S. Huntington Avenue, Boston, MA 02130, USA
- MVP Informatics, Boston—Nhan Do, M.D.; Shahpoor (Alex) Shayan, M.S.
  - VA Boston Healthcare System, 150 S. Huntington Avenue, Boston, MA 02130, USA
- MVP Data Operations/Analytics, Boston—Kelly Cho, M.P.H., Ph.D.
  - VA Boston Healthcare System, 150 S. Huntington Avenue, Boston, MA 02130, USA
- Director of Regulatory Affairs—Lori Churby, B.S.
  - VA Palo Alto Health Care System, 3801 Miranda Avenue, Palo Alto, CA 94304, USA

MVP Science

- Science Operations—Christopher J. O'Donnell, M.D., M.P.H.
- VA Boston Healthcare System, 150 S. Huntington Avenue, Boston, MA 02130, USA
- Genomics Core—Christopher J. O'Donnell, M.D., M.P.H.; Saiju Pyarajan Ph.D.
- VA Boston Healthcare System, 150 S. Huntington Avenue, Boston, MA 02130, USA
- Philip S. Tsao, Ph.D.
- VA Palo Alto Health Care System, 3801 Miranda Avenue, Palo Alto, CA 94304, USA
- Data Core—Kelly Cho, M.P.H, Ph.D.
- VA Boston Healthcare System, 150 S. Huntington Avenue, Boston, MA 02130, USA
- VA Informatics and Computing Infrastructure (VINCI)—Scott L. DuVall, Ph.D.
- VA Salt Lake City Health Care System, 500 Foothill Drive, Salt Lake City, UT 84148, USA
- Data and Computational Sciences—Saiju Pyarajan, Ph.D.

- VA Boston Healthcare System, 150 S. Huntington Avenue, Boston, MA 02130, USA
- Statistical Genetics—Elizabeth Hauser, Ph.D.
- Durham VA Medical Center, 508 Fulton Street, Durham, NC 27705, USA
- Yan Sun, Ph.D.
- Atlanta VA Medical Center, 1670 Clairmont Road, Decatur, GA 30033, USA
- Hongyu Zhao, Ph.D.
- West Haven VA Medical Center, 950 Campbell Avenue, West Haven, CT 06516, USA

Current MVP Local Site Investigators

- Atlanta VA Medical Center (Peter Wilson, M.D.)
  - 1670 Clairmont Road, Decatur, GA 30033, USA
- Bay Pines VA Healthcare System (Rachel McArdle, Ph.D.)
  - 10,000 Bay Pines Blvd Bay Pines, FL 33744, USA
- Birmingham VA Medical Center (Louis Dellitalia, M.D.)
  - 700 S. 19th Street, Birmingham, AL 35233, USA
- Central Western Massachusetts Healthcare System (Kristin Mattocks, Ph.D., M.P.H.)
  - 421 North Main Street, Leeds, MA 01053, USA
- Cincinnati VA Medical Center (John Harley, M.D., Ph.D.)
  - 3200 Vine Street, Cincinnati, OH 45220, USA
- Clement J. Zablocki VA Medical Center (Jeffrey Whittle, M.D., M.P.H.)
  - 5000 West National Avenue, Milwaukee, WI 53295, USA
- VA Northeast Ohio Healthcare System (Frank Jacono, M.D.)
  - 10701 East Boulevard, Cleveland, OH 44106, USA
- Durham VA Medical Center (Jean Beckham, Ph.D.)
  - 508 Fulton Street, Durham, NC 27705, USA
- Edith Nourse Rogers Memorial Veterans Hospital (John Wells., Ph.D.)
  - 200 Springs Road, Bedford, MA 01730, USA
- Edward Hines, Jr. VA Medical Center (Salvador Gutierrez, M.D.)
  - 5000 South 5th Avenue, Hines, IL 60141, USA
- Veterans Health Care System of the Ozarks (Gretchen Gibson, D.D.S., M.P.H.)
  - 1100 North College Avenue, Fayetteville, AR 72703, USA
- Fargo VA Health Care System (Kimberly Hammer, Ph.D.)
  - 2101 N. Elm, Fargo, ND 58102, USA
- VA Health Care Upstate New York (Laurence Kaminsky, Ph.D.)
  - 113 Holland Avenue, Albany, NY 12208, USA
- New Mexico VA Health Care System (Gerardo Villareal, M.D.)
  - 1501 San Pedro Drive, S.E. Albuquerque, NM 87108, USA
- VA Boston Healthcare System (Scott Kinlay, M.B.B.S., Ph.D.)
  - 150 S. Huntington Avenue, Boston, MA 02130, USA
- VA Western New York Healthcare System (Junzhe Xu, M.D.)
  - 3495 Bailey Avenue, Buffalo, NY 14215-1199, USA
- Ralph H. Johnson VA Medical Center (Mark Hamner, M.D.)
  - 109 Bee Street, Mental Health Research, Charleston, SC 29401
- Columbia VA Health Care System (Roy Mathew, M.D.)
  - 6439 Garners Ferry Road, Columbia, SC 29209, USA
- VA North Texas Health Care System (Sujata Bhushan, M.D.)

- o   4500 S. Lancaster Road, Dallas, TX 75216, USA
- Hampton VA Medical Center (Pran Iruvanti, D.O., Ph.D.)
  - o   100 Emancipation Drive, Hampton, VA 23667, USA
- Richmond VA Medical Center (Michael Godschalk, M.D.)
  - o   1201 Broad Rock Blvd., Richmond, VA 23249, USA
- Iowa City VA Health Care System (Zuhair Ballas, M.D.)
  - o   601 Highway 6 West, Iowa City, IA 52246-2208
- Eastern Oklahoma VA Health Care System (Douglas Ivins, M.D.)
  - o   1011 Honor Heights Drive, Muskogee, OK 74401, USA
- James A. Haley Veterans' Hospital (Stephen Mastorides, M.D.)
  - o   13000 Bruce B. Downs Blvd, Tampa, FL 33612, USA
- James H. Quillen VA Medical Center (Jonathan Moorman, M.D., Ph.D.)
  - o   Corner of Lamont & Veterans Way, Mountain Home, TN 37684, USA
- John D. Dingell VA Medical Center (Saib Gappy, M.D.)
  - o   4646 John R Street, Detroit, MI 48201, USA
- Louisville VA Medical Center (Jon Klein, M.D., Ph.D.)
  - o   800 Zorn Avenue, Louisville, KY 40206, USA
- Manchester VA Medical Center (Nora Ratcliffe, M.D.)
  - o   718 Smyth Road, Manchester, NH 03104, USA
- Miami VA Health Care System (Hermes Florez, M.D., Ph.D.)
  - o   1201 NW 16th Street, 11 GRC, Miami, FL 33125, USA
- Michael E. DeBakey VA Medical Center (Olaoluwa Okusaga, M.D.)
  - o   2002 Holcombe Blvd, Houston, TX 77030, USA
- Minneapolis VA Health Care System (Maureen Murdoch, M.D., M.P.H.)
  - o   One Veterans Drive, Minneapolis, MN 55417, USA
- N. FL/S. GA Veterans Health System (Peruvemba Sriram, M.D.)
  - o   1601 SW Archer Road, Gainesville, FL 32608, USA
- Northport VA Medical Center (Shing Shing Yeh, Ph.D., M.D.)
  - o   79 Middleville Road, Northport, NY 11768, USA
- Overton Brooks VA Medical Center (Neeraj Tandon, M.D.)
  - o   510 East Stoner Ave, Shreveport, LA 71101, USA
- Philadelphia VA Medical Center (Darshana Jhala, M.D.)
  - o   3900 Woodland Avenue, Philadelphia, PA 19104, USA
- Phoenix VA Health Care System (Samuel Aguayo, M.D.)
  - o   650 E. Indian School Road, Phoenix, AZ 85012, USA
- Portland VA Medical Center (David Cohen, M.D.)
  - o   3710 SW U.S. Veterans Hospital Road, Portland, OR 97239
- Providence VA Medical Center (Satish Sharma, M.D.)
  - o   830 Chalkstone Avenue, Providence, RI 02908, USA
- Richard Roudebush VA Medical Center (Suthat Liangpunsakul, M.D., M.P.H.)
  - o   1481 West 10th Street, Indianapolis, IN 46202, USA
- Salem VA Medical Center (Kris Ann Oursler, M.D.)
  - o   1970 Roanoke Blvd, Salem, VA 24153, USA
- San Francisco VA Health Care System (Mary Whooley, M.D.)

- 4150 Clement Street, San Francisco, CA 94121, USA
- South Texas Veterans Health Care System (Sunil Ahuja, M.D.)
  - 7400 Merton Minter Boulevard, San Antonio, TX 78229, USA
- Southeast Louisiana Veterans Health Care System (Joseph Constans, Ph.D.)
  - 2400 Canal Street, New Orleans, LA 70119, USA
- Southern Arizona VA Health Care System (Paul Meyer, M.D., Ph.D.)
  - 3601 S 6th Avenue, Tucson, AZ 85723, USA
- Sioux Falls VA Health Care System (Jennifer Greco, M.D.)
  - 2501 W 22nd Street, Sioux Falls, SD 57105, USA
- St. Louis VA Health Care System (Michael Rauchman, M.D.)
  - 915 North Grand Blvd, St. Louis, MO 63106, USA
- Syracuse VA Medical Center (Richard Servatius, Ph.D.)
  - 800 Irving Avenue, Syracuse, NY 13210, USA
- VA Eastern Kansas Health Care System (Melinda Gaddy, Ph.D.)
  - 4101 S 4th Street Trafficway, Leavenworth, KS 66048, USA
- VA Greater Los Angeles Health Care System (Agnes Wallbom, M.D., M.S.)
  - 11301 Wilshire Blvd, Los Angeles, CA 90073, USA
- VA Long Beach Healthcare System (Timothy Morgan, M.D.)
  - 5901 East 7th Street Long Beach, CA 90822, USA
- VA Maine Healthcare System (Todd Stapley, D.O.)
  - 1 VA Center, Augusta, ME 04330, USA
- VA New York Harbor Healthcare System (Scott Sherman, M.D., M.P.H.)
  - 423 East 23rd Street, New York, NY 10010, USA
- VA Pacific Islands Health Care System (George Ross, M.D.)
  - 459 Patterson Rd, Honolulu, HI 96819, USA
- VA Palo Alto Health Care System (Philip Tsao, Ph.D.)
  - 3801 Miranda Avenue, Palo Alto, CA 94304-1290, USA
- VA Pittsburgh Health Care System (Patrick Strollo, Jr., M.D.)
  - University Drive, Pittsburgh, PA 15240, USA
- VA Puget Sound Health Care System (Edward Boyko, M.D.)
  - 1660 S. Columbian Way, Seattle, WA 98108-1597, USA
- VA Salt Lake City Health Care System (Laurence Meyer, M.D., Ph.D.)
  - 500 Foothill Drive, Salt Lake City, UT 84148, USA
- VA San Diego Healthcare System (Samir Gupta, M.D., M.S.C.S.)
  - 3350 La Jolla Village Drive, San Diego, CA 92161, USA
- VA Sierra Nevada Health Care System (Mostaqul Huq, Pharm.D., Ph.D.)
  - 975 Kirman Avenue, Reno, NV 89502, USA
- VA Southern Nevada Healthcare System (Joseph Fayad, M.D.)
  - 6900 North Pecos Road, North Las Vegas, NV 89086, USA
- VA Tennessee Valley Healthcare System (Adriana Hung, M.D., M.P.H.)
  - 1310 24th Avenue, South Nashville, TN 37212, USA
- Washington DC VA Medical Center (Jack Lichy, M.D., Ph.D.)
  - 50 Irving St, Washington, D. C. 20422, USA
- W.G. (Bill) Hefner VA Medical Center (Robin Hurley, M.D.)

    o   1601 Brenner Ave, Salisbury, NC 28144, USA

-    White River Junction VA Medical Center (Brooks Robey, M.D.)

    o   163 Veterans Drive, White River Junction, VT 05009, USA

-    William S. Middleton Memorial Veterans Hospital (Robert Striker, M.D., Ph.D.)

    o   2500 Overlook Terrace, Madison, WI 53705, USA

References

1. Arnett, D.K.; Blumenthal, R.S.; Albert, M.A.; Buroker, A.B.; Goldberger, Z.D.; Hahn, E.J.; Himmelfarb, C.D.; Khera, A.; Lloyd-Jones, D.; McEvoy, J.W.; et al. 2019 ACC/AHA guideline on the primary prevention of cardiovascular disease: A report of the American College of Cardiology/American Heart Association Task Force on Clinical Practice Guidelines. *J. Am. Coll. Cardiol.* **2019**, *74*, e177–e232. [CrossRef] [PubMed]
2. Expert Panel on Detection Evaluation and Treatment of High Blood Cholesterol in Adults. Executive summary of the third report of the National Cholesterol Education Program (NCEP) Expert Panel on Detection, Evaluation, and Treatment of High Blood Cholesterol in Adults (Adult Treatment Panel III). *J. Am. Med. Assoc.* **2001**, *285*, 2486–2497. [CrossRef] [PubMed]
3. Liu, J.; Zeng, F.-F.; Liu, Z.-M.; Zhang, C.-X.; Ling, W.-H.; Chen, Y.-M. Effects of blood triglycerides on cardiovascular and all-cause mortality: A systematic review and meta-analysis of 61 prospective studies. *Lipids Health Dis.* **2013**, *12*, 159. [CrossRef] [PubMed]
4. World Health Organisation. *Global Status Report on Noncommunicable Diseases 2010: Description of the Global Burden of NCDs, Their Risk Factors and Determinants*; World Health Organisation: Geneva, Switzerland, 2011.
5. Rijkelijkhuizen, J.; Alssema, M.; Nijpels, G.; Stehouwer, C.; Heine, R.; Dekker, J. HbA1c is an independent predictor of non-fatal cardiovascular disease in a Caucasian population without diabetes: A 10-year follow-up of the Hoorn Study. *Eur. J. Prev. Cardiol.* **2012**, *19*, 23–31.
6. Singer, D.E.; Nathan, D.M.; Anderson, K.M.; Wilson, P.W.; Evans, J.C. Association of HbA1c with prevalent cardiovascular disease in the original cohort of the Framingham Heart Study. *Diabetes* **1992**, *41*, 202–208. [CrossRef] [PubMed]
7. Smith, S.A. Higher "normal" glycated hemoglobin levels were associated with increased risk for diabetes, CVD, stroke, and mortality in adults. *Ann. Intern. Med.* **2010**, *153*, JC1-13. [CrossRef] [PubMed]
8. Lind, M.; Tuomilehto, J.; Uusitupa, M.; Nerman, O.; Eriksson, J.; Ilanne-Parikka, P.; Keinänen-Kiukaanniemi, S.; Peltonen, M.; Pivodic, A.; Lindström, J. The association between HbA1c, fasting glucose, 1-hour glucose and 2-hour glucose during an oral glucose tolerance test and cardiovascular disease in individuals with elevated risk for diabetes. *PLoS ONE* **2014**, *9*, e109506. [CrossRef]
9. Higdon, J.V.; Frei, B. Coffee and health: A review of recent human research. *Crit. Rev. Food Sci. Nutr.* **2006**, *46*, 101–123. [CrossRef]
10. McKay, D.L.; Blumberg, J.B. The role of tea in human health: An update. *J. Am. Coll. Nutr.* **2002**, *21*, 1–13. [CrossRef]
11. Thorp, A.A.; Owen, N.; Neuhaus, M.; Dunstan, D.W. Sedentary behaviors and subsequent health outcomes in adults: A systematic review of longitudinal studies, 1996–2011. *Am. J. Prev. Med.* **2011**, *41*, 207–215. [CrossRef]
12. Siroux, V.; Agier, L.; Slama, R. The exposome concept: A challenge and a potential driver for environmental health research. *Eur. Respir. Rev.* **2016**, *25*, 124–129. [CrossRef] [PubMed]
13. Gaziano, J.M.; Concato, J.; Brophy, M.; Fiore, L.; Pyarajan, S.; Breeling, J.; Whitbourne, S.; Deen, J.; Shannon, C.; Humphries, D.; et al. Million Veteran Program: A mega-biobank to study genetic influences on health and disease. *J. Clin. Epidemiol.* **2016**, *70*, 214–223. [CrossRef]
14. Rotterdam, E.; Katan, M.B.; Knuiman, J.T. Importance of time interval between repeated measurements of total or high-density lipoprotein cholesterol when estimating an individual's baseline concentrations. *Clin. Chem.* **1987**, *33*, 1913–1915. [CrossRef]
15. Schreiber, M.; Malesios, C.; Psarakis, S. Exploratory factor analysis for the Hirsch index, 17 h-type variants, and some traditional bibliometric indicators. *J. Informetr.* **2012**, *6*, 347–358. [CrossRef]
16. Kang, H.S.; Ahn, I.S.; Kim, J.H.; Kim, D.K. Neuropsychiatric symptoms in Korean patients with Alzheimer's disease: Exploratory factor analysis and confirmatory factor analysis of the neuropsychiatric inventory. *Dement. Geriatr. Cogn. Disord.* **2010**, *29*, 82–87. [CrossRef]
17. Panaretos, D.; Tzavelas, G.; Vamvakari, M.; Panagiotakos, D. Factor analysis as a tool for pattern recognition in biomedical research; a review with application in R software. *J. Data Sci.* **2017**, *16*, 615–630.
18. Yong, A.G.; Pearce, S. A beginner's guide to factor analysis: Focusing on exploratory factor analysis. *Tutor. Quant. Methods Psychol.* **2013**, *9*, 79–94. [CrossRef]
19. Hendrickson, A.E.; White, P.O. Promax: A quick method for rotation to oblique simple structure. *Br. J. Stat. Psychol.* **1964**, *12*, 65–70. [CrossRef]
20. SAS Institute Inc. *SAS/STAT®15.1 User's Guide*; SAS Institute Inc.: Cary, NC, USA, 2018.
21. Fuller, W. *Measurement Error Models*; JohnWiley: New York, NY, USA, 1987.
22. Horn, J.L. A rationale and test for the number of factors in factor analysis. *Psychometrika* **1965**, *30*, 179–185. [CrossRef] [PubMed]
23. Kim, J.-O.; Ahtola, O.; Spector, P.E.; Mueller, C.W. *Introduction to Factor Analysis: What It Is and How to Do It*; Sage: Thousand Oaks, CA, USA, 1978.

24. Villalpando, S.; Zamudio, Y.L.; Shamah-Levy, T.; Mundo-Rosas, V.; Manzano, A.C.; Lamadrid-Figueroa, H. Substitution of whole cows' milk with defatted milk for 4 months reduced serum total cholesterol, HDL-cholesterol and total apoB in a sample of Mexican school-age children (6–16 years of age). *Br. J. Nutr.* **2015**, *114*, 788–795. [CrossRef] [PubMed]

25. Steinmetz, K.A.; Childs, M.T.; Stimson, C.; Kushi, L.H.; McGovern, P.G.; Potter, J.D.; Yamanaka, W.K. Effect of consumption of whole milk and skim milk on blood lipid profiles in healthy men. *Am. J. Clin. Nutr.* **1994**, *59*, 612–618. [CrossRef] [PubMed]

26. Wang, L.; Manson, J.E.; Buring, J.E.; Lee, I.-M.; Sesso, H.D. Dietary intake of dairy products, calcium, and vitamin D and the risk of hypertension in middle-aged and older women. *Hypertension* **2008**, *51*, 1073–1079. [CrossRef] [PubMed]

27. Appel, L.J.; Moore, T.J.; Obarzanek, E.; Vollmer, W.M.; Svetkey, L.P.; Sacks, F.M.; Bray, G.A.; Vogt, T.M.; Cutler, J.A.; Windhauser, M.M. A clinical trial of the effects of dietary patterns on blood pressure. *N. Engl. J. Med.* **1997**, *336*, 1117–1124. [CrossRef] [PubMed]

28. German, J.B.; Gibson, R.A.; Krauss, R.M.; Nestel, P.; Lamarche, B.; Van Staveren, W.A.; Steijns, J.M.; De Groot, L.C.; Lock, A.L.; Destaillats, F. A reappraisal of the impact of dairy foods and milk fat on cardiovascular disease risk. *Eur. J. Nutr.* **2009**, *48*, 191–203. [CrossRef] [PubMed]

29. Lichtenstein, A.H.; Appel, L.J.; Brands, M.; Carnethon, M.; Daniels, S.; Franch, H.A.; Franklin, B.; Kris-Etherton, P.; Harris, W.S.; Howard, B. Summary of American Heart Association diet and lifestyle recommendations revision 2006. *Arterioscler. Thromb. Vasc. Biol.* **2006**, *26*, 2186–2191. [CrossRef]

30. U.S. Department of Health and Human Services; U.S. Department of Agriculture. *2015–2020 Dietary Guidelines for Americans*, 8th ed.; U.S. Department of Health and Human Services: Rockville, MD, USA, 2015.

31. Djoussé, L.; Arnett, D.K.; Coon, H.; Province, M.A.; Moore, L.L.; Ellison, R.C. Fruit and vegetable consumption and LDL cholesterol: The National Heart, Lung, and Blood Institute Family Heart Study. *Am. J. Clin. Nutr.* **2004**, *79*, 213–217. [CrossRef]

32. Singh, R.B.; Rastogi, S.S.; Niaz, M.A.; Ghosh, S.; Singh, R.; Gupta, S. Effect of fat-modified and fruit-and vegetable-enriched diets on blood lipids in the Indian Diet Heart Study. *Am. J. Cardiol.* **1992**, *70*, 869–874. [CrossRef]

33. Singh, R.B.; Ghosh, S.; Singh, R. Effects on serum lipids of adding fruits and vegetables to prudent diet in the Indian Experiment of Infarct Survival (IEIS). *Cardiology* **1992**, *80*, 283–293. [CrossRef]

34. DASH Research Group. Effects on blood lipids of a blood pressure–lowering diet: The Dietary Approaches to Stop Hypertension (DASH) Trial. *Am. J. Clin. Nutr.* **2001**, *74*, 80–89. [CrossRef]

35. Ballesteros, M.N.; Cabrera, R.M.; Saucedo, M.S.; Yepiz-Plascencia, G.M.; Ortega, M.I.; Valencia, M.E. Dietary fiber and lifestyle influence serum lipids in free living adult men. *J. Am. Coll. Nutr.* **2001**, *20*, 649–655. [CrossRef]

36. Stone, N.J. Lowering low-density cholesterol with diet: The important role of functional foods as adjuncts. *Coron. Artery Dis.* **2001**, *12*, 547–552. [CrossRef]

37. Jensen, E.N.; Buch-Andersen, T.; Ravn-Haren, G.; Dragsted, L.O. Mini-review: The effects of apples on plasma cholesterol levels and cardiovascular risk—A review of the evidence. *J. Hortic. Sci. Biotechnol.* **2009**, *84*, 34–41. [CrossRef]

38. Vidal, R.; Hernandez-Vallejo, S.; Pauquai, T.; Texier, O.; Rousset, M.; Chambaz, J.; Demignot, S.; Lacorte, J.-M. Apple procyanidins decrease cholesterol esterification and lipoprotein secretion in Caco-2/TC7 enterocytes. *J. Lipid Res.* **2005**, *46*, 258–268. [CrossRef] [PubMed]

39. Lam, C.K.; Zhang, Z.; Yu, H.; Tsang, S.Y.; Huang, Y.; Chen, Z.Y. Apple polyphenols inhibit plasma CETP activity and reduce the ratio of non-HDL to HDL cholesterol. *Mol. Nutr. Food Res.* **2008**, *52*, 950–958. [CrossRef] [PubMed]

40. Ogino, Y.; Osada, K.; Nakamura, S.; Ohta, Y.; Kanda, T.; Sugano, M. Absorption of dietary cholesterol oxidation products and their downstream metabolic effects are reduced by dietary apple polyphenols. *Lipids* **2007**, *42*, 151. [CrossRef]

41. Serra, A.T.; Rocha, J.; Sepodes, B.; Matias, A.A.; Feliciano, R.P.; de Carvalho, A.; Bronze, M.R.; Duarte, C.M.; Figueira, M. Evaluation of cardiovascular protective effect of different apple varieties–correlation of response with composition. *Food Chem.* **2012**, *135*, 2378–2386. [CrossRef]

42. Gonzalez, M.; Rivas, C.; Caride, B.; Lamas, M.A.; Taboada, M.C. Effects of orange and apple pectin on cholesterol concentration in serum, liver and faeces. *J. Physiol. Biochem.* **1998**, *54*, 99–104.

43. Wang, X.; Ouyang, Y.; Liu, J.; Zhu, M.; Zhao, G.; Bao, W.; Hu, F.B. Fruit and vegetable consumption and mortality from all causes, cardiovascular disease, and cancer: Systematic review and dose-response meta-analysis of prospective cohort studies. *Br. Med. J.* **2014**, *349*, g4490. [CrossRef] [PubMed]

44. Lesack, K.; Naugler, C. An open-source software program for performing Bonferroni and related corrections for multiple comparisons. *J. Pathol. Inform.* **2011**, *2*, 52.

45. Freeland-Graves, J.H.; Nitzke, S. Position of the Academy of Nutrition and Dietetics: Total diet approach to healthy eating. *J. Acad. Nutr. Diet.* **2013**, *113*, 307–317. [CrossRef]

46. Tucker, K.L. Dietary patterns, approaches, and multicultural perspective. *Appl. Physiol. Nutr. Metab.* **2010**, *35*, 211–218. [CrossRef] [PubMed]

47. Schulze, M.B.; Hoffmann, K. Methodological approaches to study dietary patterns in relation to risk of coronary heart disease and stroke. *Br. J. Nutr.* **2006**, *95*, 860–869. [CrossRef] [PubMed]

48. Ocké, M.C. Evaluation of methodologies for assessing the overall diet: Dietary quality scores and dietary pattern analysis. *Proc. Nutr. Soc.* **2013**, *72*, 191–199. [CrossRef] [PubMed]

MDPI

St. Alban-Anlage 66

4052 Basel

Switzerland

Tel. +41 61 683 77 34

Fax +41 61 302 89 18

www.mdpi.com

Nutrients Editorial Office

E-mail: nutrients@mdpi.com

www.mdpi.com/journal/nutrients

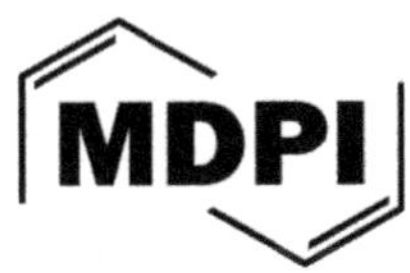

9 783036 577128